ATHEROSCLEROSIS
DRUG DISCOVERY

ADVANCES IN EXPERIMENTAL MEDICINE AND BIOLOGY

ATHEROSCLEROSIS DRUG DISCOVERY

Edited by

Charles E. Day
The Upjohn Company–Atherosclerosis Research

Springer Science+Business Media, LLC

Library of Congress Cataloging in Publication Data

Brook Lodge Symposium on Anti-atherosclerosis Drug Discovery, 1st, 1975.
  Atherosclerosis drug discovery.

  (Advances in experimental medicine and biology; 67)
  Bibliography: p.
  Includes index.
    1. Arteriosclerosis—Research—Congresses. 2. Cardiovascular agents—Research—
  Congresses. 3. Diseases—Animal models—Congresses. I. Day, Charles E. II. Title.
  III. Series [DNLM: 1. Arteriosclerosis—Drug therapy—Congresses. 2. Drug ecalua-
  tion—Methods—Congresses. W1 AD559 v. 69 1975/[WG550 B871 1075a]
  RC692.B72   1975   616.1'36   76-5395

  ISBN 978-1-4757-9309-3   ISBN 978-1-4614-4618-7 (eBook)
  DOI 10.1007/978-1-4614-4618-7

Proceedings of the First Brook Lodge Symposium on
Anti-Atherosclerosis Drug Discovery held at Brook Lodge in
Augusta, Michigan, August 13-15, 1975

©1976 Springer Science+Business Media New York
Originally published by Plenum Press, New York in 1976
Softcover reprint of the hardcover 1st edition 1976

United Kingdom edition published by Plenum Press, London
A Division of Plenum Publishing Company, Ltd.
Davis House (4th Floor), 8 Scrubs Lane, Harlesden, London NW10 6SE, England

PREFACE

     Although atherosclerosis is the leading cause of death in the
so-called affluent societies, there is presently no drug in our
pharmacologic armamentarium against disease to either prevent or
reverse this insidious killer and debilitant of human lives.
Because of this void the First Brook Lodge Symposium on Anti-
Atherosclerosis Drug Discovery was convened at Brook Lodge in
Augusta, Michigan, August 13-15, 1975. The symposium was sponsored
by The Upjohn Company and was international in scope, with investigators attending from such countries as England, Japan, Belgium,
and Italy.

     The symposium focused on the problems associated with the
discovery and evaluation of new drugs effective in preventing
or reversing atherosclerosis. The thrust of material is centered
around animal models useful as tools in the search and evaluation
of new drugs. Broadly categorized, the models are nonhuman
primates, rabbits, rodents, quail, and tissue culture. The
material is a mix of studies on serum lipids and, more importantly,
of studies on the artery, irrespective of serum lipid levels. The
prevention of arterial lesions, not reduction of serum lipids, is
emphasized. A review of all anti-atherosclerotic agents, with the
exception of hypolipidemic agents, is included in this volume of
the proceedings of the symposium.

     Data are reported on the utility of selectively bred SEA
Japanese quail for random screening for anti-atherosclerosis drugs,
at the arterial level, in the pharmaceutical industry. The small
size and cost of the animal coupled with its susceptibility to
atherosclerosis induction make it a good model to detect, initially,
agents that prevent lesion development in the artery itself. After
screening large numbers of compounds in quail, active leads can be
further evaluated in a nonhuman primate animal model such as
Macaca fascicularis, which is well described in this volume. The
quail and nonhuman primate system also has the potential for detection and evaluation of agents active in reversing the atherosclerotic process.

Although finding agents active against atherosclerosis directly at the arterial level is emphasized, a consideration of serum lipids and, especially, lipoproteins is not excluded. A new class of lipoprotein modifying agents is reported on for the first time. These compounds, such as 1-[p-(1'-adamantyloxy)phenyl]-piperidine, have the unique ability to markedly reduce atherogenic lipoproteins while concomitantly increasing nonatherogenic ones in hypercholesterolemic animals such as the rat. A detailed system for large scale screening for such agents is presented. The approach of attacking atherogenesis through modification of specific atherogenic lipoproteins appears more promising than the nonselective reduction of serum total cholesterol. The goal is to reduce atherogenic low density lipoproteins and increase nonatherogenic high density lipoproteins.

The potential utilization of tissue culture techniques for the detection and evaluation of anti-atherosclerotic agents is presently a popular area of research. Some potential uses are explored in this volume. It should be recognized, however, that any agent possessing a desired activity in tissue culture must ultimately be tested in a whole animal system in vivo. As illustrated by one report in the tissue culture section, agents active in tissue culture may not be active in whole animals because of problems in absorption, distribution, metabolism, or excretion of drug.

Because of the relative lack of drugs effective against atherosclerosis, even in experimental animals, the first Brook Lodge symposium was necessarily concerned with means to discover and evaluate such agents. I hope that the tools reported here for drug discovery and evaluation will be applied so that the second Brook Lodge symposium will deal specifically with promising anti-atherosclerosis drugs.

Charles E. Day

The Upjohn Company
Kalamazoo, Michigan
November 20, 1975

CONTENTS

SECTION 1
PRIMATE MODELS

SECTION 2
RABBIT MODELS

SECTION 3
RODENT MODELS

SECTION 4
AVIAN MODELS

SECTION 5
TISSUE CULTURE

SECTION 1

PRIMATE MODELS

A MODEL FOR THERAPEUTIC INTERVENTIONS ON ESTABLISHED CORONARY ATHEROSCLEROSIS IN A NONHUMAN PRIMATE

M. R. Malinow, Phyllis McLaughlin, Lynne Papworth,
H. K. Naito, Lena Lewis, and W. P. McNulty
Oregon Regional Primate Research Center, Beaverton,
Oregon 97005; University of Oregon Health Sciences Center,
Portland, Oregon 97207; and Cleveland Clinic, Cleveland,
Ohio 44106

Modern medicine is faced with the challenge of helping hundreds of millions of individuals with undetected coronary atherosclerosis, many of whom will eventually develop ischemic heart disease and probably die as a consequence. To reduce the incidence of clinically unrecognized coronary atherosclerosis, a risk-free, noninvasive, and so far nonexistent method of detecting the progress of coronary atherosclerosis in man is long overdue. Until such a method becomes available, the most feasible alternative is to substitute an animal model in which coronary atherosclerosis can be induced and to study its progression, regression, or arrest. Nonhuman primates are a natural choice since spontaneous atherosclerotic lesions have been described in all species so far studied (1). But our knowledge of the incidence and prevalence of atherosclerosis in these models is limited because most reports are based on only a few animals (1). Furthermore, such spontaneous lesions are generally minimal (2,3) and do not impair normal arterial functions as they do in man. A priori, not every species of nonhuman primate appears to meet all the requirements for determining the effect of therapeutic interventions on the course of coronary atherosclerosis. However, monkeys had to be selected on the basis of availability, and the lesions induced were more advanced than the spontaneous type (1). Although particular aspects of atherogenesis have been determined in squirrel monkeys (4,5,6), rhesus (7), and stumptailed macaques (8) (to name just a few), progress toward finding the "ideal" nonhuman primate model has been impeded. Sometimes, as in the squirrel monkey, the distribution of the coronary lesions has differed from that in man. More recently, the increasing unavailability of some species, like the rhesus and stumptailed macaques, has slowed the search considerably. Since the pioneer work of Kramsch and Hollander,

3

who first described the dietary induction of atherosclerosis in
cynomolgus monkeys (Macaca fascicularis) (9), we have performed a
series of experiments which suggest that this species has several
characteristics which recommend it as a model for studying therapeutic interventions on coronary atherogenesis. Our studies have
been limited to adult female animals and are not yet completed,
but we present here an interim report on the experiments in progress. Although we have not compared the incidence and severity of
atherosclerosis in males and females, our observations agree in
the main with those reported by Kramsch and Hollander (9) in male
cynomolgus monkeys. In this respect, cynomolgus monkeys seem to
be like rhesus monkeys in which cholesterol-induced atherosclerosis
showed no sex-related differences (10). Thus experimental atherosclerosis in monkeys is similar to the "spontaneous" atherosclerosis
observed in several ethnic groups which do not have the predominance
of male coronary atherosclerosis reported in white populations (11).

AVAILABILITY

The Government of India's recent embargo on exports of rhesus
monkeys has severely limited the world supply of these monkeys for
medical research (12). Moreover, more recently, the stumptailed
macaque (M. speciosa), in which Pick et al. (8) confirmed the
aggravating effect of hypertension on atherosclerosis, may be
placed on the endangered species list, and its availability may be
curtailed (13). Since shipments of South American monkeys from
Peru and Colombia have been curtailed (14), the difficulty of
obtaining them has increased. Though large monkeys like baboons
are still available in adequate numbers, certain limitations such
as the higher cost of caging and maintenance make them unsuitable.
Others like the great apes are practically unavailable for experiments that require a considerable number of animals. Fortunately,
a large number of cynomolgus monkeys, which range from Southeast
Asia to Polynesia, are still available, can be obtained with
relative ease and at reasonable cost, require small cages, and
consume considerably less food than larger animals.

ACCEPTANCE OF SPECIAL DIETS AND OF DRUGS

The fact that with proper handling most nonhuman primates,
including cynomolgus monkeys, accept diets high in saturated fat
and cholesterol facilitates the induction and acceleration of
atherogenesis. A semipurified diet (Table I) well accepted by
different species of monkeys and with a fat content similar to
that consumed in the U.S. was designed by Dr. O. W. Portman and
has been in use at our Center for several years. We have added
cholesterol at levels ranging from 34 to 120 mg/100 Kcal, which

TABLE I

Composition of Semipurified Diet (Percent)*

Casein	25.0
Butter	25.5
Sucrose	43.0
Cholesterol	0.5**
Salt Mix IV	4.0
Vitamin Mix	2.0

*Values/kg of diet: Vitamin A-acetate, 20,000 U; α-tocopherol, 0.1 g; crystalline vitamin D3, 100 µg (4,000 U); menadione, 0.04 g; ascorbic acid, 0.5 g; inositol, 1.0 g; choline chloride, 5.0 g; niacin, 0.049 g; riboflavin, 0.01 g; thiamine, 0.01 g; pyridoxine, 0.01 g; Ca-pantothenate, 0.03 g; biotin, 0.2 mg; folic acid, 1.0 mg; and vitamin B_{12}, 0.02 mg. Calories percent: protein 21, carbohydrate 36, fat 43.

**The amount of cholesterol in mg/100 Kcal including that found in butter (280 mg/100 g) is: BC 0%, 14; BC 0.1%, 34; BC 0.2%, 52; BC 0.3%, 68; BC 0.5%, 120. In all diets except BC 0.5%, 2.5% corn oil replaces 2.5% of the butter.

are comparable to those ingested by man in the western world (Table I). Figure 1 shows that over a period of six months cynomolgus monkeys on the semipurified diet underwent changes in body weight that were similar to those in monkeys on regular chow; the monkeys remained in good health during more than 4 years on the diet. Despite the difficulty of measuring exactly the food intake of monkeys, we have weighed the semipurified diet of six cynomolgus monkeys during 7 days and have estimated and subtracted the weight of the discarded food. The approximate intake of the diet shown in Table I (referred to hereafter as the butter-cholesterol or BC 0.5% diet) was 28 g/kg/day or 133 cal/kg/day. The monkeys also accepted BC diets with different cholesterol content (see below, Fig. 4) as well as the addition of various drugs and nutrients to the BC 0.5% or BC 0.1% diets* (Table II).

*Semipurified BC diet with 0.1% cholesterol added (w/w). BC diet refers to the same diet without specification of the amount of cholesterol added.

TABLE II

Drugs and Nutrients Accepted by Cynomolgus Monkeys
when Mixed with the Semipurified Diet

% cholesterol of BC diet	Drug or nutrient	Dosage (g/100 gm food)
0.5%	Sodium D-thyroxine [1]	0.0075; 0.003
	PDC, 2-6 pyridine-dimethanol-bis (N-methylcarbamate) Pyridinolcarbamate [2]	0.04; 0.12; 0.20
	Cholestyramine [3]	2.0; 5.0
	Lignin* (Orzan) [4]	5.0; 4.0
	Alfalfa	51.0
	4-chloro-(2,5-xylidine)-2 pyrimi-dinylthio acetic acid (Wy-14, 643) [5]	0.045
0.1%	9-hydroxy-18, 19-bisnor-prostanoic acid (Compound C83) [6]	0.25; 0.50
	Wheat bran	49.0
	Rice bran	50.0
	Soya bran	46.0
	Levodopa (Larodopa) [7]	0.175; 0.350+
	Isocarboxazid (Marplan) [8]	0.0175
	Imipramine hydrochloride (Tofranil HCl) [9]	3 mg/day (with fruit)

*Diarrhea observed after 30 days. +Diminished appetite in some animals.

(1) Flint Laboratories; (2) Banyu Pharmaceutical Co.; (3) Merck, Sharp and Dohme; (4) Crown Zellerbach; (5) Wyeth Laboratories; (6) Istituto Biochimica Italiano; (7) Roche Laboratories; (8) Hoffman-La Roche; (9) Geigy.

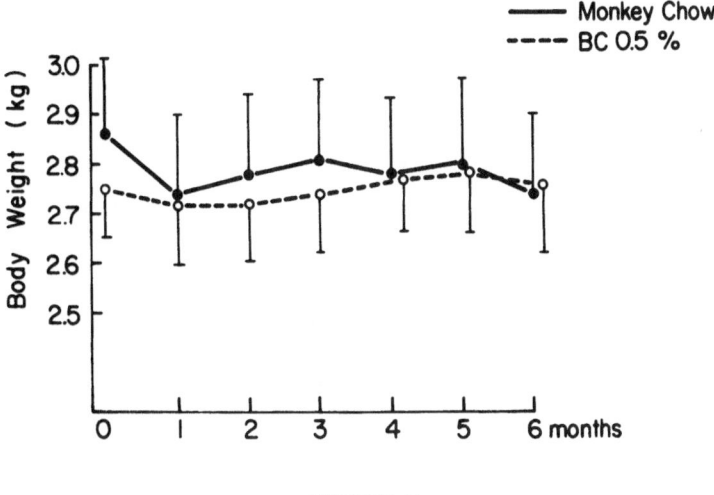

FIGURE 1

Body weight changes in <u>M</u>. <u>fascicularis</u> maintained on the BC 0.5%
diet for 6 months. Average of six monkeys per group; bars, S.E.

PLASMA LIPID CHANGES

    Animals differ widely in their plasma cholesterol levels even
when they ingest similar amounts of cholesterol. Fillios and
Mann, who observed such differences in rabbits, suggested that
they be classified as hypo-responders, normal, and hyper-responders,
depending upon the cholesterol level after the ingestion of choles-
terol-containing diet (15). This variability of plasma cholesterol
levels in animals on diets with added cholesterol has been documented in several species, including rabbits (15,16), rats (17),
rhesus (18), squirrel monkeys (5), and cynomolgus monkeys (see
below). Recent advances in our understanding of the factors
responsible for this responsiveness stem mainly from studies on
squirrel monkeys (5,6).

    Plasma cholesterol levels (19) in cynomolgus monkeys maintained
on Purina monkey chow (25% protein) and occasional fresh fruits
ranged from 80 to 195 mg/100 ml and rose when the semipurified
diets were ingested. Figure 2 shows the continuous distribution
of plasma cholesterol observed in 236 cynomolgus monkeys on the BC
0.5% diet for 30 days. The monkeys were arbitrarily separated
into hypo-, normo-, and hyper-responders, depending on the plasma
cholesterol level; the dividing concentration was 290 and 990 mg/
100 ml, respectively. The number of monkeys in each classification
and the average level of plasma cholesterol, as well as their
plasma cholesterol level when they were eating regular chow, are

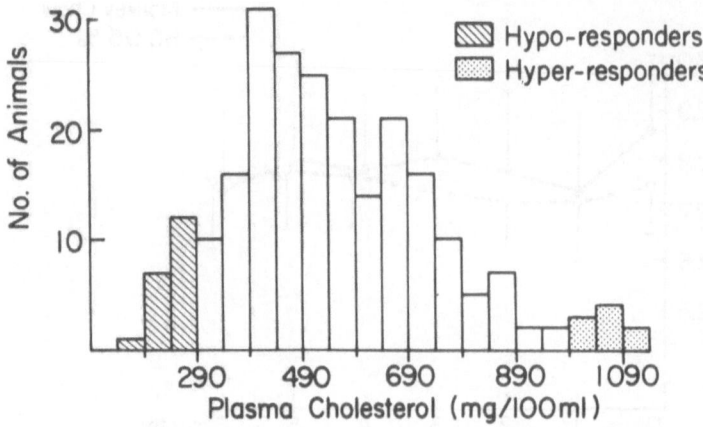

FIGURE 2

Distribution of plasma cholesterol in 236 M. fascicularis maintained for 1 month on the BC 0.5% diet.

TABLE III

Plasma Cholesterol in Cynomolgus Monkeys Fed a Semipurified
Diet (BC 0.5%) for One Month (Mean $\pm$ S.E.)

Group	Plasma Cholesterol (mg/100 ml)	
	Chow diet	Semipurified diet
Hypo-responders	126 $\pm$ 6 (8)*	254 $\pm$ 7 (20)
Normo-responders	140 $\pm$ 7 (36)	554 $\pm$ 11 (207)
Hyper-responders	161 $\pm$ 9 (8)	1076 $\pm$ 23 (9)
p ("t" test) (hypo-vs hyper)	< 0.01	< 0.001

*Number of animals

shown in Table III. It is clear that hypo- and hyper-responders differ greatly in their response to dietary cholesterol and that, when they ingest a diet almost free of cholesterol, their basal cholesterolemia is also lower in the former than in the latter.

Cynomolgus monkeys also exhibit hypo- and hyper-response when fed lower amounts of cholesterol. Another group of monkeys on the BC 0.1% diet for 25 days was separated into only two subgroups depending on whether the plasma cholesterol level was below or above 290 mg/100 ml. In retrospect, we could determine that the plasma cholesterol level was already different when the two subgroups of monkeys were on regular chow, and the difference was maintained throughout the 5 1/2 month feeding of the BC 0.1% diet (Fig. 3).

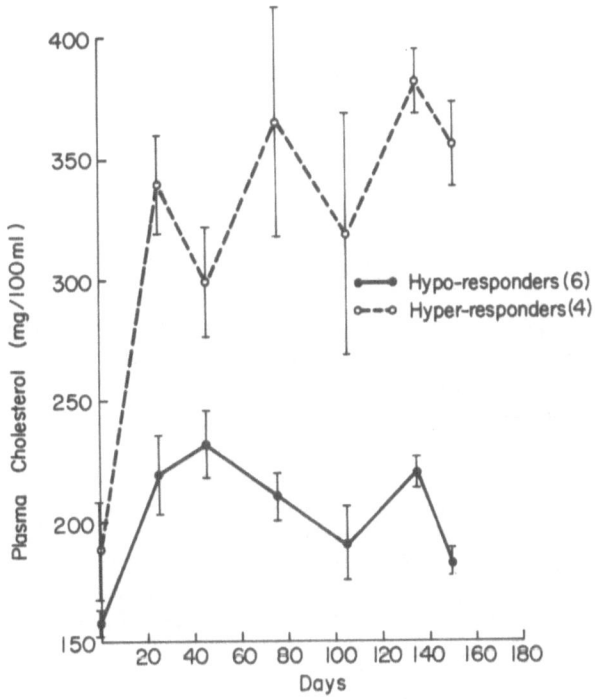

FIGURE 3

Plasma cholesterol in M. fascicularis maintained on the BC 0.1% diet for 5 1/2 months. The animals were segregated after 25 days into two groups according to their plasma cholesterol; the dividing level was 290 mg/100 ml. No. of animals between parentheses. Bars, S.E.

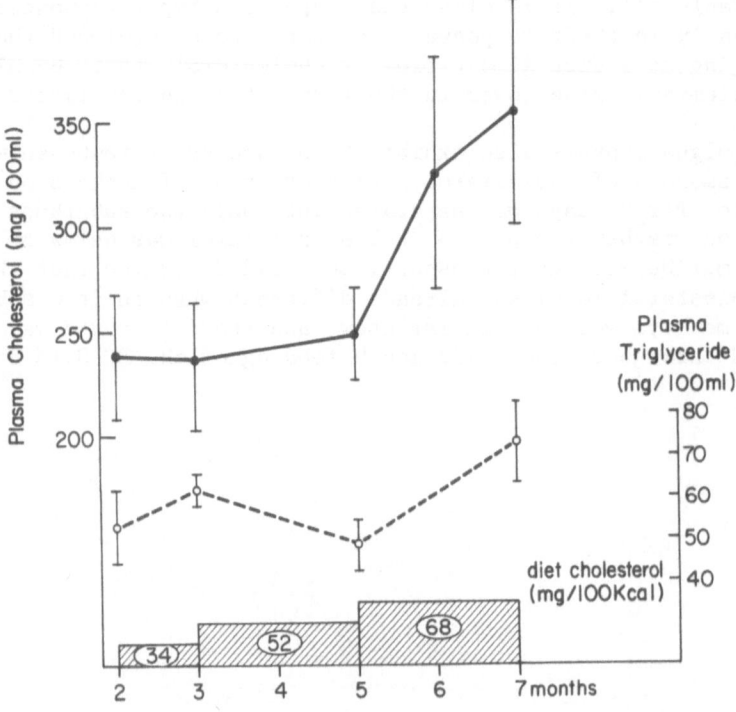

FIGURE 4

Plasma cholesterol and triglyceride levels in M. fascicularis
maintained on BC diets containing different amounts of cholesterol.
Average of six animals; bars, S.E.

In animals within a given response group, the level of plasma
cholesterol can be modified by the amount of dietary cholesterol.
Figure 4 shows the plasma cholesterol and triglyceride levels
observed in six normal responders receiving different amounts of
cholesterol in the BC diet. As can be observed, plasma cholesterol
rose with increasing levels of dietary cholesterol, while triglyceride concentrations remained low.

The normal triglyceride levels (Fig. 4 and Table IV) suggest
that the hypercholesterolemia induced by the BC diets was associated with hyperlipoproteinemia type IIA. However, triglycerides
were higher with the BC 0.5% than with the BC 0.1% diet. Lipoprotein electrophoresis showed faint staining of the prebeta region
in only a few monkeys as well as an increase in beta lipoprotein
in the hypercholesterolemic monkeys.

TABLE IV

Triglyceride Levels in Cynomolgus Monkeys Fed
on Semipurified Diets (Mean $\pm$ S.E.)

Monkey	# of animals	Diet	# of months on diet	TG (mg/100 ml)
Normo-responders	18	BC 0.5%	6	115 $\pm$ 18 [1]
Normo-responders	6	BC 0.1%	3	62 $\pm$ 4 [1]
Hypo-responders	8	BC 0.5%	1	54 $\pm$ 11 [2]
Hyper-responders	8	BC 0.5%	1	68 $\pm$ 13 [2]

[1] Autoanalyzer method file, Triglyceride AAII-23, 1971.
Technicon Inst. Corp., Tarrytown, N.Y. 10591.

[2] Young and Eastman, S. Afr. J. Lab. Clin. Med. 9:28, 1963.

We have attempted to modify diet-induced hypercholesterolemia
by the addition of different brans or the administration of cholestyramine or D-thyroxine. Table V shows the results and indicates
that only cholestyramine controlled hypercholesterolemia.

ATHEROSLCEROSIS

Most of our anatomical studies have been performed in animals
after 6 months on the BC 0.5% diet; the results will be compared
with those of earlier or later studies.

Atherosclerotic changes in the aorta, the common, external
and internal carotids, the subclavian, the mesenteric, and the
coronary arteries were observed in most of the animals on the BC
0.5% diet for 6 months. Some of the coronary lesions became
apparent as early as 4 months after the diet began (Fig. 5) and
progressed as time went by, but no coronary arterial occlusions

TABLE V

Plasma Cholesterol in Cynomolgus Monkeys on Semipurified Diet (Mean $\pm$ S.E.)

Diet	Drug or nutrient (g/100 g food)	No. of monkeys	Months on diet			
			1	2	3	6
BC 0.1%		6	260 $\pm$ 21	238 $\pm$ 30	236 $\pm$ 29	
BC 0.1% + Cholestyramine	5.0	6	160 $\pm$ 16**	148 $\pm$ 11*	136 $\pm$ 13*	
BC 0.1% + Soya Bran	46.0	6	278 $\pm$ 23	250 $\pm$ 11	241 $\pm$ 25	
BC 0.1% + Rice Bran	50.0	6	272 $\pm$ 23	310 $\pm$ 33	276 $\pm$ 20	
BC 0.1% + Wheat Bran	48.0	6	322 $\pm$ 24	322 $\pm$ 29	280 $\pm$ 24	
BC 0.5%		11				756 $\pm$ 88
BC 0.5% + D-thyroxine	0.003	12				625 $\pm$ 82

p ("t" test) vs controls, * < 0.02; ** < 0.01.

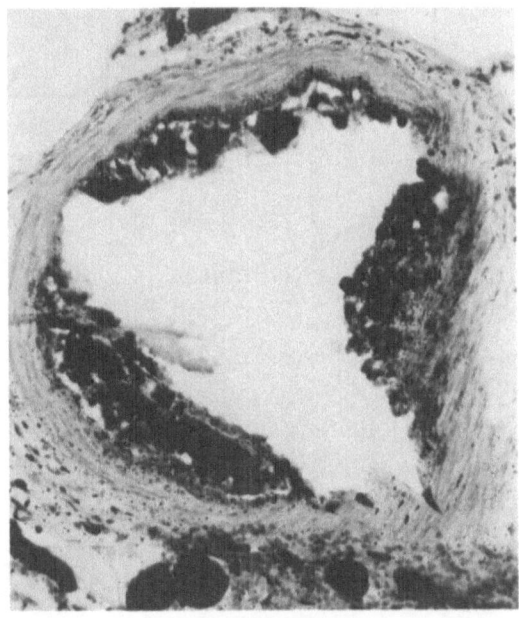

FIGURE 5

Frozen section of wall of right coronary artery a few mm from the
origin in a M. fascicularis fed the BC 0.5% diet for 4 months.
Three intimal plaques contain intra- and extracellular lipids.
Oil Red 0-hematoxylin, 190x. (Reduced 10% for reproduction.)

have been observed even after 4 years. Segmental raised lesions
stained with Sudan IV in irregular patches have involved the
aorta, the carotid, and the common iliac arteries. The intima was
thickened by a proliferation of foam cells, the elastic lamellae
became reduplicated, and lipids were found inside and in between
cells. Up to 60-70% of the lumen in the subepicardial branches of
the coronary arteries have been obstructed, and the intramyocardial
branches were somewhat infiltrated with sudanophilic material. In
the subepicardial branches, the lumen was diminished by the proliferation of foam cells which invaded the media and the adventitia.
The internal elastic lamina was frequently reduplicated, broken,
or absent in irregular spots, and collagen fibers appeared (Fig.
6). Intensely Oil Red O positive material was observed within and
between cells, cholesterol crystal clefts were present, and mucopolysaccharides were increased. In monkeys on this diet for 4
years, the arterial lesions contained much less lipids, a fibrous
cap covered a deeply situated gruel, and the subintima and media
were occasionally calcified and necrosed (Figs. 7 and 8). Occasionally, intramural hemorrhages developed in a thickened plaque

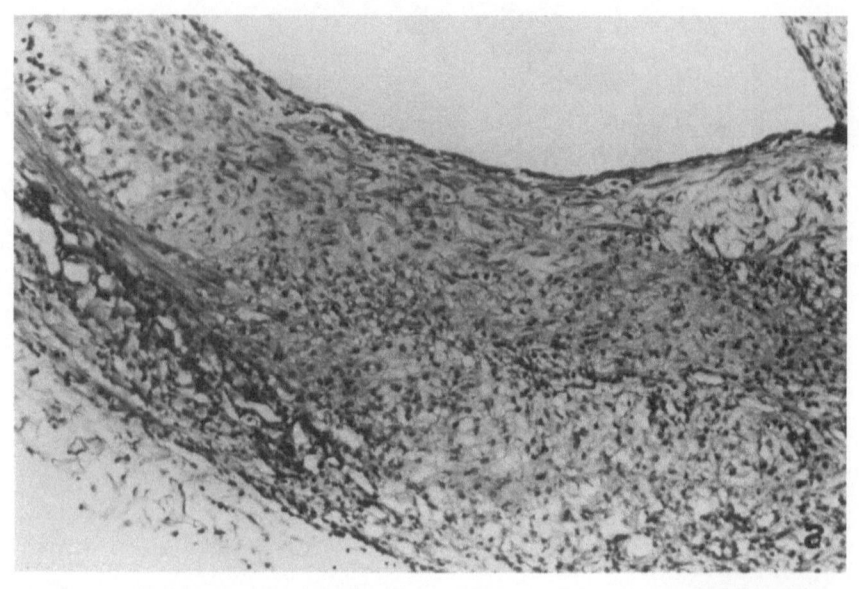

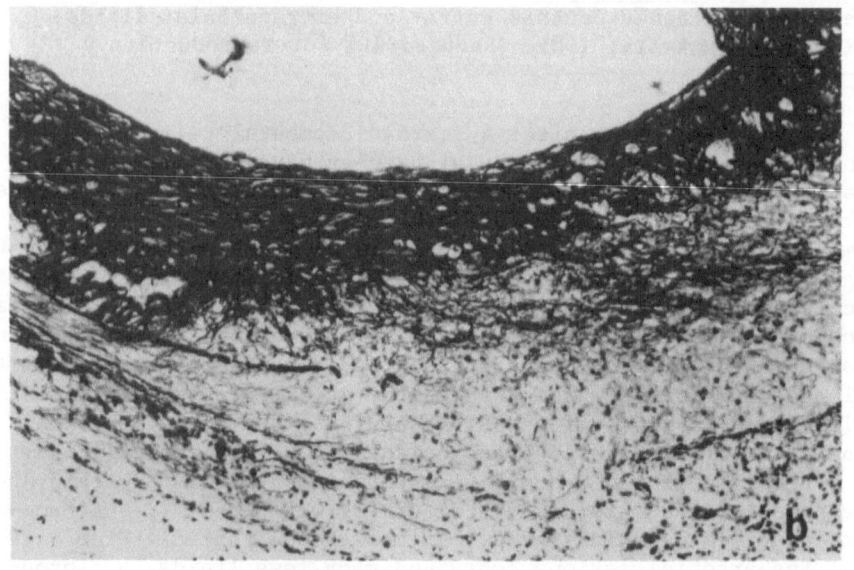

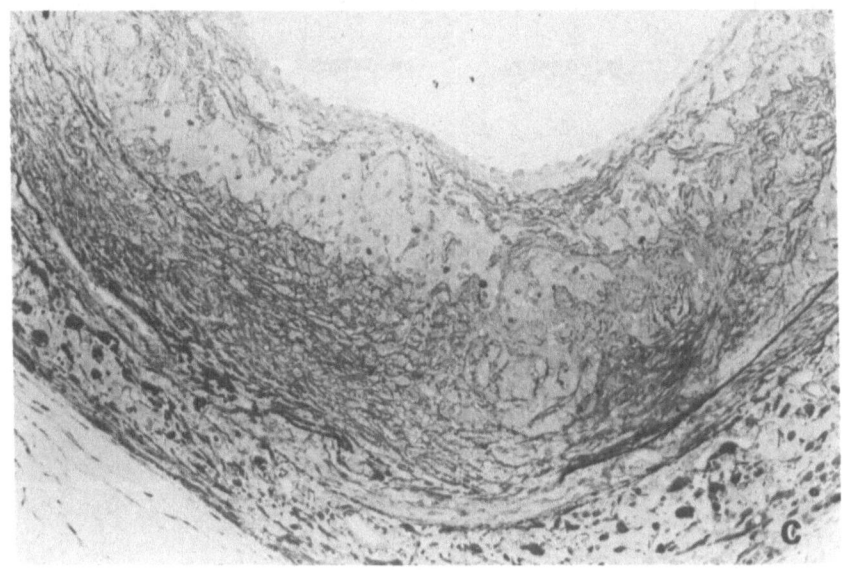

FIGURE 6

a.- Wall of right coronary artery a few mm from the origin, in a
M. fascicularis fed the BC 0.5% diet for 6 months. On the left a
portion of the muscularis is recognizable beneath a greatly thickened intima. On the right the identity of the muscularis is lost
in a mass of foam cells. H and E, 40x. b.- Adjacent section,
showing interruption of both internal and external elastic lamellae,
spreading of foam cells into the adventitia, and dense masses of
new elastic tissue in the intima. Aldehyde-fuchsin-trichrome, 40x.
c.- Semithin (1μ) epoxy section from adjacent block, showing in
more detail foam cells and proliferation of fine elastic fibers in
the thickened intima. Methylene blue-basic fuchsin, 40x. (Reduced
10% for reproduction.)

(Fig. 9). Thus these chronic lesions exhibit some of the complications observed in man, including occlusion (see below), and are
microscopically very similar to those in human atherosclerosis,
whereas the changes observed in monkeys on the BC 0.5% diet for 4
to 6 months are much more cellular and the lipid deposition is
more marked than in man.

    Lesions in the vessels of the circle of Willis can be observed
as early as 4 months after the BC 0.5% diets, and small plaques
have been present in the vertebral, basilar, and middle and anterior
cerebral arteries (Fig. 10). The plaques consisted of slightly
thickened intima, with reduplication of the underlying elastic
lamina and increased mucopolysaccharides, while Oil Red O positive
material was observed occasionally. In one instance, a plaque had

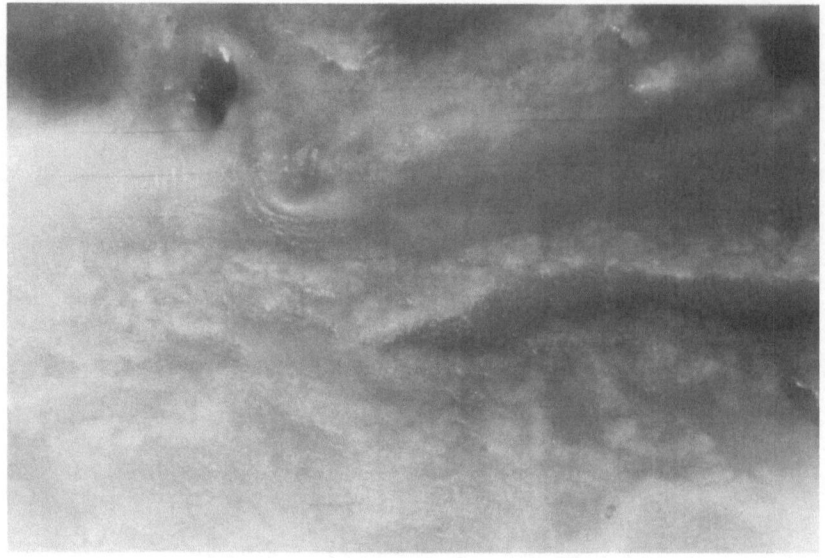

FIGURE 7

Intimal surface of thoracic aorta of a M. fascicularis on the BC
0.1% diet for 4 years. The surface is nearly covered with irregular pearly plaques. 3.2x.(Reduced 10% for reproduction.)

occluded a posterior cerebral artery in a monkey maintained for 4
years on the BC 0.1% diet (Figs. 11 and 12). Throughout this
interval, the monkey was used in several drug studies, but no
drugs had been given in the last 2 years. The plaque consisted of
proliferated foam cells, with numerous cholesterol clefts and
increased mucopolysaccharides. The internal elastic lamina was
well-preserved, but numerous strands of apparently newly formed
elastic fibers were interspersed with the cellular content of the
plaque.

     To compare the results of therapeutic interventions in several
groups of monkeys, we quantified the lesions and used the usual
statistical methods for testing the differences; the procedure has
already been described (20). All evaluations are performed "blind-
ly." The aorta is removed and a cannula is inserted in the arch
to fix the coronary arteries with 10% formalin at 120 mm Hg overnight. The aorta with its adventitia stripped away is fixed in
10% formalin, stained with Sudan IV, sewn on paper cards, and
classified (Fig. 13):
     (1+) No lesions. The substitution of the usual 0 for 1+ was
          done to facilitate computer handling of the data since
          "0" is used as "no data available";

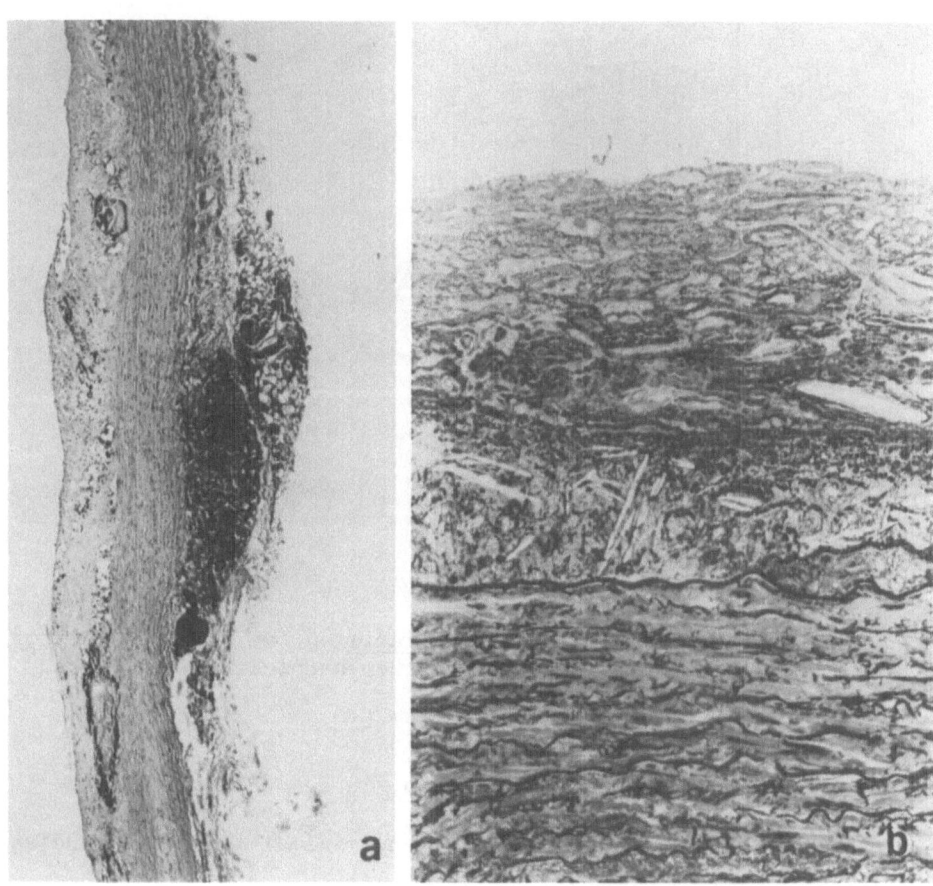

FIGURE 8

a.- Longitudinal section of thoracic aorta in a M. fascicularis on
the BC 0.1% diet for 4 years. The intima (left) is thickened,
fibrous, and partly calcified. A lymphocytic infiltration is observed in the adventitia (right), probably not related to the
atherosclerotic process. H and E, 10x. b.- Semithin (1μ) epoxy
section of same aorta. A dense fibroelastic cap overlies an almost
acellular mass containing cholesterol clefts. The internal elastic
lamella is partly reduplicated. Methylene blue-basic fuchsin, 100x.
(Reduced 10% for reproduction.)

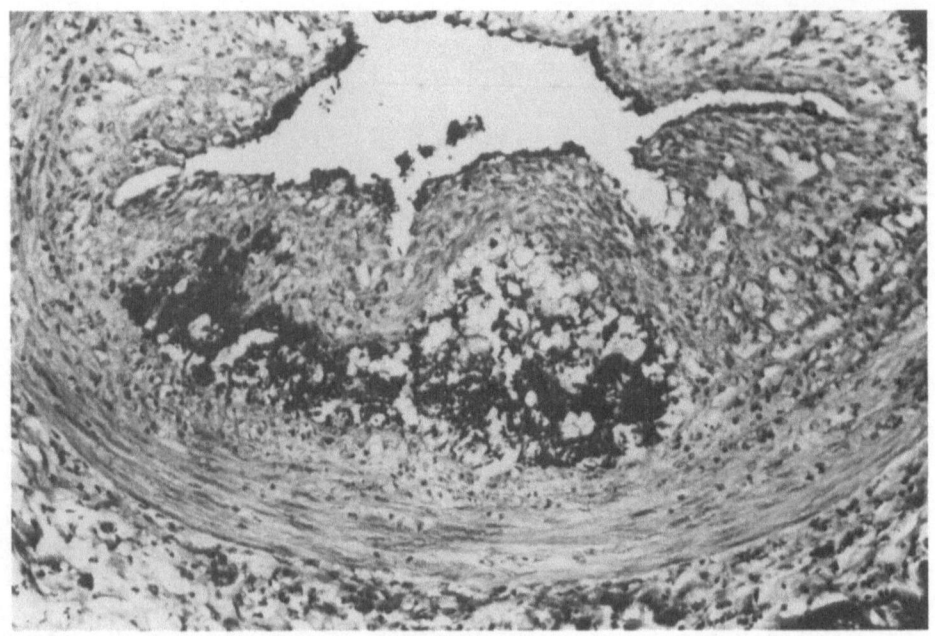

FIGURE 9

Right coronary artery of a M. fascicularis on the BC 0.1% diet for
4 years. A recent hemorrhage lies within a thickened and fibrous
intima. H and E, 40x.

     (2+) Minimal sudanophilia at arch, in descending aorta, or
          both;
     (3+) Moderate sudanophilia at arch, minimal in the descending
          aorta;
     (4+) Moderate sudanophilia at arch, marked in descending
          aorta, with or without minimal fibrosis;
     (5+) Extensive sudanophilia at arch, marked to extensive in
          descending aorta, with or without severe fibrosis.

    The coronary arteries are dissected free and five segments
are selected (Fig. 14), embedded in paraffin, sectioned transverse-
ly, and stained with H and E and with Gomori's orcein stain for
elastic fibers. Some 30 random sections from each segment are
mounted and the more involved section of each segment is projected
with a camera lucida on paper and traced. The area of the lumen
is then determined by planimetry and its ratio to that of the area
limited by the internal elastic lamella is determined. Including
the 5 coronary arterial segments studied, the percent encroachment
of the lumen is averaged for each animal and these results are
averaged for each group.

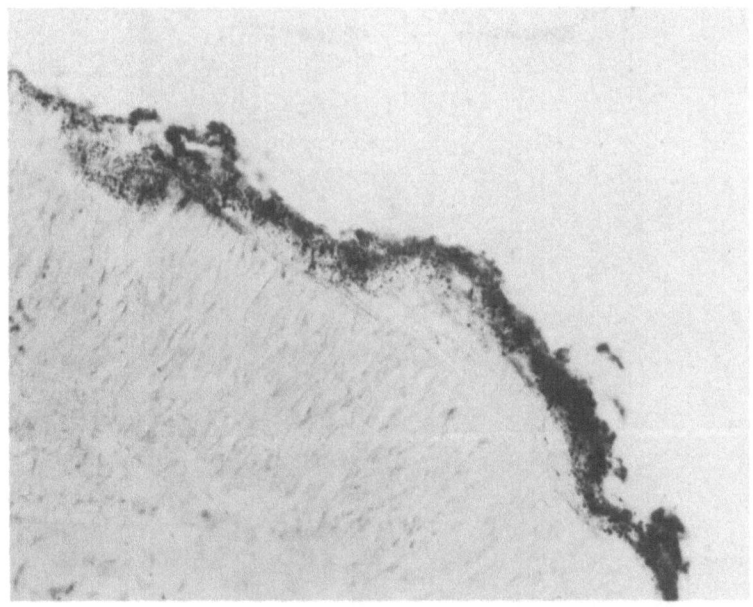

FIGURE 10

Frozen section of basilar artery of a M. fascicularis on the BC
0.5% diet for 4 months. Lipid material observed in the endothelium;
the intima is slightly thickened. Oil Red O-hematoxylin, 190x.

Relation between Plasma Cholesterol and Arterial Lesions

The extent of aortic and coronary atherosclerosis in monkeys
on the BC 0.5% diet for 6 months has been plotted as a function of
the plasma cholesterol concentration determined before death
(Figs. 15 and 16). Although arterial involvement correlates well
with plasma cholesterol (aorta r = 0.610; p < 0.01; coronary r =
0.742; p < 0.01), the intragroup variation is such that some animals
which have the most advanced lesions have the same terminal plasma
cholesterol levels (800-900 mg/100 ml) as animals with only minimal
aortic and coronary involvement. Assuming that the final plasma
cholesterol levels reflect those present throughout the observation,
we have called these animals hyper- and hypo-reactive to plasma
cholesterol, respectively; a similar pattern of arterial "reactivity" was reported previously in cholesterol-fed rabbits (21). It
is evident from Figures 15 and 16 that aortic and coronary "reactivity" does not always correspond in the same animal; in other
words, the aorta can be hypo-reactive in an animal with a hyper-
reactive coronary artery and vice versa. The same lack of corres-
pondence is illustrated in Figure 17 which depicts the cholesterol

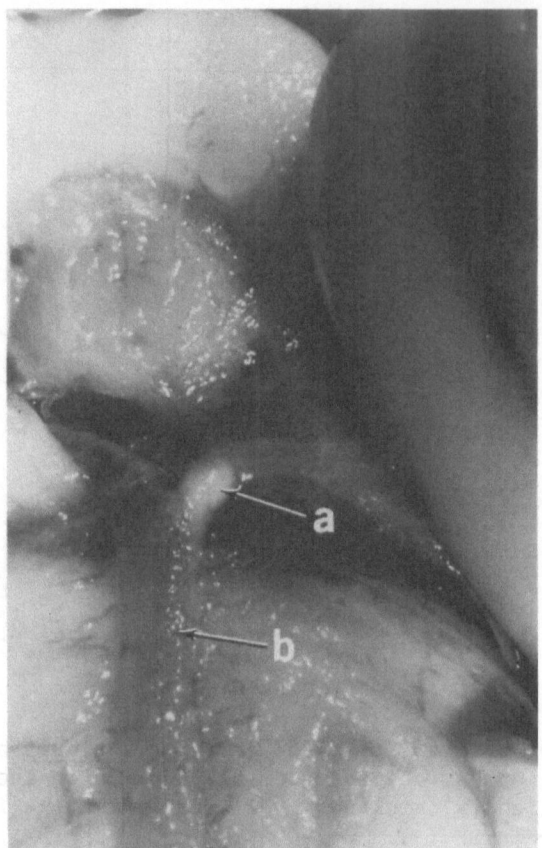

FIGURE 11

Inferior view of bifurcation of the basilar artery in a M. fascicularis on the BC 0.1% diet for 4 years. A pale mass distends the
left posterior cerebral artery just beyond its origin (a); (b),
basilar artery. 3.2x. (Reduced 10% for reproduction.)

---

content of the arch vessels and of the abdominal aorta in cynomolgus monkeys on the BC 0.5% diet for 6 months. The vessels were
freed of the adventitia and homogenized with a Brinkmann Polytron
homogenizer in a medium containing TRIS buffer pH 7.5, 0.05 M;
sucrose, 0.23 M; dithiothreitol, 9 μM; EDTA, 22 μM; and phenomethyl-
sulfanilfluoride, 0.5 mg/ml. The suspension was centrifuged at
10,000 g for 25 min. The pellet was dried, weighed, and saponified
with 2 ml of 33% alcoholic KOH at 70°C for 60 min and the lipids
were extracted into 2 volumes of petroleum ether (B.P. 30-60°C).
Cholesterol was determined in an aliquot by the $FeCl_3$ method
modified by Rudel and Morris (19). Figure 17 shows that the

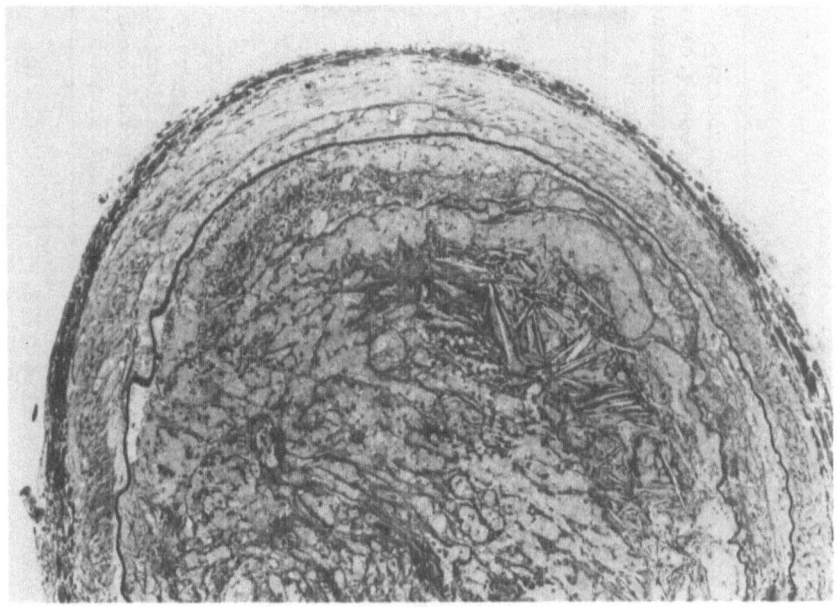

FIGURE 12

Semithin (1μ) epoxy section of occlusion of left posterior cerebral
artery in a M. fascicularis on the BC 0.1% diet for 4 years. The
lumen is completely filled with foam cells, fine elastic fibers,
and masses of lipid containing cholesterol clefts. Methylene
blue-basic fuchsin, 40x.(Reduced 10% for reproduction.)

cholesterol content in the arch vessels (carotids and subclavian
arteries) is higher than in the abdominal aorta, and it correlates
well (r = 0.869; p < 0.01) with the terminal plasma cholesterol
levels; moreover, the concentration in the abdominal aorta does
not correlate with cholesterolemia (r = 0.329; p, N.S.). The
anatomical and chemical discrepancies suggest that observations
conducted in some given arteries should be extrapolated to different
ones only with utmost caution.

Coronary Atherosclerosis in Hypo- and Hyper-responder Animals

The relation between plasma cholesterol and the extent of
atherosclerotic involvement augurs that despite individual variations, hypo-responder animals as a group will have less coronary
atherosclerosis than hyper-responders. Such, at any rate, is the
case in monkeys on the BC 0.1% diet (Table VI). The lack of
statistical significance is probably due to the small number of
animals studied and to the fact that, as a consequence, only two
groups were considered. That is, the normo-responders were probably

TABLE VI

Plasma Cholesterol, Preβ- and β-Lipoprotein Cholesterol, and Coronary
Atherosclerosis in Cynomolgus Monkeys Fed on a Semipurified Diet
(BC 0.1%) for 5 1/2 Months (Mean ± S.E.)

Group	No. of animals	Total cholesterol (mg/100 ml)	Preβ- and β-lipoprotein cholesterol (mg/100 ml)(1)	Coronary atherosclerosis (% encroachment of lumen)
Hypo-responders	6	181 ± 7	97 ± 7	1.2 ± 0.5
Hyper-responders	4	305 ± 19**	201 ± 20*	7.2 ± 3.6***

*p ("t" test) < 0.01; **p < 0.001; ***0.2 > p > 0.1.
(1)Cornwell and Kruger, J. Lipid Res. 2:110-134, 1961 (dextran sulfate precipitation).

TABLE VII

Findings in 18 Normo-responder Cynomolgus Monkeys Fed on a
Semipurified Diet (BC 0.5%) for 6 Months

Body weight (kg)		Terminal plasma cholesterol (mg/100 ml)	Lens wt (mg)	Aortic atherosclerosis (1+ to 5+)	Coronary atherosclerosis (% encroachment of lumen)
Initial	Final				
2.55 ± 0.064	2.57 ± 0.062	701 ± 51	69.84 ± 1.88	3.81 ± 0.26	28 ± 6

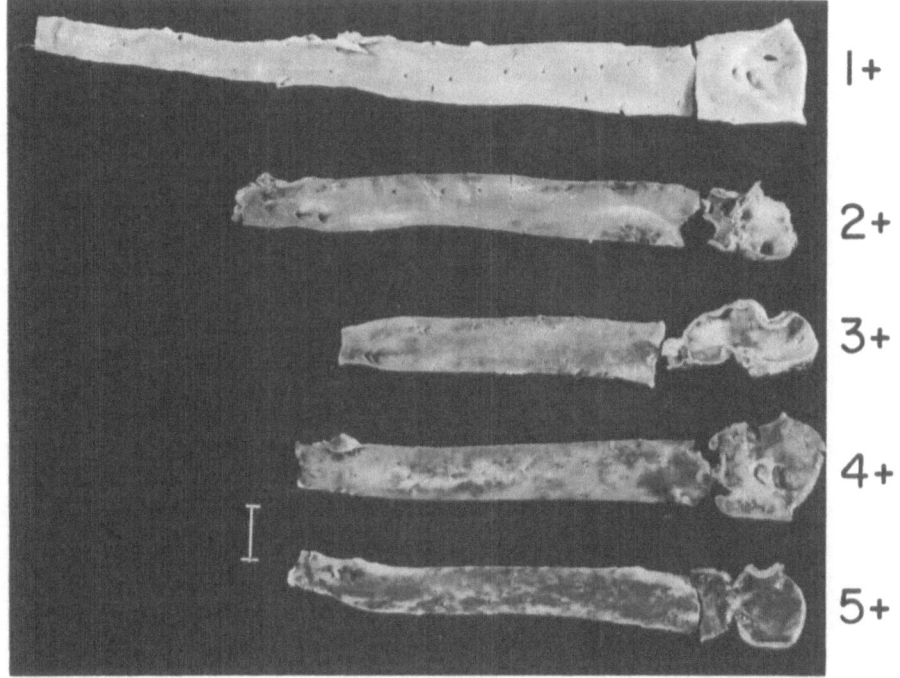

FIGURE 13

Aortas from M. fascicularis on the BC 0.5% diet for 6 months (2+
through 5+) and from a cynomolgus monkey on standard laboratory
chow (1+). The aortas have been stained with Sudan IV and graded
as described in the text. White line, 1 cm.

included among the hyper-responders as well as hypo- and hyper-
reactive animals in both groups.

Atherosclerosis in Normo-responder Animals

Table VII shows the extent of aortic and coronary atherosclerosis in 18 monkeys on the BC 0.5% diet for 6 months, which had a
cholesterolemia ranging from 499 to 816 mg/100 ml after 1 month on
the diet. The monkeys maintained their body weight throughout the
observation and had a terminal plasma cholesterol around 700 mg/
100 ml. The lens weight--an indication of age (21)--was similar
to that found in other adult cynomolgus monkeys studied previously
(20). The dispersion of aortic and coronary atherosclerosis data
in the group is relatively small, probably because of the attempt
to choose monkeys within a given range of cholesterol level.

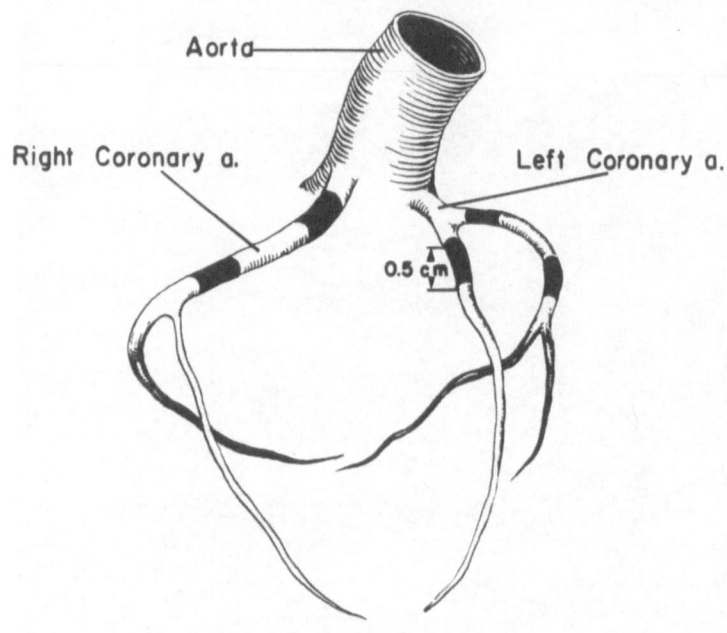

FIGURE 14

Coronary arterial tree in M. fascicularis. The black areas represent the segments removed for histologic study and quantitation,
see text. (From Malinow et al. Atherosclerosis 15:31-36, 1972).

Influencing Atherosclerotic Regression with D-Thyroxine

Because of the well-documented hypocholesterolemic effect of
thyroxine and its analogs (23), there is a great deal of speculation
about whether these substances also have antiatherogenic effects.
The reports so far are conflicting. For example, the development
of aortic atherosclerosis was retarded in rabbits on an atherogenic
diet by the administration of dessicated thyroid (24) but not of
thyroxine (24,25). Moreover, neither dessicated thyroid nor
thyroxine consistently prevent atherosclerosis in cholesterol-fed
chicks (26). In cholesterol-fed rabbits, conflicting results
followed the administration of thyroid hormone analogs which had
lower calorigenic activity than the thyroid hormones (27).
Injection of D-thyroxine in rabbits increased the severity of
aortic atherosclerosis (28) and reduced it in the aortic arch but
not in the abdominal aorta (29). Moreover, neither thyroid hormones
nor their analogs affected the regression of diet-induced aortic
atherosclerosis in chicks (26) or rabbits (29).

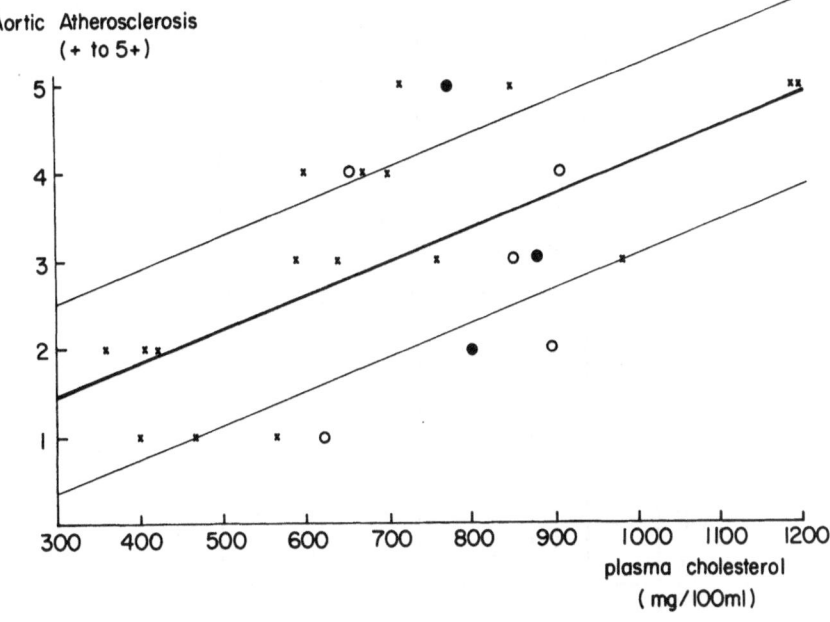

FIGURE 15

Aortic atherosclerosis and terminal plasma cholesterol in M.
fascicularis maintained on the BC diet for 6 months. Grading of
lesions, see text. The heavy line shows the regression function;
thin line, one S.E. Circles, see Figure 16.

We have studied regression of atherosclerosis and the possible
effects of D-thyroxine in cynomolgus monkeys as a part of a more
extensive experiment not yet reported. Monkeys on the BC 0.5%
diet for 6 months were assigned randomly to four groups: (a) for
immediate post mortem study (N=11) or for study 10 months later
after being on (b) chow diet (N=20); (c) chow diet with 7.5 mg of
D-thyroxine/kg food (N=18); or (d) chow diet with 30.0 mg of
D-thyroxine/kg of food (N=21). At monthly intervals plasma cholesterol was determined in certain animals according to a strict
random procedure, as well as before termination in all cases. The
monkeys receiving D-thyroxine tended to return more rapidly to
normo-cholesterolemic levels than the others, but the differences
between them and the monkeys without D-thyroxine were not consistent during the various intervals. The extent of aortic and
coronary atherosclerosis determined at the end of 10 months is
shown in Table VIII. D-thyroxine did not decrease the extent of
the lesions. However, in monkeys on the cholesterol-free

TABLE VIII

Aortic and Coronary Atherosclerosis in Cynomolgus Monkeys (Mean $\pm$ S.E.).

Group	D-T4 (mg/kg food)	# of Animals	Aortic Grade (1+ to 5+)	Coronary artery lumen encroachment (%)	
				Left Coronary	Right Coronary
6 months of BC 0.5% diet	0	11	3.27 $\pm$ 0.38	19.7 $\pm$ 6.7	12.0 $\pm$ 4.5
6 months of BC 0.5% diet + 10 months on standard diet	0	20	1.81 $\pm$ 0.15**	11.2 $\pm$ 2.1 +	10.9 $\pm$ 2.6 +
	7.5	18	1.67 $\pm$ 0.16***	15.6 $\pm$ 2.8 (17) +	12.6 $\pm$ 2.3 (16) +
	30.0	21	1.95 $\pm$ 0.11**	13.2 $\pm$ 2.1 +	10.1 $\pm$ 2.3 +

p ("t" test) vs 6 months of BC 0.5% diet; ** < 0.01; *** < 0.001; + N.S.; number of animals between parentheses.

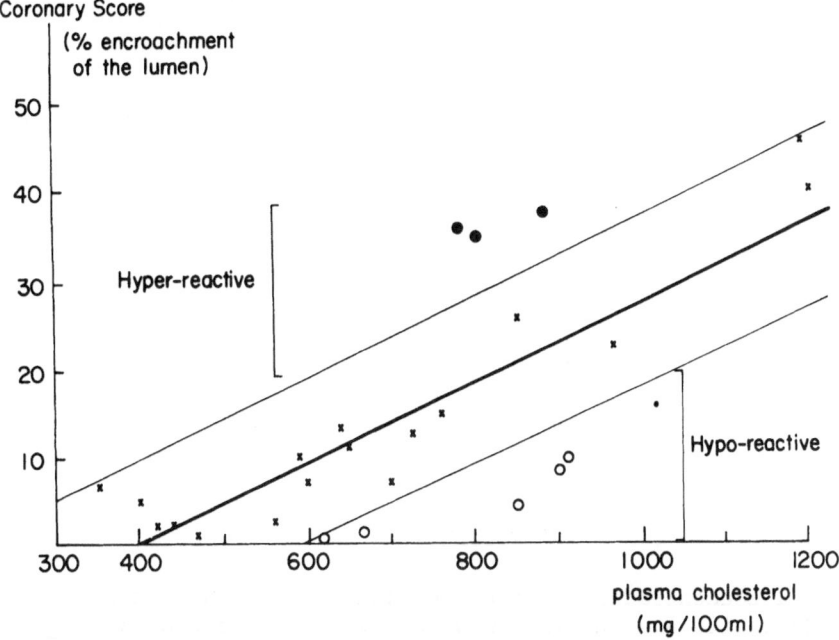

FIGURE 16

Coronary atherosclerosis and terminal plasma cholesterol in the animals shown on Figure 15. The regression function and one S.E. have been calculated. Cases removed by more than one S.E. from the regression line are tentatively identified as hypo-reactive (circles) and hyper-reactive (solid circles); these symbols are used for the same animals in Figure 15.

---

diet, the lesions have apparently regressed in the aorta but not in the coronary arteries. Studies performed on rhesus monkeys (30) suggest that regression in the coronary arteries should be evident 24 months after the atherogenic diet is discontinued.

CONCLUSIONS

The observations so far conducted in cynomolgus monkeys on semipurified diets containing butter and cholesterol suggest that this nonhuman primate is an excellent model for studying the therapy of established coronary atherosclerosis.

(1) This species is available at a reasonable cost and can be kept in captivity in good health for prolonged periods of time.

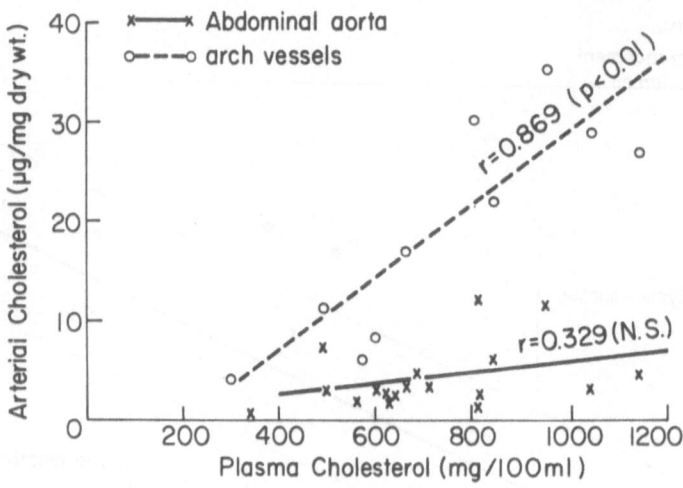

FIGURE 17

Cholesterol concentration in the abdominal aorta and in arch
vessels (carotids and subclavian arteries) in normo-responder M.
fascicularis maintained on the BC 0.5% diet for 6 months. The
regression functions and index of correlation "r" are shown.
N.S., nonsignificant.

----

    (2) It readily accepts semipurified diets with a percentage
composition similar to that of human diets in the U.S.
    (3) Ingestion of these diets leads quite rapidly (around 6
months) to moderate coronary atherosclerosis. More prolonged
feeding leads to lesions which are histologically very similar to
those in man.
    (4) The distribution of lesions in the main coronary arteries
is similar to that in man.
    (5) Methods to quantify the coronary lesions are available.
    (6) The diets can be so modified that cholesterol levels
closely resemble those in hypercholesterolemic man.
    (7) The monkeys are amenable to several therapeutic regimens
which show promise of arresting the progress or inducing the
regression of the coronary lesions.

ACKNOWLEDGMENTS

    Publication #806 of the Oregon Regional Primate Research
Center. Aided by NIH grants RR-00163, HL-16587 and HL-6835, and
American Heart Association, Northeast Ohio Affiliates Inc. grant
#3084-R.

REFERENCES

1. McNulty, W.P. and M.R. Malinow. 1972. The cardiovascular system. In: _Pathology of Simian Primates_. Ed. by R.N. T-W-Fiennes, Karger, Basel, pp. 756-808.

2. Malinow, M.R. and C.A. Maruffo. 1965. Naturally-occurring atherosclerosis in howler monkey (_Alouatta caraya_). J. Atheroscler. Res. 6:368-380.

3. Malinow, M.R. and C.A. Storvick. 1968. Spontaneous coronary lesions in howler monkeys (_Alouatta caraya_). J. Atheroscler. Res. 8:421-431.

4. Malinow, M.R., A. Perley and P.A. McLaughlin. 1968. The effects of pyridinolcarbamate on induced atherosclerosis in monkeys. J. Atheroscler. Res. 8:455-561.

5. Clarkson, T.B., H.B. Lofland, Jr., B.C. Bullock and H.O. Goodman. 1971. Genetic control of plasma cholesterol: Studies on squirrel monkeys. Arch. Pathol. 92:37-45.

6. Lofland, H.B., Jr., T.B. Clarkson, R.W. St. Clair and N.D.M. Lehner. 1972. Studies on the regulation of plasma cholesterol levels in squirrel monkeys of two genotypes. J. Lipid Res. 13:39-47.

7. Taylor, C.B., P. Manalo-Estrella and G.E. Cox. 1963. Atherosclerosis in rhesus monkeys. Arch. Pathol. 76:239-249.

8. Pick, R., P.J. Johnson and G. Glick. 1974. Deleterious effects of hypertension on the development of aortic and coronary atherosclerosis in stumptail macaques (_Macaca speciosa_) on an atherogenic diet. Circ. Res. 35:472-482.

9. Kramsch, D.M. and W. Hollander. 1968. Occlusive atherosclerotic disease of the coronary arteries in monkey (_Macaca irus_) induced by diet. Exp. Molec. Pathol. 9:1-22.

10. Taylor, C.G., G.E. Cox, P. Manalo-Estrella, J. Southworth, D.E. Patton and C. Cathcart. 1962. Atherosclerosis in rhesus monkeys. II. Arterial lesions associated with hypercholesterolemia induced by dietary fat and cholesterol. Arch. Pathol. 74:16-34.

11. Malinow, M.R. 1963. Hormones and atherosclerosis. Adv. Pharmacol. 2:211-242.

12. 1975. Rhesus monkey prices double. Nat. Soc. Med. Res. Bull. 26(5):1.

13. 1975. International Primate Protection League issues appeal
     for moratorium on purchase of stumptailed monkeys. Lab.
     Primate Newslett. 14(3):37.

14. Muckenhirn, N. 1975. Trends in primate imports into the
     United States. ILAR News 18(3):2.

15. Fillios, L.C. and G.V. Mann. 1956. The importance of sex in
     the variability of the cholesteremic response of rabbits fed
     cholesterol. Circ. Res. 4:406-412.

16. Connor, W.E. and S.L. Connor. 1972. The key role of nutri-
     tional factors in the prevention of coronary disease. Prev.
     Med. 1:49-83.

17. Imai, Y. and H. Matsumara. 1973. Genetic studies on induced
     and spontaneous hypercholesterolemia in rats. Atherosclero-
     sis 18:59-64.

18. Cox, G.E., C.B. Taylor, L.G. Cox and M.A. Counts. 1958.
     Atherosclerosis in rhesus monkeys. I. Hypercholesterolemia
     induced by dietary fat and cholesterol. Arch. Pathol.
     66:32-52.

19. Rudel, L.L. and M.D. Morris. 1973. Determination of choles-
     terol using o-ophthalaldehyde. J. Lipid Res. 14:364-366.

20. Malinow, M.R., P. McLaughlin and A. Perley. 1972. The
     effect of pyridinolcarbamate on induced atherosclerosis in
     cynomolgus monkeys. Atherosclerosis 15:31-36.

21. Malinow, M.R., A.A. Pellegrino and E.H. Ramos. 1958. Chemi-
     cal and anatomical correlations in cholesterol-fed rabbits.
     Acta Physiol. Latino Amer. 8:37-46.

22. Malinow, M.R. and A. Corcoran. 1966. Growth of the lens in
     howler monkeys (Alouatta caraya). J. Mammal. 47:58-63.

23. Boyd, G.S. and M.F. Oliver. 1960. The effect of certain
     thyroxine analogues on the serum lipids in human subjects.
     J. Endocrinol. 21:33-43.

24. Turner, K.B. 1933. Studies on the prevention of cholesterol
     atherosclerosis in rabbits. Effects of whole thyroid and of
     potassium iodide. J. Exper. Med. 58:115-125.

25. Moyer, A.W., D. Kritchevsky, W.C. Tesar, J.B. Logan, R.F.J.
     McCandless, R.A. Brown and H.R. Cox. 1956. Effect of
     varying dosages of potassium iodide in experimental athero-
     sclerosis. Proc. Soc. Exp.   Biol. Med. 92:416-418.

26. Katz, L.N. and R. Pick. 1961. Experimental atherosclerosis as observed in the chicken. J. Atheroscler. Res. 1:93-100.

27. Selenkow, H.A. and S.P. Asper, Jr. 1955. Biological activity of compounds structurally related to thyroxine. Physiol. Rev. 35:426-474.

28. Fisher, E.R. 1964. Thyroidal influence on experimental cholesterol atherosclerosis. Am. J. Path. 45:21-39.

29. Kritchevsky, D., J.L. Moynihan, J. Langan, S.A. Tepper and M.L. Sachs. 1961. Effects of D- and L-thyroxine and of D- and L-3,5,3"-triiodo-thyronine on development and regression of experimental atherosclerosis in rabbits. J. Atheroscler. Res. 1:211-221.

30. Armstrong, M.L., E.D. Warner and W.E. Connor. 1970. Regression of coronary atheromatosis in rhesus monkeys. Circ. Res. 27:59-67.

THE NONHUMAN PRIMATES AS MODELS FOR STUDYING HUMAN ATHEROSCELROSIS:

STUDIES ON THE CHIMPANZEE, THE BABOON AND THE RHESUS MACACUS

V. BLATON and H. PEETERS

Simon Stevin Instituut voor Wetenschappelijk Onderzoek

Jerusalemstraat 34, B-8000 BRUGGE (Belgium)

This work was supported by grants from the National Institutes of Health, Bethesda, Md (USA), Public Health Service Grant n° HE9969, the World Health Organization, the NFGWO (Belgium) Grants n° 1153, 1206, the Franqui Foundation and the RUCA-ZOO (Antwerpen).

The main objective of experimental atherosclerosis is to start in animals an atherogenic process in such a way as to be able to study the origin, the development and the effects. Many species exhibit spontaneous arterial disease of the aorta and coronary arteries, and these provide useful models for study (1).

Over several years non human primates have become of interest as animal models for research on human atherosclerosis because of their phylogenetic relationship to man and the hope that atherosclerosis induced in them would have more similarities to man than that induced in lower animals. Of approximately 200 species of non human primates, 12 have been examined for the prevalence of naturally occurring lesions, and in seven of these species diet-induced atherosclerosis has been studied. Although numerous genera of monkeys have not been completely evaluated, those appearing to have the most potential usefulness as biomedical models in studying human atherosclerosis research are the New World Genera Saimiri (2-3), Cebus (4-6) and Pan Troglodytes (Chimpanzees) (7-9) and the Old World Genera Papio (10-13) and Macacus (14).

Among the New World monkeys that have been studied, the Squirrel monkeys develop naturally occurring atherosclerosis most frequently (15). Atherosclerosis in these species can be induced by diets, and the lesions developed in the aorta are morphologically similar to those of humans. Coronary atherosclerosis is however more often seen

in the small intramyocardial arteries (16). Although naturally
occurring sudanophilic lesions of the aorta are uncommon in the
Cebus monkeys (C. albifrons), diet-induced coronary atherosclerosis
in these species resembles that of squirrel monkeys but, in contrast,
these animals have only slight lesions of the aorta and extensive
lesions of the carotid bifurcation (5, 15, 17). Spider monkeys
(Ateles sp.) are another group of New World Monkeys that have been
reported to develop naturally occurring atherosclerosis but have been
used very little in atherosclerosis research (18). These animals
became only slightly hypercholesterolemic when fed diets containing
1 mg of cholesterol / Kcal, which produce marked cholesterolemia in
most species of non human primates. Both control and experimental
spider monkeys had aortic fatty streaks and occasional lesions of the
major branches of the coronary arteries (19).

    Phylogeny, anatomy and cholesterol metabolism bring the chimpan-
zee (Pan Troglodytes) closer to man than any other subhuman primate.
In their natural habitat, chimpanzees feed on an omnivorous diet, comparable in many aspects to the human diet (20). Atheromatous coronary lesions similar to those of man were found by Vastesaeger et al.
(21), and more spontaneous aortic and cerebral atherosclerosis was
found in adult chimpanzees than in any other non human primates (22).
Manning (23) demonstrated coronary atherosclerosis and thrombosis
leading to the death of an 8 year old ape - presumably a chimpanzee.
One more similarity between man and the chimpanzee may be found in the
precociousness of the first alterations of intimal sclerosis, which
are systematically present in the coronary arteries of the newborn in
man and chimpanzee.

    The mean plasma lipids in 63 captive chimpanzees are higher than
in any group of captive monkeys, and the dispersion of the individual
cholesterol (120 - 470 mg %) values is as wide as in a western human
population (24, 25). It seems also highly probable that besides
dietary factors, stress has a non negligible influence on plasma
cholesterol in chimpanzees as well as in man (26). Feeding chimpanzees 2% cholesterol in maize or cotton seed oil does not influence
significantly either free or esterified cholesterol (24), which
is in analogy with human behaviour under the same conditions (27).
High caloric diets, however, supplemented with 2.5 % cholesterol induced
a hyperbetalipoproteinemia in chimpanzees which is in many aspects
identical to human type IIa (8).

    Mann (29) demonstrated furthermore that chimpanzees are about
five times more sensitive to dietary cholesterol than rabbits are.
Evidence of hereditary hyperbetalipoproteinemia has been provided in
other species of non human primates (30). The presence   of the
spontaneous cerebral lesions in a hypercholesterolemic female chimpanzee makes plausible the hypothesis of essential hypercholesterolemia in this animal (31). There are several reasons to believe that
genotype IIa exists in the chimpanzee, and if genetic studies on a

large scale would confirm the reality of familial hypercholesterolemia in chimpanzees, then perhaps some breedings could be more or
less arbitrarily selected as suitable and others excluded as unfit
for experimental atherosclerosis

The striking resemblance of the biochemical and pathological
data to that of human type IIa (8) makes of this ape a most valuable tool for experimental atherosclerosis.

Among the Old World non human primates similar differences can
be found. The rhesus monkey (Macaca mulatta) has been the most
commonly used in the study of human atherosclerosis. Naturally
occurring aortic and coronary atherosclerosis is infrequent in rhesus but may occur and be quite severe in some aged animals (32).
Under an atherogenic diet the rhesus monkey becomes markedly hypercholesterolemic and develops arterial lesions particularly of the
aorta and proximal main branches of the coronary arteries (14, 33,
34).

Baboons (Papio cynocephalus) appear to be resistant and develop only slight aortic lesions. However, in the wild these animals
develop diffuse fatty streaks and some adult animals show lesions in
the aorta complicated by hemorrhage into the plaque (35, 36).
Although the baboon plasma lipids expressed in mg % and in percentage are similar to man, the plasma lipoprotein profiles are quite
different especially in the ratio of high and low density lipoproteins (37, 38). Experimental work demonstrated that atherosclerosis can be induced in baboons by a cholesterol rich diet, containing
egg yolk and butter (39, 40). Type II hyperlipoproteinemia that
occurs in man, was induced to a certain similar extent in the baboon
by an atherogenic diet (11, 13, 41-44).

The search for a completely satisfactory animal model is not
finished, but in most studies there are not enough detailed biochemical data available to distinguish one species from another. In this
communication the properties that the ideal animal should possess
for studying the effect of the plasma hyperlipoproteinemia on the
development of atherosclerosis will be discussed in the following way:
1. The circulating plasma lipoproteins must have near identical phy-
sico-chemical and physiological properties of the human plasma lipoproteins, 2. The animal model must be accessible for inducing the
hyperlipoproteinemia resembling the human hyperlipoproteinemia, and
3. The arterial lesions produced experimentally by diet should closely resemble those seen in the human.

ANIMALS AND DIETS

Ten chimpanzees (white faced, Pan troglodytes) of mixed sexes
(7 males, 3 females) 2-3 years of age at the beginning of the experiment were divided in two groups. Four animals were given a control
diet and six animals were fed an atherogenic diet. These animals
were being investigated as part of a long term study on the effect
of high cholesterol diets on atherosclerosis in the chimpanzee and
had been consuming the diets for 7-8 years. The control group received 10 gm basic control diet per kg body weight / day, supplemented
with two apples, two bananas and one-half orange. Vegetables (400 g/
day), one egg, and half a liter of skimmed milk a day were also
given. The atherogenic diet contained the control diet, 2.5 % cholesterol and 14 % butter. The daily dietary intake was 12 gm basic
atherogenic diet per kg body weight per day supplemented with one
liter of milk a day. Supplements of fruits, one egg and vegetables
were the same as for the control group. Vitamins and minerals were
added to the diet. In table 1 a detailed analytical composition of
the chimpanzee control and atherogenic diet is given.

The total intake of the fat diet corresponds to a cholesterol
intake of 0.25 gm/kg body weight/day. The daily caloric intake
amounted to 1750 kcal/day for the control group and to 2900 kg/day
for the atherogenic group. Both groups of animals at the beginning
of the experiment showed the same body weight. During the experiment
there was a $\pm$ 8 % weight gain of the animals under atherogenic diet
over the control animals.

The control diet had a lipid content of 3 gm % with 0.15 gm %
cholesterol and a protein content of 17 gm %. The atherogenic wet
diet contained 24 gm % lipid with 3.3 gm % cholesterol and 14 gm %
protein. Palmitic (22 %), oleic (31 %) and linoleic (30 %)
were the chief fatty acids in the control diet. In the fat diet
there was a relative increase of myristic (Δ 9 %) and palmitic
(Δ 9 %) and a relative decrease of linoleic acid (Δ 22 %).

Four chimpanzees of mixed sexes (2 males and 2 females) 8-10
years of age, eating a control diet for several years, were given
a sucrose enriched diet during 110 days. The composition of the
diet is completely described in table 1. The sucrose diet consists
of 200 g control diet supplemented with 300 g sucrose, one egg, half
a liter of skimmed milk, fruit and vegetables. The sucrose diet contains 85 % carbohydrates and the fatty acid profile of the control
diet consists of 57 % saturated, 33 % mono-unsaturated and 10 % polyunsaturated fatty acids.

Eighteen young baboons (Papio cynocephalus), three females and
15 males, 12-18 months of age, were divided in equal groups and given
either a control or an atherogenic diet. These animals were also
part of a long term study of the effect of hypercholesterolemic diets

TABLE I

Chimpanzee Diet Composition

DIET	INTAKE/DAY and COMPOSITION	LIPIDS g/100 g (dry)			FATTY ACIDS %			DIET SUPPLEMENT	Kcal/DAY and % ORIGIN
		TG	Chol	PL	Δ:0	Δ:1	Δ:p		
CONTROL (C)	10 g/kg	2.2	0.2	0.5	33	33	34	2 apples 2 bananas 1/2 orange 400 g veget. 1 egg 1/2 1 skim milk vitamins	+ 1750 Kcal 24 % protein 8 % lipid 68 % CHO
FAT	12 g/kg 83.5 % (C) 2.5 % Chol 14.0 % butter	19.8	3.3	0.6	57	33	10	idem (C) + milk	+ 2900 Kcal 17 % protein 37 % lipid 46 % CHO
SUCROSE	12 g/kg 40 % (C) 60 % sucrose	0.9	0.1	0.2	33	33	34	idem (C)	+ 2600 Kcal 11 % protein 4 % lipid 85 % CHO

on atherosclerosis in the baboon and had been consuming the diets
for 1.5 - 3 years.

The control diet consisted of rat cake supplemented with Vitamin C. The atherogenic diet contains the control diet supplemented
with 15 % egg-yolk and 15 % butter and contains 20 % lipid with
0.55 % cholesterol. Palmitic (27 %), oleic (23 %) and linoleic
(31 %) are the chief fatty acids in the control diet. In the
atherogenic diet there was a relative increase of oleic acid to 39 %
and of saturated fatty acids, concomitant with a large and simultaneous decrease of the linoleic and arachidonic acid content.

The total intake of the atherogenic diet amounted to approximately 25 g/kg body weight/day and corresponds to a cholesterol intake
of 0.14 g/kg of body weight/day. Animals were of different body
weight (4 - 8 kg) and given food ad libitum. Weight gain in the
two groups was the same.

Sixteen male rhesus monkeys (Macaca mulatta), 1 year old were
divided into two groups. 12 were on a control diet and 4   were fed
the high cholesterol rich diet as described for the chimpanzee. Each
animal ate an average of 110 g of the fresh diet put in the cage
daily. As in the other non human primates, such as chimpanzees and
baboons, the diet induces within about 6 months a marked hyperbetalipoproteinemia with elevated plasma cholesterol levels reaching
600 mg % with normal triglyceride levels.

SAMPLES

Human Plasma Samples

For comparative work on the induced hyperlipoproteinemia in the
non human primates, after an overnight fast plasma was taken from
5 male subjects (45-55 years of age) with angina pectoris or hyper-
tensive vascular disease, who had type II hyperlipoproteinemia.
Other plasma samples were obtained from different patients with type
IV hyperlipoproteinemia and also from 4 normal young men aged 21-25
years old.

The EDTA (1 mg/ml) plasma samples were kept at 4°C prior to
analyses which were performed within a few days of taking the blood.

Plasma Samples   from   Non Human Primates

All animals were tranquilized with Sernylan® (Parke Davis)   and
Ptalamonal® (Janssen Pharmaceuticals), and fasting blood into EDTA

(1 mg/ml) was taken from the femoral artery as previously described (46). Plasma was obtained after centrifugation at 3,000 g
and used within 6 hr for lipoprotein isolation. For lipid and fatty
acid analysis samples were kept at 4°C.

METHODS

Biochemical Methods for Lipid Analysis

Most of the methods and techniques used in the separation and
characterization of the plasma lipoproteins and plasma lipids are
fully described in earlier papers.
Integrated procedure of lipoprotein and lipid analysis : All
biochemical methods and techniques used in the separation and characterization of the electrochromatographic plasma lipoprotein fractions
were described by Blaton et al. (11) and Peeters et al. (12).
The lipid and fatty acid composition of the individual plasma lipoproteins are not altered by the integrated procedure (47). The
beta lipoprotein concentration could be expressed in Macklagan units
according to the method of Walton and Scott (48).

The lipoprotein patterns obtained by electrochromatography have
previously been compared with those obtained by paper electrophoretic
and ultracentrifugal fractionation procedures. Immunological, ultracentrifugal and electrochromatographic comparisons were made (43,
49). No significant differences were found in lipid distribution
among the lipoproteins obtained by centrifugation or by electrochromatography (43).

Lipid fatty acids were analyzed by gas liquid chromatography
after saponification in 3 % potassium hydroxide in methanol at 70°C
and after esterification in BF_3-CH_3OH (250 mg/l) by heating for
30 min. at 80°C in a sealed tube. Column temperature was programmed
from 195-225°C at 2°C/min after an isothermal period of 5 min (43).

Biochemical determination of lipids in plasma and low and high
density lipoproteins : Plasma lipids were extracted with chloroform/
methanol (2/1, V/V) in a ratio of organic phase to plasma of 24:1.
Total lipids, cholesterol and triglycerides were determined according to De la Huerga (50), Rozenthal (51) and Van Handel and
Zilversmith (52). Phospholipids were analyzed according to a
modified method of Rouser (12). Lipids from lipoproteins separated by electrochromatography were extracted from the curtain fragments twice with $CHCl_3-CH_3OH$ (1/1, V/V) for 15 hr with constant
stirring and the last traces of phospholipids were extracted with
CH_3OH-CH_3COOH (99/1, V/V). Recovery of all lipids by elution from
paper was 99.2 %.

Lipids in plasma and in the alpha and beta lipoproteins were
further differentiated by thin layer chromatography on Silicagel G

plates in PE (40-60)/(CH_2H_5)$_2O/CH_3COOH$ (80/20/1, V/V/V). For
fatty acid analysis the detection was performed with a solution of
42 mg/100 ml Rhodamine B and 14 mg/100 ml 2,7-dichlorofluoresceine
in (C_2H_5)$_2O/C_2H_5OH/H_2O$ (63/30/7, V/V/V).

Biochemical Methods for Isolation and Characterization of Plasma
              Lipoproteins and their Apolipoproteins

     Most of all methods and techniques used in the separation and
characterization of the plasma apolipoproteins are described in earlier papers (7, 38).

     Preparation and delipidation of plasma lipoproteins : After
an initial centrifugation at 9,000 g for 30 min. at 4°C (IEC ultracentrifuge, A 321 rotor) chylomicron free plasma was layered with
a d = 1.006 g/ml of NaCl and VLDL was isolated at 70,488 g for 26 hr
at 16°. Low density lipoprotein classes (LDL_1 and LDL_2) and high
density lipoprotein classes (HDL_2 and HDL_3) are centrifuged according to the method of Blaton et al. (7). Densities were adjusted
by adding solid NaCl-KBr. The high density lipoprotein samples (400
mg% protein), dialyzed against 0.1 M NaCl, were delipidated according
to a slightly modified method of Sodhi and Gould (53). The precipitates were solubilized in $NaHCO_3$, pH 9.1, finally lyophilized and
stored at -20°C. The low density lipoproteins were delipidated
after incubation in 1 % SDS according to Koga et al. (54).

     Electrophoresis of plasma lipoproteins and of the apopolypep-
tides :

     Agarose gel electrophoresis : The homogeneity of isolated plas-
ma lipoproteins was characterized on a modified agarose gel system
as previously described by Lindgren (55) and Van Melsen et al.(56).
The agarose electrophoretic method of Hatch et al. (57) was used
for the quantitative evaluation of lipoprotein patterns.

     Polyacrylamide gel electrophoresis : Analytical polyacrylamide
gel electrophoresis was performed in 10.9 % acrylamide and 0.3 %
N.N'-methylenebisacrylamide (2.7 % cross-linking) in the presence
of 8 M urea using the modified method of Davies (58). In our
procedure however the proteins were fixed in 20 % trichloroacetic
acid (TCA) for 2 hr and further destained in 7.5% HAc and stored
in 5 % HAc.

Sodium dodecyl sulphate - polyacrylamide molecular weight determinations : Apolipoproteins were preincubated in 1 % SDS betamercaptoethanol, and 0.01 M sodium phosphate (pH 7.0) at 37° for 2 hr and
were further dialyzed against 0.1 % SDS 0.1 % betamercaptoethanol
in the same buffer. Gels were prepared according to Weber and
Osbron (59). More details were previously described (7, 38).
Preparative and analytical isoelectric focusing : Preparative iso-

electric focusing was performed according to the method of Vesterberg and Svensson (60) with the LKB instruments. Apopolypeptides
from HDL were isolated based on their isoelectric points and collected in a preparative manner for further identification according to
an adapted method (7). Analytical polyacrylamide gel isoelectric
focusing was performed according to Awdeh et al. (61) on a Multyphor
(LKB) equipment. The microheterogeneity and the individual isoelectric points of the polymorphic forms of apolipopolypeptides were
determined by an adapted method (7, 38).

Isolation and identification of apopolypeptides from plasma
lipoproteins :

Chromatography of plasma apolipoproteins : Sephadex G-200 gel
filtration. The apolipoproteins were fractionated by a modification of the procedure of Scanu et al. (62), on two sequentially
connected columns (2.5 x 100 cm) equilibrated with 0.01 M tris-
HCl buffer (pH 8.6) - 8 M urea - 0.001 M EDTA in the presence of
sodium azide (20 mg %). The apopolypeptides were isolated from
apoHDL by chromatography on DEAE cellulose in 6 M urea using a modification of the method of Shore and Shore (63). Whatmann DE-52
cellulose was equilibrated with 0.01 M tris-HCl pH 8.2, containing
6 M urea. The column (0.9 x 60 cm) was eluted with a 1,600 ml
linear gradient of 0.01 M Tris HCl, pH 8.2, 6 M urea, to 0.10 M
Tris HCl, pH 8.2, 6 M urea. Both methods were completely described
(7, 38).

Terminal amino acid residues : NH_2-terminal residues were determined by the dansylation procedure as described by Gros and Labouesse (64), and the dansyl amino acids were identified by TLC on
silica gel plates according to Zanetta et al. (65). For the COOH-
terminal analysis, di-isopropyl fluorophosphate treated carboxypep-
tidase A, obtained from Sigma, was prepared according to Ambler (66).
Sodium bicarbonate buffer instead of N-ethylmorpholine acetate buffer,
pH 8.5, was used. The released amino acids were identified and quantitated on a Beckman Model 121 automatic amino acid analyzer as previously described (7).

Amino acid analysis : The quantitative amino acid analysis was
performed by the method of Spackman et al. (67) on a Beckman model
121 amino acid analyzer equipped with an automatic sample injector.
Half-cystine and methionine were determined as cysteic acid and methionine sulfone after performic acid oxidation of the protein (68).
Tryptophan was determined after p-toluene sulphonic acid hydrolysis
for 22 hr at 110°C according to Liu and Chang (69).

Biophysical Methods for Characterization of Apolipoproteins

Microcalorimetry : Calorimetric measurements were carried out
at 27.5° in an LKB batch microcalorimeter with gold plated cells.
The calibration of the calorimeter was performed electrically and
checked by measuring the dilution heat of sucrose solution (70).

Sequence of apopolypeptides : The amino acid sequence of baboon
apo-A-I and apo-A-II was established from the cyanogen bromide fragments. The sequences were determined by conventional methods and
involved the isolation of the tryptic peptide (71).

HISTOLOGICAL EXAMINATIONS OF ARTERIES

Upon death by myocardial infarction the heart in two chimpanzees and representative tissue segments of the main arterial trunks
were stored in 10 % buffered formalin. Paraplast sections (4 μ
thick) were made after routine embedding in a tissue processor.
Other frozen sections (15 μ thick) of adjacent tissue were cut with
the ice microtome for the demonstration of lipids. The following
stains were used : Hematoxyline - eosin, Van Gieson, Orecin, PAS
after manus, Alcian blue at pH 2.5 and Scarlet red. For fluorescence
microscopy fresh mounted sections in Uvak and after acriflavine orange stain. The observations were made in blue light making use of
BG 38 and BG 12 filter, and in UV making use of BG 38 and two UGI
filters. Polariscopy was used for birefringence. The presence of
plasma low and high density lipoproteins in the arterial intima was
investigated in deepfrozen material fixed in alcohol and rehydrated
in physiological saline by immunohistological examination in the
presence of apoA and apoB. Coronary arteries of baboons and rhesus
monkeys under control and hypercholesterolemic diet were macroscopically and microscopically examined.

RESULTS

Comparative Properties of the Circulating Plasma Lipoproteins

Plasma lipid and lipoprotein spectra : Table II describes the
main plasma lipids of the chimpanzee as compared to the baboon and
the rhesus values. Low lipid values were obtained for the baboon,
but in a similar percentage composition as in the other species and
in man. Total cholesterol is mainly transported by LDL in the chimpanzee and in the rhesus. In the baboon however HDL is the chief
carrier of cholesterol. The percentage distribution of the phospholipid subclasses are given in Table III. As for man and chimpanzee
phosphatidylcholine (PC) (72 %) is the predominant phospholipid
component in the baboon and the rhesus, followed by sphingomyelin

TABLE II

Normal Plasma Lipid Values in Non-Human Primates

Normal Plasma Lipid Levels

mg%	chimp. n=4	baboon n=8	rhesus n=4
TC	259	116	132
FC	65	23	31
CE	326	156	170
TG	60	36	39
PL	295	119	230

TABLE III

Normal Plasma Phospholipid Levels in Human and Non-Human Primates

Normal Plasma PL-Levels

%	human n=12	chimp. n=4	baboon n=3	rhesus n=4
OH-PC	5.2	4.1	6.2	4.8
Sph	18.5	16.6	7.3	7.5
PC	72.1	70.1	73.9	79.4
PI	0.5	1.8	3.7	1.9
PS	0.2	1.4	1.2	0.2
PEt	3.5	6.0	5.7	6.2

(Sph) which is much higher in the new world species (10 %).
The minor phospholipid subclasses as phosphatidylethanolamine (PE),
inositol (PI) and phosphatidyl serine (PS) are identical in the
non human primates and higher in concentration (mg %) than in man.
Differences observed in the PL subclasses are related to structural
and compositional differences in the individual apolipoproteins,
which contain potential differences in functional aspects. Detailed
fatty acid analyses showed linoleic acid ($\pm$ 30 %) and oleic acid
($\pm$ 20 %) as the main fatty acid components in the observed species.

     The analytical ultracentrifugal analyses of human and non human
primate plasma lipoproteins were performed as described by Ewing et
al. (72). The agarose electrophoretic lipoprotein patterns are
shown in fig. 1 and the analytical ultracentrifugal data are given
in Table IV. The baboon plasma contained no VLDL (Sf 20), and compared to the human pattern decreased low density lipoproteins
(Sf 0-20) were observed. As a result the % concentration of the
baboon total HDL (74 %) and the rhesus HDL (68 %) were much higher than in man (32 %) and chimpanzee (53 %). In comparison to
man the non human primates showed an inverse HDL_2/HDL_3 ratio.

Chemical and immunological analysis of the plasma lipoproteins :
In earlier reports no differences were described for the percentage
lipid composition of the plasma lipoprotein subclasses in the non
human primates with a high ressemblance to the human values (43).

     With regard to the plasma samples the immunological relation-
ship was examined between the non human primates and human lipoproteins using the antisera which were available, specific for human
apo-A, apo-B and apo-C and also for Lp(a) lipoprotein and human Ag

NORMAL PLASMA LIPOPROTEINS

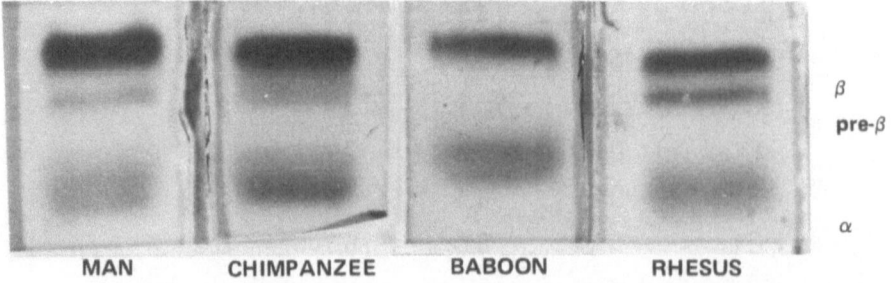

Figure 1. The agarose electrophoretic lipoprotein patterns in man and
          non human primates.

TABLE IV

The UCF Lipoprotein Pattern in Man, Chimpanzee, and Baboon in Mg%

mg/100ml	Sf >20	Sf 12-20	Sf 0-12	F° 1.20 3.5-9	0 -3.5
human [a]	173	57	380	62	226
chimp.	40	14	324	268	156
baboon [b]	0	3	118	211	134

a : Nichols   b : Howard

lipoprotein allotypes.   All chimpanzee plasma reacted with sheep and rabbit anti-human antiserum specific for the apolipoproteins A, B and C, which suggest that human and chimpanzee apopolypeptides are very closely related.   After absorption of this antisera no residual precipitin reactivity could be detected against human serum.   A surprising finding was that all chimpanzee specimens reacted with human Lp(a) lipoprotein, again giving an apparent reaction of identity. Furthermore in the chimpanzee, the human Ag allotypes Ag(t), Ag(y) and Ag(g) were identified.   The baboon and the rhesus plasma lipoproteins are immunologically quite different. For apo(A) and apo(B) similar results were observed, apo(C) however was, in more than 50 % of the samples, absent, and furthermore Lp(a) was never detected. Chimpanzee plasma adsorbed with anti-baboon plasma lipoprotein gives still a residual immunoprecipitin reactivity against human plasma lipoproteins.   This suggests that chimpanzee plasma lipoproteins, very closely related to man, have higher immunological properties than the representatives of the old world (73).

The purified THDL (d = 1.063-1.210) from the non human primates yielded a percentage protein-lipid distribution similar to the normal data in man and had a protein content of 47.5 %.   Surprising findings were in the percentage distribution of the phospholipid classes.   As for man and as described for plasma, PC is the major phospholipid, but the baboon and the rhesus have higher values.   Differences in the non human primates were in the higher percentage PC and the lower Sph content for the old world representatives (Table V).   The chimpanzee phospholipid subclasses are identical to man.

TABLE V

The Phospholipid Subclasses in HDL (d=1.063-1.210 g/ml)

HDL (1.063-1.210)	PC	OH-PC	Sph	PI	PS´	PEt	other PL
human [a]	74.4	2.9	13.2	2.4	0.8	3.1	3.1
chimp.	79.8	0.4	12.5	0.7	0.2	6.4	-
baboon	81.2	0.7	5.9	3.6	0.4	8.3	-
rhesus [b]	87.7	3.6	3.8	-	1.1	3.8	-

a: Skipski   b: Scanu

The apoHDL polypeptides from the chimpanzee and the baboon were analyzed by polyacrylamide gel electrophoresis in SDS medium with and without the reducing agent beta-mercaptoethanol and are compared to man (fig. 2). The chimpanzee has a similar peptide pattern as in man, with apo-A-I as the main component, but with a lower apoA-II resulting in a higher apo-A-I/apo-A-II ratio (5/1). The dimeric apo-A-II, absent in the baboon and in the rhesus (74) is replaced by a monomeric peptide of M.W. 11,000, characterized by the absence of histidine, cystine, tryptophan and isoleucine.

The low density lipoprotein classes (LDL_2, d= 1.019-1.063), which are similar in the percentage distribution of polar and apolar lipids (43), have also an identical amino acid composition in all species (Table VI) and established again an identical apoB for human and non human primates. The amino acid composition however from LDL_1 (d = 1.006-1.019), similar for man and chimpanzee, is quite different for the baboon, which is related to differences in the apoC peptides as was shown immunologically (Table VII).

Structural and functional aspects of the high density lipoproteins in human and non human primates : The apoHDL peptides from human and non human primates were fractionated on DEAE-cellulose columns (fig. 3). The major component A-I identical for all species, appears in different polymorphic forms and shows an identical amino acid composition (Table VIII). The human dimeric peptide apo-A-II is present in the chimpanzee and completely absent in the other

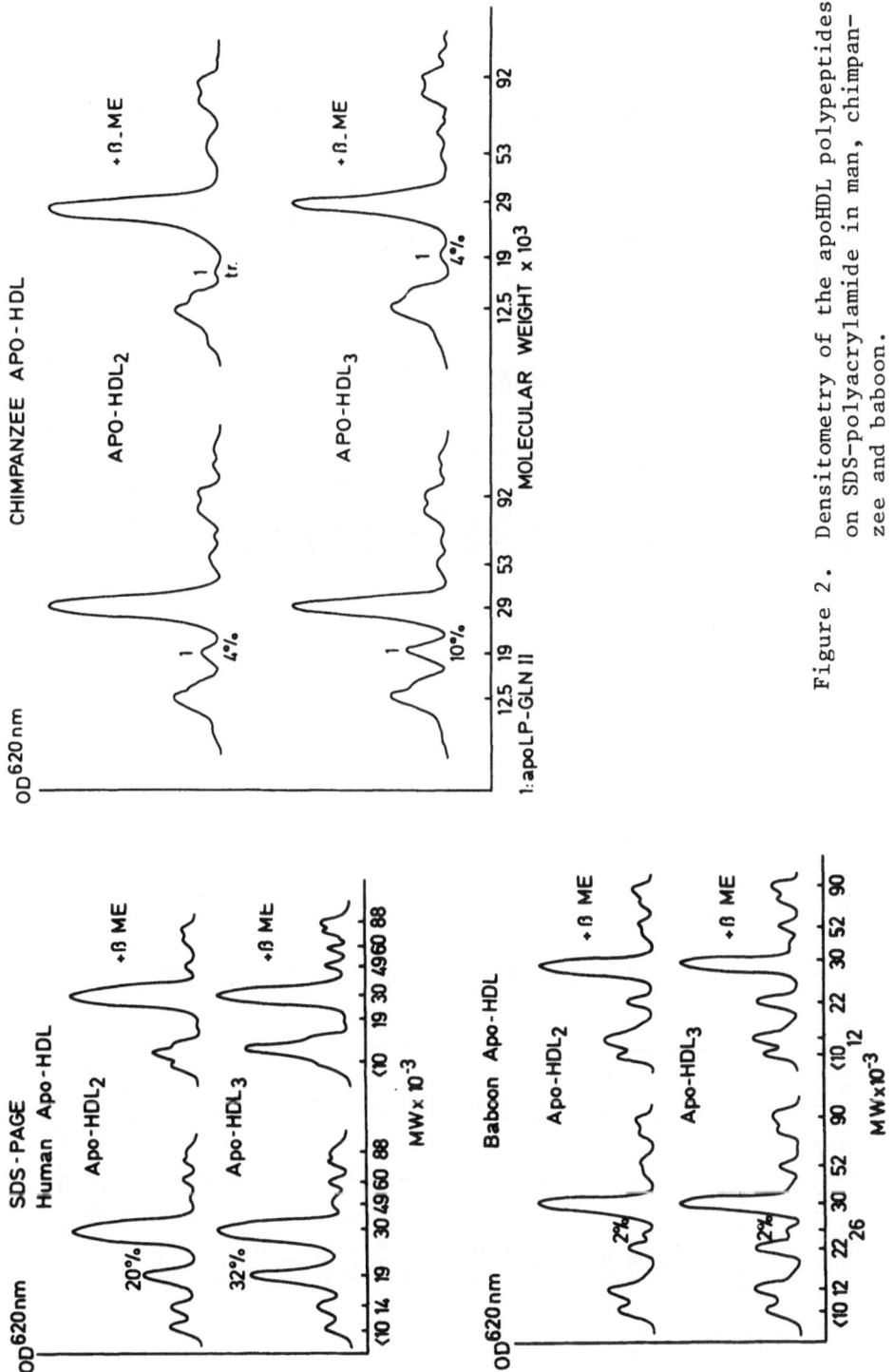

Figure 2.   Densitometry of the apoHDL polypeptides on SDS-polyacrylamide in man, chimpanzee and baboon.

TABLE VII

Comparative Amino Acid Composition of Plasma LDL1 (d=1.006–1.019) in Man, Chimpanzee, and Baboon.

amino acid	human	chimp.	baboon
LYS	70 *	73	65
HIS	19	20	22
ARG	39	54	34
TRP	nd**	nd	nd
ASP	98	91	104
THR	65	63	68
SER	100	90	128
GLU	133	163	121
PRO	38	36	49
GLY	56	54	89
ALA	82	79	75
CYS/2	8	nd	nd
VAL	62	63	45
MET	22	nd	nd
ILE	39	40	42
LEU	102	112	91
TYR	27	23	25
PHE	40	39	42

* mol/1000 mol of amino acids

** not determined

TABLE VI

Comparative Amino Acid Composition of Plasma LDL2 (d=1.019–1.063) in Man, Chimpanzee, and Baboon.

amino acid	human	chimp.	baboon
LYS	79 *	78	74
HIS	25	25	26
ARG	35	36	37
TRP	nd**	5	3
ASP	103	100	105
THR	61	63	65
SER	90	85	84
GLU	126	122	134
PRO	36	32	36
GLY	46	45	49
ALA	62	63	62
CYS/2	nd	11	7
VAL	49	53	54
MET	17	24	27
ILE	60	56	46
LEU	126	120	118
TYR	33	31	28
PHE	52	51	45

* mol/1000 mol of amino acids

** not determined

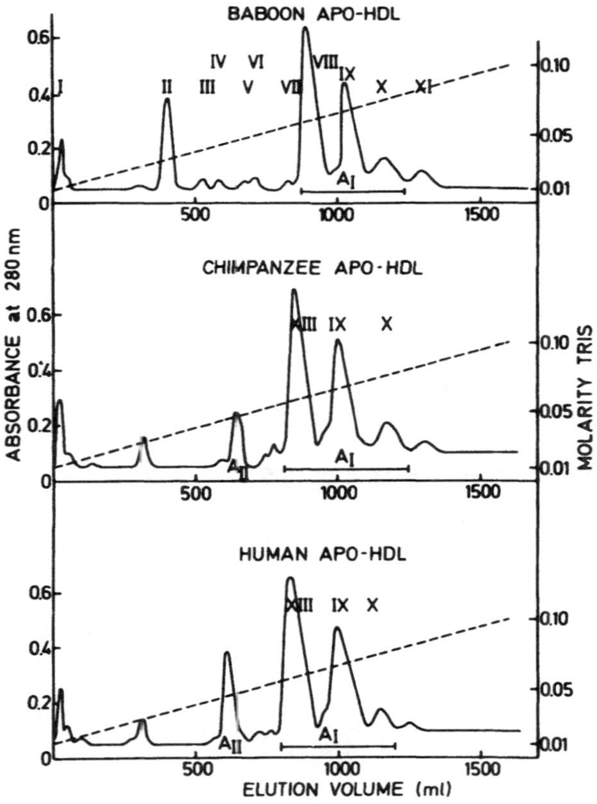

TABLE VIII

The Amino Acid Composition of Apo-A-I in Human and Non Human Primates.

amino acid	human [a]	chimp	baboon	rhesus [b]
LYS	78 *	91	83	87
HIS	23	20	30	26
ARG	68	62	63	57
TRP	30	11	13	22
ASP	98	85	79	79
THR	38	42	45	44
SER	62	57	65	57
GLU	181	196	189	192
PRO	37	40	42	44
GLY	44	44	45	44
ALA	76	80	74	74
CYS/2	0	0	0	0
VAL	51	54	61	61
MET	15	17	12	9
ILE	0	0	0	0
LEU	148	149	152	157
TYR	28	27	26	26
PHE	23	25	21	22

* mol /1000mol of amino acids
a Shore and Shore (1968)
b Edelstein et al (1972)

Figure 3.

Chromatography of apoHDL on DEAE-cellulose columns.

two species. The baboon and rhesus HDL contain an identical monomeric peptide completely different in amino acid composition from
human apo-A-II (Table IX).

The amino acid sequence of the macacus rhesus is known, and work
is in progress on the determination of the structure of the baboon
DEAE-fraction II (fig. 4). From the amino acid analysis of CNBr
fraction I and II, it was possible to show a complete identity for
the amino acid sequence in the COOH-terminal portion of the molecule
and in the two tryptic peptides from CNBr-fraction I.

With the exception of two changes, the sequence of the baboon
apo-A-I is identical to human apo-A-I through the first 30 residues.
The changes are at residue 15 (ala - val) and residue 21 (val -
ala).

From the recombination studies of the apo polypeptides with sonicated phospholipid emulsions structural and functional aspects are
related. Baboon apo-A-I and human apo-A-I bind phospholipids in the
same way without any difference.

TABLE IX

The Amino Acid Composition of Apo-A-II
in Human and Non Human Primates

amino acid	human [a]	chimp. [b]	baboon [c]	rhesus [d]
LYS	115 *	117	96	104
HIS	0	0	0	0
ARG	0	0	13	13
TRP	0	0	0	0
ASP	41	65	55	52
THR	82	78	76	78
SER	82	65	81	65
GLU	198	195	221	221
PRO	52	52	51	52
GLY	43	39	27	26
ALA	68	65	80	78
CYS/2	15	13	0	0
VAL	77	65	84	91
MET	15	26	18	13
ILE	15	13	0	0
LEU	103	104	104	104
TYR	45	52	45	52
PHE	50	52	49	52

* mol/1000 mol of amino acids
a Shore and Shore (1968)
b Scanu et al. (1974)
c DEAE-fraction II
d Edelstein et al. (1972)

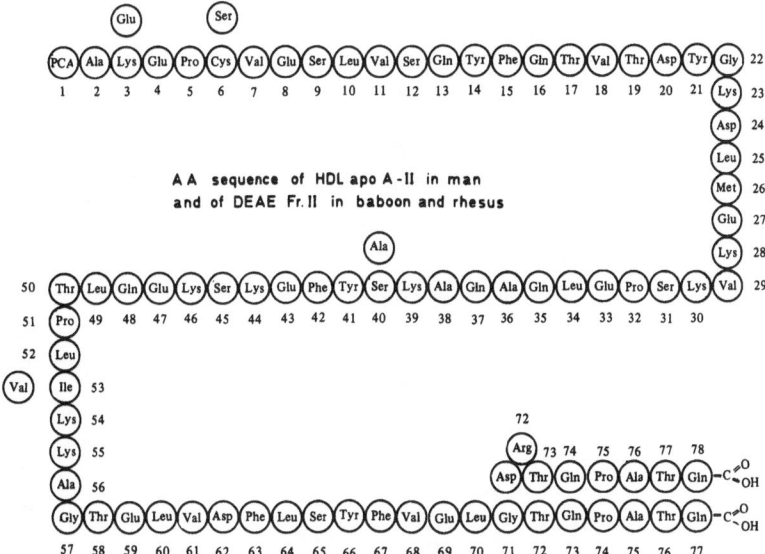

Figure 4.   The amino acid sequence of HDL apo-A-II in man, baboon
and rhesus macacus. (76)

Comparative Properties of the Induced Hyperlipoproteinemia

After 6 months feeding of a high fat high cholesterol diet a
hyperbetalipoproteinemia was induced in the non human primates comparable to the human type II hyperbetalipoproteinemia (Table IX).
The chimpanzee and the rhesus showed a marked increase of cholesterol,
while in the baboon cholesterol as well as phospholipids is increased
to a similar extent.   In all species triglycerides are low and were
unchanged under the regime.   The S/PC ratio, a prerequisite of atherogenicity, is significantly increased in human type IIa, and similar
data were observed for the chimpanzee and the rhesus. The baboon,
however, was unchanged.

In the chimpanzee and the rhesus the hyperbetalipoproteinemia
pattern showed a marked increase of beta lipoproteins and no increase
of VLDL (fig. 5, 6).

Only after a long period of high cholesterol diet was there a
lipoprotein profile of the atherogenic baboon comparable to human
type II.

The chief effects of the atherogenic diet in the baboon were
the increase in total cholesterol, in phosphatidylcholine (PC)
especially in the beta lipoproteins, an unexpected decrease of
C/PL in the beta lipoproteins and an increase of cholesterol oleate.

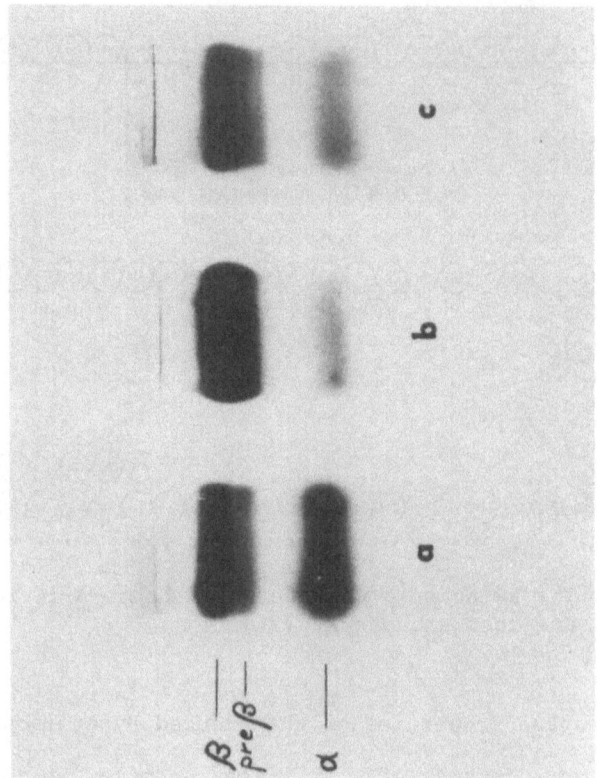

Figure 6. Agarose electrophoresis of rhesus hyperbetalipoproteinemic plasma (b) compared to normal plasma (a).

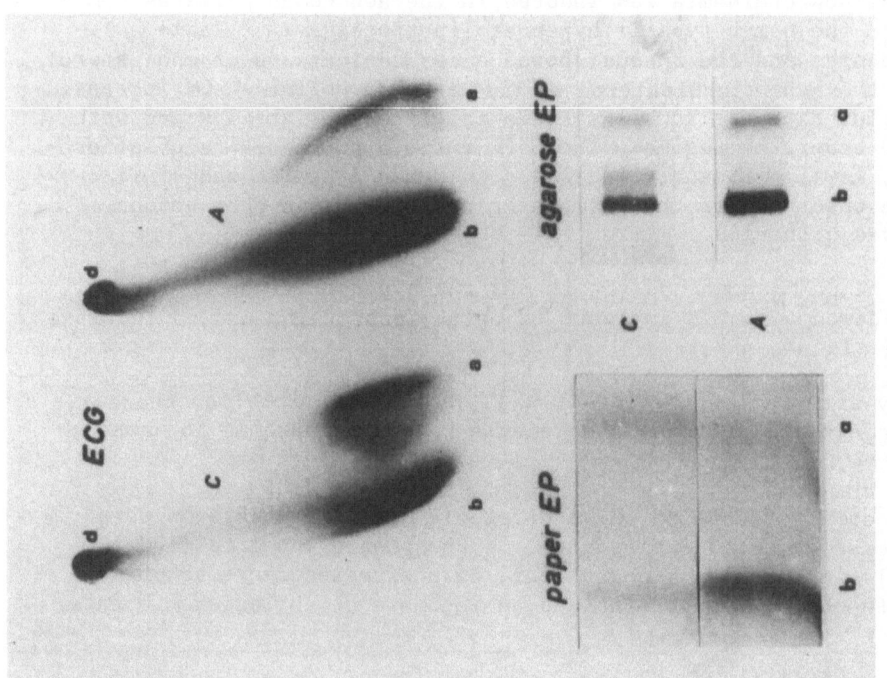

Figure 5. Agarose and paper electrophoresis, and electrochromatography (ECG) of chimpanzee hyperbetalipoproteinemic plasma (A) compared to normal plasma (C).

TABLE IX

The Plasma Lipid Composition of a Hyperlipoproteinemia
in Man and Non Human Primates.

Plasma - hyperbetalipoproteinemia

mg%	human		chimp.		baboon		rhesus	
	C	IIa	C	A	C	A	C	A
TC	151	332	259	606	116	196	132	388
TG	31	108	60	65	36	33	39	18
PL	163	283	295	459	119	203	230	243
C/PL	0.92	1.18	0.88	1.31	0.97	1.01	0.57	1.59
S/PC	0.25	0.30	0.24	0.29	0.14	0.13	0.10	0.18

The most conspicuous differences to type II in man however are the
cholesterol/phospholipid decrease in the beta lipoproteins and the
increase of PC in beta lipoproteins (11, 12, 13).

As in the other non human primates, such as chimpanzees and baboons, the diet induces in the rhesus monkey within about 6 months
a marked hyperbetalipoproteinemia with elevated plasma cholesterol
levels reaching 600 mg % and normal triglyceride levels. Moreover,
increased oleic to linoleic acid (18:1/18:2) and sphingomyelin
to lecithin (S/PC) ratios were obtained.

The cholesterol induced lipoprotein changes in the chimpanzees
and those obtained in human hyperbetalipoproteinemia are identical.

In man aswell as in the chimpanzee there is a tremendous increase of beta lipoproteins and of free and esterified cholesterol
(fig. 7). Triglycerides were practically unchanged, and there
was no change in the VLDL concentration as proved by agarose gel
electrophoresis before and after centrifugation (fig. 8). The
phospholipids were increased but less than cholesterol, and this
lipid abnormality is almost completely confined to beta lipoproteins. The oleic to linoleic acid ratio of both lipoproteins was
increased because of changes in the cholesterol esters. As in human
hyperbetalipoproteinemia similar changes in the phospholipids are
observed and are characterized by an increase of the sphingomyelin
to phosphatidylcholine ratio especially in the betalipoproteins (8).

The results reported here indicate that the chimpanzee also produces hyperprebetalipoproteinemia under influence of a sucrose diet. UCF analyses showed an increase of the Sf 20-400 range (fig. 7),and the agarose gel electrophoresis confirms the increase of floating VLDL. In some cases however the increase of VLDL was accompanied by an increase of sedimenting VLDL (fig. 8).

Unpublished data of our work indicate however that the rapid changes in lipoproteins, lipids and fatty acid profiles are only obtained if a relative high quantity of sucrose is given to the animals (75).

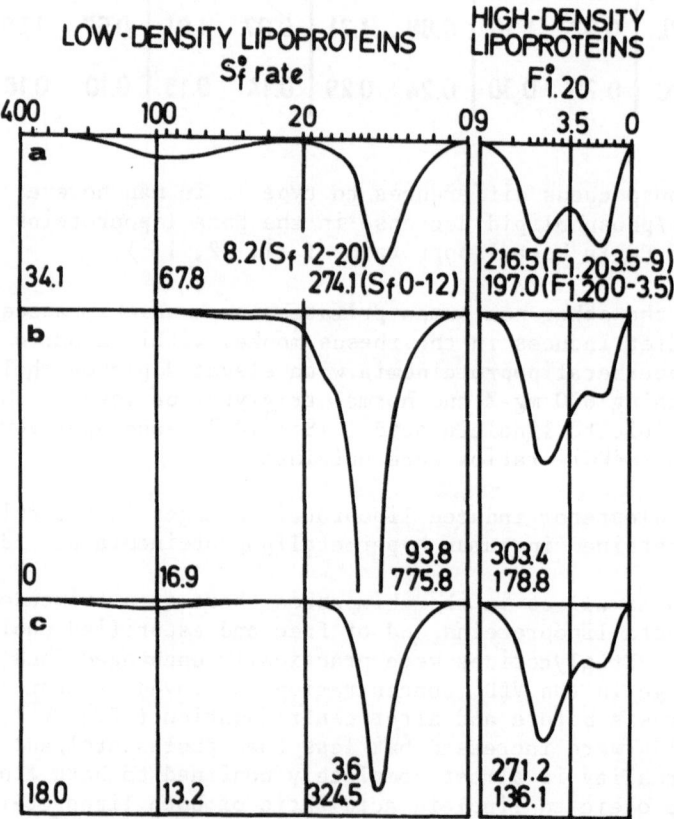

Figure 7. Ultracentrifugal plasma lipoprotein patterns of chimpan-
            zees under control (c), under fat (b) and under high
            carbohydrate diets (a).

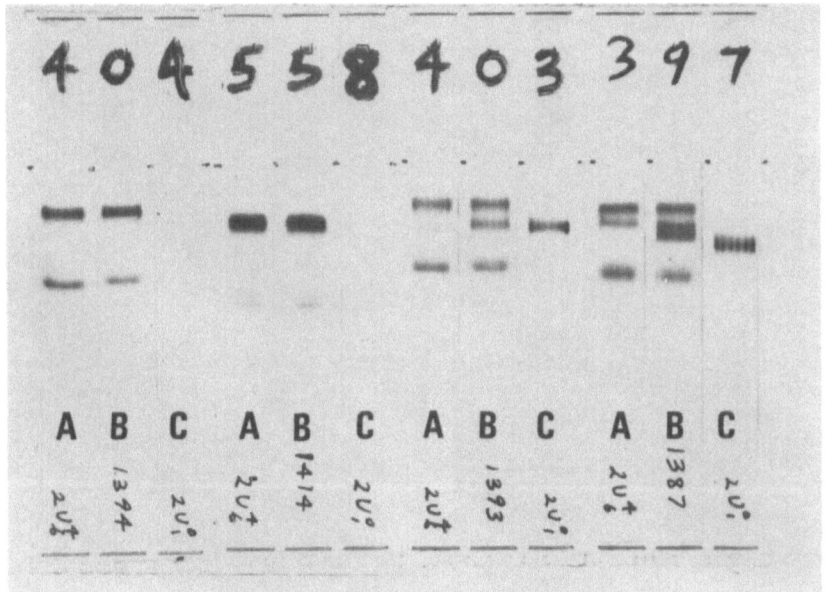

Figure 8.   Agarose electrophoresis of chimpanzee plasma lipoproteins
            a : VLDL free plasma ; b : whole plasma ; c : plasma VLDL.
            404 is a normal chimpanzee ; 558 a hypercholesterolemic
            animal ; 403 and 397 two chimpanzees under high carbohy-
            drate diet.

The Arterial Lesions in the Non Human Primates

As little as 18 months after starting the dietary regime it was
possible to find fatty streaks in the aorta, strikingly similar to
those found in man (45). It is important to emphasize that coronary and cerebral lesions were never seen during this long period of
investigation. On the other hand the control animals not subjected to atherogenic diets also demonstrated frequent artery lesions.

Similar results were observed for the rhesus monkeys. Grossly
visible coronary artery plaques were seen after 18 months diet.

Two chimpanzees of the animal group under a 5 to 6 years atherogenic diet died unexpectedly. Autopsy and macroscopic examination
revealed that the cause of the death was a large fresh infarction of
the wall of the left ventricle due to occluding thrombus on
stenosing lesions of the arterial branches of the coronary artery.
Numerous atherosclerotic plaques were also seen in the aorta subclavia and in the abdominal aortas (fig. 9). Microscopic examination
showed that all the examined histological sections had lesions, even

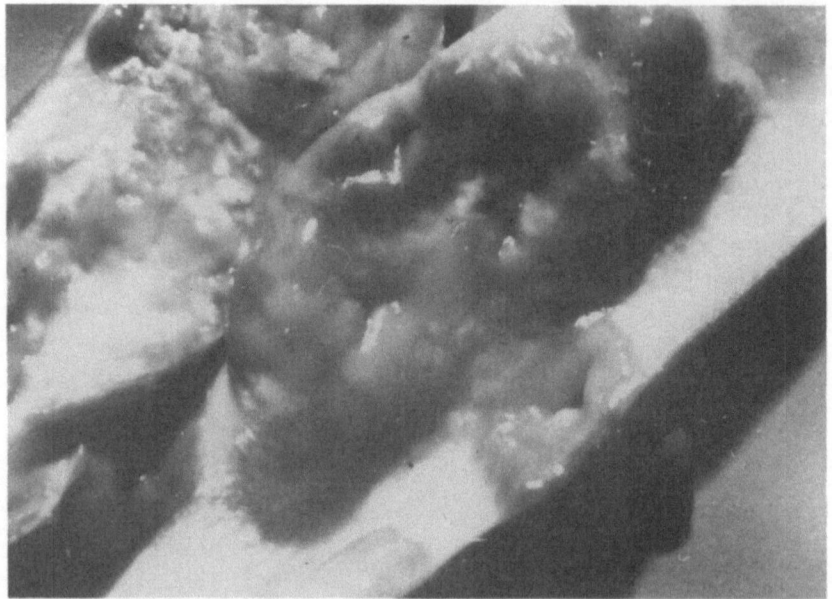

Figure 9.   The atherosclerotic plaques in the aorta subclavia.

those segments which were macroscopically noted as normal. Complete
occlusion with revascularisation was found twice in two different
vessels from the A. praeventricularis.   In the present animals inflammatory reactions ,although of low grade, could be observed. A few
other changes could be favorably compared to those described in
dogs and rabbits, but most of the encountered lesions remarkably
simulate the atheromatous lesions described in man (8).

CONCLUSIONS

There is no dearth of experimental techniques for producing the
hyperlipoproteinemia resulting in atherosclerotic complications and
for myocardial infarction in the non human primates. Most of the
recent experiments which have given information of great value have
been studied with relatively expensive animals for a long period of
time up to 6-7 years.

It is evident that no animal model perfectly duplicates the human disease or satisfies all desirable requirements.

The chimpanzees, representatives of the New World monkeys, have
circulating plasma lipoproteins identical to man in composition as
well as in function. The results reported above indicate that the

compositional changes of chimpanzee plasma lipoproteins in response
to dietary changes reflect the appearance of type II and type IV
hyperlipoproteinemia similar to the human disease. Moreover, there
are more indications about the existence of genotype IIa in the
chimpanzee, and also on the influence of stress on the plasma lipids,
so that the developed intimal lesions similar to the human pathology
are in this sense multifactorially influenced.

From a phylogenetic point of view the chimpanzee is closer to man
than any other non human primate. Furthermore, the chimpanzee lipoproteins are useful models for understanding the relationship between function and structure of the plasma lipoproteins in health and
disease.

Baboon and rhesus monkeys show similar results, but more differences to the human lipoproteins in health and disease were observed.

At present it appears that the most useful models of human atherosclerosis are those induced in the non human primates, especially
in the chimpanzee.

ACKNOWLEDGEMENT

We wish to thank Dr. R.L. Jackson and Dr. R. Roth (Baylor
College of Medicine, Houston) for the preliminary results on the sequence of baboon apo-A-I and apo-A-II.

Microcalorimetric studies are in progress and are made by
Dr. M. Rosseneu (Simon Stevin Instituut, Brugge).

The analytical ultracentrifugal data on the chimpanzees were
obtained by Dr. F. Lindgren (Donner Laboratories, Berkeley, Ca.).

Histopathological work was done at Janssen Pharmaceutica,
Belgium (Mr. R. Vandesteene, Dr. Thienpont).

Mr. W. Vandenbergh and Dr. Mortelmans are acknowledged for
their collaboration with the animal study.

We are indebted to Mr. B. Declercq, Mr. D. Vandamme, Mr. R.
Vercaemst, Mrs. N. Vandecasteele, Mr. H. Caster for their technical
assistance.

REFERENCES

1. CLARKSON, T.B.(1972).
   Animal models of atherosclerosis. In : Advances in Veterinary
   Science and Comparative Science, ed. C.A. Brandly and C.E.
   Cornelius, Academic Press, New York, pp. 151-173.

2. PORTMAN, O., and S.B. ANDRUS (1965).
   Comparative evaluation of three species of New World Monkeys
   for studies of dietary factors, tissue lipids and atherogenesis.
   J. Nutr., 87, 429-438.

3. MIDDLETON, C.C., T.B. CLARKSON, H.B. LOFLAND and R.W. PRICHARD
   (1967).
   Diet and atherosclerosis of squirrel monkeys·
   Arch. Pathol., 83, 145-153.

4. MANN, G.V., S.B. ANDRUS, A. McNALLY and F.J. STARE (1953).
   Experimental atherosclerosis in cebus monkeys
   J. Exp. Med., 98, 195-218.

5. WISSLER, R.W., L.E. FRAZIER, and R.A. RASMUSSEN (1962).
   Atherogenesis in the cebus monkey : I. A comparison of three
   food fats under controlled dietary conditions·
   Arch. Pathol., 74, 312-322.

6. BULLOCK, B.C., T.B. CLARKSON, N.D. LEHNER, H.B. LOFLAND and
   R.W. ST.CLAIR (1969).
   Atherosclerosis in cebus albifrons monkeys. III. Clinical and
   pathological studies.
   Exp. Mol. Pathol., 10, 39-62.

7. BLATON, V., R. VERCAEMST, N. VANDECASTEELE, H. CASTER and
   H. PEETERS (1974).
   Isolation and partial characterization of chimpanzee plasma high
   density lipoproteins and their apolipoproteins·
   Biochemistry, 13, 1127-1135.

8. BLATON, V., D. VANDAMME, M. VASTESAEGER, J. MORTELMANS and
   H. PEETERS (1974).
   Dietary induced hyperbetalipoproteinemia in chimpanzees : compa-
   rison to the human hyperlipoproteinemia.
   Exp. Mol. Pathol., 20, 132-146.

9. VASTESAEGER, M., V. BLATON, B. DECLERCQ, J. VERCRUYSSE, D. VAN-
   DAMME, H. PEETERS and J. MORTELMANS (1973)·
   Comparative treatment of hyperlipoproteinemias in chimpanzees·
   Acta Zool. Antverpiensia, nr 53, 81.

10. STRONG, J.P., and H.C. McGILL (1967)·
    Diet and experimental atherosclerosis in baboons·
    Am. J. Pathol., 50, 669-690.

11. BLATON, V., A.N. HOWARD, G.A. GRESHAM, D. VANDAMME, and
    H. PEETERS (1970).
    Lipid changes in the plasma lipoproteins of baboons given an
    atherogenic diet. I. Changes in the lipids of total plasma and
    of alpha and beta lipoproteins.
    Atherosclerosis, 11, 497-507.

12. PEETERS, H., V. BLATON, B. DECLERCQ, A.N. HOWARD, and
    G.A. GRESHAM (1970).
    Lipid changes in the plasma lipoproteins of baboons given an
    atherogenic diet. II. Changes in the phospholipid classes of
    total plasma and of alpha and beta lipoproteins.
    Atherosclerosis, 12, 283-290.
13. HOWARD, A.N., V. BLATON, D. VANDAMME, N. VAN LANDSCHOOT, and
    H. PEETERS (1972).
    Lipid changes in the plasma lipoproteins of baboons given an
    atherogenic diet. III. A comparison between the plasma of the
    baboon and chimpanzee given atherogenic diets and lipid changes
    in human plasma lipoproteins of type II hyperlipoproteinemia.
    Atherosclerosis, 16, 257-272.
14. MANNING, P.J. and T.B. CLARKSON (1972).
    Distribution and lipid content of diet-induced atherosclerotic
    lesions of rhesus monkeys.
    Exp. Mol. Pathol., 17, 38-54.
15. NEWMAN, W.P., C.C. MIDDLETON, T.B. CALRKSON, J. ROSAL and
    J.P. STRONG (1974).
    Naturally occurring arterial lesions in New World Primates.
    Am. Med. Assoc., 98, 173-176.
16. MIDDLETON, C.C., J. ROSAL, T.B. CLARKSON, W.P. NEWMAN and
    H.C. Mc.GILL (1967).
    Arterial lesions in squirrel monkeys
    Arch. Pathol., 83, 352-358.
17. CLARKSON, T.B., H.B. LOFLAND, B.C. BULLOCK, N.D. LEHNER,
    R.W. ST. CLAIR and R.W. PRICHARD (1969).
    Atherosclerosis in some species of New World Monkeys
    Ann. N.Y. Acad. Sci., 162, 103-109.
18. LOFLAND, H.B., R.W. ST. CLAIR, J.C. McNINTCH and R.W. PRICHARD
    (1967).
    Atherosclerosis in New World Primates
    Arch. Pathol., 83, 211-214.
19. PUCAK, G.J., N.D. LEHNER, T.B. CLARKSON, B.C. BULLOCK and
    H.B. LOFLAND (1973).
    Spider Monkeys (Ateles sp.) as animal models for atherosclero-
    sis research.
    Exp. Mol. Pathol., 18, 32-49.
20. GOODALL, J. (1963).
    My life among wild chimpanzees.
    Nat. Geographic, 124.
21. VASTESAEGER, M.M., and R. DELCOURT (1961).
    Spontaneous atherosclerosis and diet in captive animals.
    Nutr. Diet, 3, 174-177.
22. STARE, F.J., S.B. ANDRUS, and R. OSTWALD (1963).
    Primates in medical research with special reference to new
    world monkeys.
    In : Proc. Conf. on Research with Primates, Tektronix Foundation,
    Beaverton, Wash., 59.

23. MANNING, G.W. (1942).
    Coronary disease in the ape.
    Am. Heart J., 23, 719-724.
24. VASTESAEGER, M.M., and R. DELCOURT (1966).
    Spontaneous atherosclerosis in chimpanzees
    Acta Cardiol., 11, 283.
25. PEETERS, H., and V. BLATON (1972).
    Comparative lipid values of human and non human primates. In:
    Medical Primatology III. Ed. M. Jankowski and G. Goldsmith,
    Karger, Basel, 336-342.
26. DELCOURT, R., G. NISSANE, P. OSTERRIETH, and M. VASTESAEGER
    (1964).
    Acta Cardiol., 19, 531.
27. KEYS, A., J.J. ANDERSON, F. FIDANZA, M.H. KEYS, and B. SWAHN
    (1955).
    Effects of diet on blood lipids in man.
    Clin. Chem., 1, 34.
28. PEETERS, H. (1959).
    Paper electrophoresis : Principles and techniques
    Adv. Clin.   Chem., 2, 2-134.
29. MANN, G.V., S.B. ANDRUS, A. McNALLY, and F.J. STARE (1963).
    Diet and cholesterolemia in chimpanzees.
    Fed. Proc., 22, 642.
30. MORRIS, M.D., and W.E. GEER (1970).
    Familial hyperbetalipoproteinemia in the rhesus monkey.
    In : Atherosclerosis, ed. R. Jones, Springer Verlag, N.Y., 192.
31. VASTESAEGER, M.M., J. VERCRUYSSE and J.J. MARTIN (1972).
    Pitfalls of experimental atherosclerosis in the chimpanzee
    In : Medical Primatology III Ed. M. Jankowski and G. Goldsmith.
32. LINDSAY, S., and I.L. CHAIKOFF (1966).
    Naturally occurring arteriosclerosis in non human primates.
    J. Atheroscler. Res., 6, 36-61.
33. SCOTT, R.F., E.S. MORRISON, J. LARNOLYCH, S.C. NAM and F.
    CARLSTRON (1967).
    Experimental atherosclerosis in rhesus monkeys. I. Gross and
    microscopic features and lipid values in serum and aorta.
    Exp. Mol. Pathol., 7, 11-33.
34. WISSLER, R.W., R.H. HUGHES, L.E. FRAZIER, G.S. GETZ, and
    D. TURNER (1965).
    Aortic lesions and blood lipids in rhesus monkeys fed "table
    prepared : human diets"
    Circulation, 32, 220-222.
35. LINDSAY, S., and I.L. CHAIKOFF (1957).
    Atherosclerosis in the baboon.
    Arch. Pathol., 63, 460-471.
36. McGILL, H.C., J.P. STRONG, R.L. HOLMAN, and N.T. WERTHESSEN
    (1960).
    Arterial lesions in the kenya baboon.
    Circ. Res.   8, 670-679.

37. PEETERS, H., and V. BLATON (1969).
    Comparison of lipid and lipoprotein patterns in primates.
    Acta Zool. et Pathol. Antverpiensia, 48, 221-231.
38. BLATON, V., R. VERCAEMST, N. VINAIMONT, and H. PEETERS (1975).
    Isolation and characterization of baboon plasma high density
    lipoproteins and their apolipoproteins : Comparison to human
    and non human primates.
    J. Biol. Chem., in press.
39. GRESHAM, G.A., and G.A. HOWARD (1965).
    Vascular lesions in primates.
    Ann. N.Y. Acad. Sci., 127, 694-701.
40. STRONG, J.P., and H.C. McGILL (1967).
    Diet and experimental atheroslcerosis in baboons
    Am. J. Pathol., 50, 669-690.
41. BLATON, V., and H. PEETERS (1969).
    Lipid and fatty acid modifications in plasma lipoproteins of
    baboons under atherogenic diet.
    Acta Zool. et Pathol. Antverpiensia, 48, 223-242.
42. BLATON, V., D. VANDAMME, and H. PEETERS (1972).
    Chimpanzee and baboon as biochemical models for human athero-
    sclerosis.
    Medical Primatology III. Ed. M. Jankowski and G. Goldsmith,
    Karger, Basel, 306-312.
43. BLATON, V., and H. PEETERS (1971).
    Integrated approach to plasma lipid and lipoprotein analysis
    In : Blood Lipids and Lipoproteins, Ed. G. Nelson, J. Wiley
    and Sons, New York, 369-431.
44. HOWARD, A.N., V. BLATON, G.A. GRESHAM, D. VANDAMME, and
    H. PEETERS (1971).
    The lipoproteins in hyperlipidaemic primates as a model for
    human atherosclerosis.
    Protides of the Biological Fluids, 19, 341-344, Pergamn Press.
45. GRESHAM, G.A., A.N. HOWARD, J. McQUEEN, and D.E. BOWYER (1965).
    Atherosclerosis in primates.
    Brit. J. Exp. Path., 66, 94-103.
46. MORTELMANS, J. (1969).
    Tranquilization and anaesthesia.
    In : Primates in Medicine, Ed. W.   Beveridge, Karger, 2,113-122.
47. BLATON, V., H. PEETERS, W. DE KEERSGIETER, B. DECLERCQ,
    D. DEPICKERE, and D. VANDAMME (1965).
    Differential fatty acid composition of alpha 1 and beta lipo-
    proteins.
    Protides of the Biological Fluids, 13, 315-319, Elsevier.
48. WALTON, K.W., and P.J. SCOTT (1964).
    Estimation of the low density lipoproteins of serum in health and
    disease using large molecular weight dextran sulphate.
    J. Clin. Pathol., 17, 627-643.

49. PEETERS, H., and E. LAGA (1962).
Influence des mucopolysaccharides sur la résorption des graisses
par le tube digestif.
3e Rencontre sur les Lipides Alimentaires, Rimini, 825–839.
ed. La Nutrizione, Roma.

50. DE LA HUERGA, J., C. YESININCK, and H. POPPER (1953).
Estimation of total serum lipids by a turbidimetric method.
Am. J. Clin. Pathol., 23, 1163–1167.

51. ROZENTHAL, H.L., M.L. PFLUKE, and G. BUSCAGLIA (1957).
A stable iron reagent for determination of cholesterol.
J. Lab. Clin. Med., 50, 318–322.

52. VAN HANDEL, E., and D.B. ZILVERSMIT (1957).
Micromethod for the direct determination of serum triglycerides.
J. Lab. Clin. Med., 50, 152–157.

53. SODHI, H.S., GORDON R. GOULD (1967).
Combination of delipidized high density lipoproteins with lipids.
J. Biol. Chem., 242, 1205–1210.

54. KOGA, S., L. BOLIS, and A.M. SCANU (1971).
Isolation and characterisation of subunit polypeptides from
apoproteins of rat serum lipoproteins.
Biochim. Biophys. Acta, 236, 416–430.

55. LINDGREN, F.T., and L.C. JENSEN (1972).
The isolation and quantitative analysis of serum lipoproteins
In : Blood Lipids and Lipoproteins, Ed. G. Nelson,
J. Wiley and Sons, New York, 181–274.

56. VAN MELSEN, A., Y. DE GREVE, F. VANDERVEIKEN, M. VASTESAEGER,
V. BLATON, and H. PEETERS (1974).
A modified method for phenotyping of hyperlipoproteinemia on
agarose electrophoresis.
Clin. Chim. Acta, 55, 225–234.

57. HATCH, F.T., F.T. LINDGREN, L.C. JENSEN, G.L. ADAMSON, A.W. WONG,
and R.I. LEVY (1973).
Quantitative agarose gelelectrophoresis of plasma lipoproteins :
A simple technique and two methods for standardization.
J. Lab. Clin. Med., 81, 946–960.

58. DAVIES, B.J. (1964).
Method and application to human serum proteins.
Ann. N.Y. Acad. Sci., 121, 404–427.

59. WEBER, K., and M. OSBORN (1969).
The reliability of molecular weight determinations by dodecyl
sulphate-polyacrylamide gelelectrophoresis.
J. Biol. Chem., 244, 4406–4412.

60. VESTERBERG, O. (1972).
Isoelectric focusing of proteins in polyacrylamide gels.
Biochim. Biophys. Acta, 257, 11–19.

61. AWDEH, Z.L., A.R. WILLIAMSON, and B.A. ASKONAS (1968).
Isoelectric focusing in polyacrylamide gel and its application
to immunoglobulins.
Nature, 219, 66–67.

62. SCANU, A., J. Toth, C. Edelstein, S. Koga and E. Stiller (1969).
    Fractionation of human serum high density lipoproteins in urea
    solutions. Evidence for polypeptide heterogeneity
    Biochemistry, 8, 3309-3316.
63. SHORE, V., and B. SHORE (1967).
    Some physical and chemical studies on the protein moiety of a
    high density (1.126-1.195 g/ml) lipoprotein fraction of human
    serum.
    Biochemistry, 6, 1962-1969.
64. GROS, C., and B. LABOUESSE (1969).
    Study of the dansylation reaction of amino acids, peptides and
    proteins.
    Eur. J. Biochem., 7, 463-470.
65. ZANETTA, J.P., G. VINCENDON, P. MANDEL, and G. GOMBOS (1970).
    The utilisation of 1-dimethylaminonaphthalene-5-sulphonyl chlo-
    ride for quantitative determination of free amino acids and par-
    tial analysis of primary structure of proteins.
    J. Chromatog., 51, 441.
66. AMBLER, G. (1964).
    Enzymic hydrolysis with carboxy peptidases. Methods Enzymol.,
    11, 155-166.
67. SPACKMAN, D.H. (1967)
    Accelerated amino acid analysis.
    Methods Enzymol., 11, 3-15.
68. HIRS, C.H.W. (1967).
    Determination of cystine as cysteic acid.
    Methods Enzymol., 11, 59-62.
69. LIU, T.Y., Y.H. CHANG (1971).
    Hydrolysis of protein with p-toluenesulfonic acid. Determination
    of tryptophan.
    J. Biol. Chem., 246, 2842-2848.
70. ROSSENEU, M.Y., F. SOETEWEY, V. BLATON, J. LIEVENS, and
    H. PEETERS (1974).
    Microcalorimetric study of phospholipid binding to human apoHDL.
    Chem. Phys. Lipids, 13, 203-214.
71. DELAHUNTY, T., H. NORDEAN BAKER, A.M. GOTTO, and R.L. JACKSON
    (1975).
    The primary structure of human plasma high density apolipopro-
    tein Glutamine I (apo-A-I).
    J. Biol. Chem., 2718-2724.
72. EWING, A.M., N.K. FREEMAN, and F.T. LINDGREN (1965).
    The analysis of human serum lipoprotein distributions.
    In : Advances in Lipid Research, ed. R. Paoletti and D.
    Kritchevsky, 3, 25-61, Acad. Press, New York.
73. WALTON, K., V. BLATON, and H. PEETERS (1975).
    Immunological properties of the plasma lipoproteins in the non
    human primates.
    Biochim. Biophys. Acta, in press.

74. SCANU, A.M., C. EDELSTEIN, L. VITELLO, R. JONES, and
    R. WISSLER (1973).
    The serum high density lipoproteins of macacus rhesus. I.
    Isolation, composition and properties.
    J. Biol. Chem., 248, 7648-7652.
75. PEETERS, H., V. BLATON, and F.T. LINDGREN (1973).
    Dietary induced hyperlipoproteinaemia in chimpanzees.
    Circulation, 48, Suppl. 4, p. IV-203.
76. SCANU, A. (1975).
    Polypeptide A-II of serum high density lipoproteins: A
    lipophilic protein of phylogenetic interest. PAABS Revista,
    4, 1-11.

PHYLOGENETIC VARIABILITY OF SERUM LIPIDS AND LIPOPROTEINS IN NON-

HUMAN PRIMATES FED DIETS WITH DIFFERENT CONTENTS OF DIETARY CHOLES-

TEROL

S. R. Srinivasan, C. C. Smith, B. Radhakrishnamurthy,
R. H. Wolf and G. S. Berenson

Dept. of Medicine, LSU School of Medicine and The Delta
Primate Center of Tulane University, New Orleans, La.

ABSTRACT

The response of serum lipids and lipoproteins to different
levels of dietary cholesterol (0.05% to 1.5% w/w) was measured in
six nonhuman primate species. Relative response of serum cholesterol in different species, measured in terms of response index,
varied with dietary cholesterol concentration. The overall response
for the different diets allowed ranking of the species as follows:
Squirrel > green > spider ≃ rhesus ≃ patas > chimpanzee. The serum
cholesterol response was reflected not only in an increase in β +
pre-β-lipoprotein cholesterol but also in α-lipoprotein cholesterol,
with significant differences among species in the amount of cholesterol transported in the lipoprotein classes.

INTRODUCTION

Diet-induced atherosclerosis has been studied extensively in
many animal models. The use of primates in these studies has gained
importance because of their close phylogenetic relationship to man.
Of the many primate species available, only a few, e.g., rhesus,
baboon, squirrel, and cebus, have been widely used (1-9). Perhaps
no single species will be best suited for the study of all aspects
of atherosclerosis (10), therefore a systematic examination of
response of different species to diet might provide a basis for
selecting the most appropriate species for any study.

Since an increase in serum lipids is closely related to the
development of experimental atherosclerosis, and since differences

among species in response of serum lipids to atherogenic diets may
be more apparent during the transient phase following transition
from basal to atherogenic diet, we have examined variations within
and among species in the early response of serum lipids to different
levels of dietary cholesterol. This paper presents results of some
preliminary analyses of the data obtained.

MATERIALS AND METHODS

Animals

    Five adults of mixed sex of each of six species [Pan troglodytes
(chimpanzee), Macaca mulatta (rhesus), Cercopithecus aethiops
(green), Erythrocebus patas (patas), Saimiri sciurea (squirrel), and
Ateles sp. (spider)] were housed in individual cages at the Delta
Regional Primate Research Center.

Diet

    The animals were fed diets similar to one described by Malinow
et al. (5), containing by weight: Purina Monkey Chow® 25, 51.0%;
banana, 12%; butter, 5.0%; water, 32%; and cholesterol, < 0.005%,
(basal), 0.05%, 0.2%, 0.5%, 1.0% or 1.5%. The estimated caloric
density of the food was 2.72 cal/gm. The calories per kilogram of
body weight consumed by each species was determined by observations
of intake for one week prior to the experiment with the following
results: rhesus, green, and spider, 85; patas, 65; squirrel, 200;
and chimpanzees, 122.

    There were no significant changes in the body weight of the
monkeys during the course of the study.

Design

    Diets were fed for 3 week periods in the following sequence:
Basal, .05% cholesterol, basal, .20% cholesterol, basal, .50%
cholesterol, basal, 1.0% cholesterol, basal, 1.5% cholesterol. One
squirrel monkey and one chimpanzee became ill for unknown reasons
early in the study and were removed from the study. During the
initial basal period and for each subsequent non-basal diet period
blood specimens (14 h fasting) were obtained twice a week under
sedation with Sernylan® (Bio-Ceutic Laboratories Inc., St. Joseph,
Mo.). Serum was prepared and analyzed for serum lipoproteins and
lipid concentration.

Serum Lipid Measurements

Serum total cholesterol and triglyceride concentrations were measured using a Technicon Auto Analyzer II (Technicon Instruments Corp., Tarrytown, N.Y.) with standardization by the U.S. Center for Disease Control (Atlanta, Ga.). Cholesterol content of combined serum β and pre-β-lipoproteins was determined by a heparin-calcium precipitation method (11,12). The relative proportions of β and pre-β-lipoproteins were obtained by a densitometric scan of agar-agarose gel electrophoresis (13,14). α, β, and pre-β-lipoprotein concentrations were then calculated from cholesterol content of lipoproteins (13,14). The validity of this method for lipoprotein quantitation has been established by comparing the results with those obtained by analytical ultracentrifugation (12).

Cholesterol Response Index

The serum cholesterol response to a given amount of dietary cholesterol was measured by a cholesterol response index as described by Bowyer et al. (15) with some modification. This index was obtained by dividing the area under the curve of serum cholesterol concentration, (c) above the basal level, (b) by the duration of feeding (t_2-t_1):

$$\text{Cholesterol response index:} \quad \frac{\int_{t_1}^{t_2} (c-b)dt}{(t_2-t_1)} \quad \text{mg/100 ml.}$$

The basal value (b) used for this calculation was the mean of three determinations obtained at days 14, 17, and 21 of the initial basal diet period. Similar indices were calculated for combined β-plus preβ-lipoprotein cholesterol and α-lipoprotein cholesterol.

RESULTS

The serum cholesterol responses to different levels of dietary cholesterol are given for the six species in Figure 1. The various species responded differently at different levels of dietary cholesterol. For instance at 0.05% dietary cholesterol, patas and squirrel monkeys showed very little response (2.0 and 1.9 mg% respectively); on the other hand green, spider, rhesus and chimpanzee responded well to this low dietary level of cholesterol with a mean value of 18.4, 18.1, 17.7 and 14.6 mg% respectively. Although subsequent increase in dietary intake of cholesterol produced greater varia-

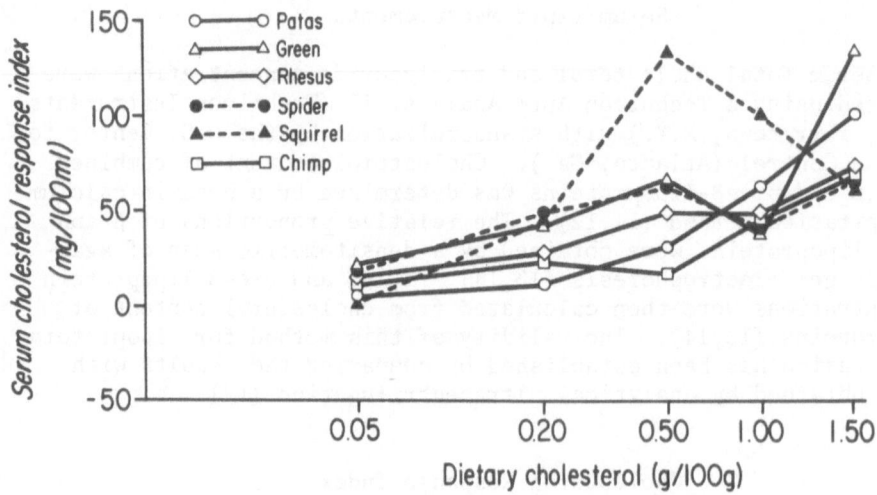

Fig. 1. Serum cholesterol response to variations in dietary cholesterol in different nonhuman primate species. (Dietary cholesterol is plotted in logarithmic scale).

tions among different species, significant and maximum interspecies differences were observed only at 0.5% cholesterol level. Analysis of variance at this level of cholesterol intake indicated a highly significant interspecies difference ($p < .0001$). The response index increased most for squirrel monkeys (130.8 mg%), followed by green (64.6 mg%), spider (62.5 mg%), rhesus (48.5 mg%), patas (30.1 mg%) and chimpanzees (15.5 mg%). At 1.0% cholesterol level squirrel, green, spider and rhesus showed a somewhat lower response than at 0.5%, whereas chimpanzee and patas showed an increase in response. A further increase in dietary cholesterol to 1.5% level induced an increase in response in green, patas, rhesus and chimpanzees (in that order). Squirrel monkeys registered a lowering in response at this dietary cholesterol level. The unexpected decrease by the squirrel monkeys at very high dietary cholesterol levels cannot be explained and could have been due to illness in this group. The overall mean serum cholesterol response index for different levels (0.05 to 1.5%) cholesterol intake showed a significant interspecies differences (variance analysis; $p < .0001$).

As expected, in addition to differences among species there were considerable variations among individuals of a given species during all diet periods.

Table 1 shows the cholesterol response of β + pre-β-lipoprotein cholesterol and α-lipoprotein cholesterol (measured in terms of response index) with 0.5% cholesterol in the diet. The response of serum cholesterol to dietary cholesterol was reflected not only in an increase of β + pre-β-lipoprotein cholesterol but also of α-lipoprotein cholesterol (except in chimpanzees). In chimpanzees, patas, and to a lesser extent in rhesus monkeys, the increase was due predominantly to β + pre-β-lipoprotein cholesterol. These observations suggest that during this transient period the distribution of cholesterol among the lipoprotein fractions varies differently for different species.

Table 2 shows the mean serum lipid and lipoprotein concentrations after three weeks of basal diet containing 0.5% cholesterol. The initial lipid and lipoprotein concentration differed significantly among the six species. Chimpanzees and squirrel monkeys had the highest mean serum cholesterol concentration, and patas monkeys had the lowest. The serum triglyceride and pre-β-lipoprotein concentrations were relatively low in all the species except chimpanzee. On basal diet chimpanzees and spider and squirrel monkeys had high concentrations of β-lipoprotein and patas had the lowest. Three weeks of 0.5% dietary cholesterol increased the serum total cholesterol significantly in all species. Though β-lipoprotein concentration increased in all species except spider monkeys the α-lipoprotein increased even more (except in chimpanzees). Cholesterol feeding seemed to decrease the serum triglyceride and pre-β-lipoprotein concentrations in all species.

DISCUSSION

The present study demonstrates differences in serum cholesterol response to variations in dietary cholesterol among six species of nonhuman primates. For the short diet periods used here, the method of integrating the area above the baseline serum cholesterol concentration gives a more precise measure of response to a given dose of dietary cholesterol than a single point determination, especially since other investigations show that it takes several months to reach a steady state after changing diet conditions.

Earlier studies in which several species were fed the same diet showed a) differences among rhesus, baboons, and spider monkeys (16); b) no differences among cebus, squirrel, and woolly monkeys, (7); and c) differences among juvenile squirrel, cynomolgus, cebus, and spider monkeys (17). In this study the mean serum cholesterol

TABLE 1

SERUM LIPOPROTEIN CHOLESTEROL RESPONSES

IN SIX NONHUMAN PRIMATE SPECIES FED 0.5% DIETARY CHOLESTEROL

Species	Cholesterol Response Index, mg/100 ml	
(no. animals)	β + pre-β-LP	α-LP
Patas	23.8[*]	6.3
(4)	± 9.0	± 4.0
Green	42.3	22.2
(5)	± 4.9	± 2.9
Rhesus	38.5	10.0
(5)	± 10.8	± 11.1
Spider	20.8	41.7
(5)	± 8.4	± 7.0
Squirrel	71.3	62.4
(4)	± 8.1	± 21.7
Chimpanzee	21.7	-6.1
(4)	± 9.3	± 5.3

P for differences among species

(by analysis of variance)   .0054   .0021

[*] Mean ± S.E.

TABLE 2

SERUM LIPID AND LIPOPROTEIN CHANGES IN SIX NON-HUMAN PRIMATE SPECIES FED 0.5% CHOLESTEROL DIET FOR 21 DAYS

mg/100 ml	Dietary Cholesterol gm/100 gm	Patas	Green	Rhesus	Spider	Squirrel	Chimpanzee	Significance of Differences among species (P)
Total Cholesterol	0	95.2 ± 6.8(5)†	172.6 ± 23.7(5)	147.6 ± 7.3(5)	160.2 ± 14.6(5)	225.0 ± 17.7(4)	282.0 ± 26.7(4)	< .0001
	0.5	162.8 ± 31.4(4)[a]	322.2 ± 32.2(5)[a]	241.8 ± 31.8(5)[b]	212.8 ± 13.2(5)[a]	362.5 ± 23.9(4)[a]	291.0 ± 29.9(4)[c]	.0011
Triglyceride	0	24.3 ± 3.6(4)	42.8 ± 12.1(4)	40.3 ± 7.5(4)	74.0 (1)	50.8 ± 4.6(4)	98.8 ± 10.7(4)	.0011
	0.5	46.8 ± 7.3(4)	50.6 ± 14.1(5)	45.0 ± 16.6(5)	70.2 ± 10.4(5)	50.0 ± 6.6(4)	154.0 ± 40.2(4)	.0046
β-LP	0	98.9 ± 11.2(5)	195.8 ± 24.6(5)	139.3 ± 13.7(5)	280.0 ± 24.7(5)	235.7 ± 23.6(4)	289.5 ± 24.8(4)	< .0001
	0.5	135.1 ± 47.6(4)	334.4 ± 54.1(5)[c]	264.8 ± 45.2(5)[b]	213.6 ± 22.9(5)	275.9 ± 34.3(4)	311.3 ± 28.8(4)	.0344
Pre-β-LP	0	21.7 ± 6.8(5)	22.4 ± 4.7(5)	77.8 ± 25.0(5)	46.3 ± 9.0(5)	57.2 ± 18.0(4)	119.3 ± 26.5(4)	.0034
	0.5	11.5 ± 4.8(4)	14.3 ± 9.3(5)	70.3 ± 10.6(5)	38.0 ± 18.2(5)	11.7 ± 4.4(4)	62.0 ± 16.0(4)	.0054
α-LP	0	259.6 ± 6.7(5)	447.2 ± 76.1(5)	383.5 ± 53.7(5)	109.7 ± 32.6(5)	600.3 ± 70.6(4)	706.5 ± 75.6(4)	< .0001
	0.5	576.7 ± 70.7(4)[b]	957.0 ± 63.7(5)[a]	601.8 ± 84.1(5)	614.8 ± 58.0(5)[a]	1360.0 ± 109.6(4)[b]	774.4 ± 118.8(4)	< .0001

† Mean ± S.E. (number of monkeys)

[a] Paired t-test for diet, p < .01
[b] Paired t-test for diet, p < .05
[c] Paired t-test for diet, p < .10

response at 0.5% dietary cholesterol and the overall mean response
for the different concentrations of dietary cholesterol intake
(0.05% to 1.5%) rank the six species in the following order:
squirrel > green > spider ≃ rhesus ≃ patas > chimpanzees. (It
should be mentioned that based on total serum cholesterol concentration a different order would be obtained.) In some of the
earlier studies it is difficult to relate the hypercholesterolemic
effects to the dietary cholesterol per se because percent of calories
from saturated fat also varied and this is known to have a synergistic effect on serum cholesterol response; this synergistic effect
also seems to differ among species (17).

The differences in response among these species must be
associated with their cholesterol metabolism, i.e., synthesis,
absorption, mobilization to and from tissues, and excretion (18-22).
These observations are preliminary to the identification of control
mechanisms influencing species susceptibility to atherosclerosis.
Whereas the dietary response of chimpanzees, patas, and to some
extent rhesus monkeys, was reflected predominantly in the β-
lipoproteins, the spider, squirrel, and green monkeys showed a
significant increase in both β- and α-lipoproteins.

Earlier studies on cholesterol feeding indicated a decrease
in α-lipoprotein in primates (23, 24); however, these observations
were based on prolonged feeding of high cholesterol diets (3 to
18 months). Studies on cholesterol metabolism in baboons have
indicated that both exogeneous and endogeneous cholesterol are
generally transported nonpreferentially by serum α- and β-lipoproteins (25). Our recent studies of spider monkeys (26) and the
studies by Calvert and Scott of pigs (27) showed a significant
increase in α-lipoproteins during three weeks of cholesterol feeding.
Morris and Greer (28) reported a transitory hyper-α-lipoproteinemia
in rhesus monkeys fed cholesterol. In view of the precursor-product
relationship between these lipoprotein classes and the role of α-
lipoprotein in lipid clearing through lipoprotein lipase and in
view of cholesterylester transport through lecithin-cholesterol-
acyltransferase   (29), the observed differences in lipoprotein
response among species needs further attention. Though the interspecies differences may be mainly due to genetic factors, identification of the physiologic basis for these species differences
should provide a better understanding of hyperlipoproteinemia
induced by diet.

REFERENCES

1. Scott, R. F., E. S. Morrison, J. Jarmolych, S. C. Nam, M. Kroms, and F. Coulston. 1967. Experimental atherosclerosis in rhesus monkeys. I. Gross light microscopy features and lipid in serum and aorta. Exp. Mol. Pathol. 7:11-33.

2. Taylor, C. B., G. E. Cox, P. Manalo-Extrella, and J. Southworth. 1962. Atherosclerosis in rhesus monkeys. II. Arterial lesions associated with hypercholesteremia induced by dietary fat and cholesterol. Arch. Path. 74:16-34.

3. Wissler, R. W., G. S. Getz, D. Vesselinovitch, L. E. Frazier, and R. H. Hughes. 1966. Acute severe experimental atherosclerosis in rhesus monkeys. Fed. Proc. 25:597.

4. Strong, J. P. and H. C. McGill. 1967. Diet and experimental atherosclerosis in baboons. Am. J. Pathol. 50:669-690.

5. Malinow, M. R., C. A. Maruffo, and A. M. Perley. 1966. Experimental atherosclerosis in squirrel monkeys (Saimiri sciurea). J. Pathol. Bacteriol. 92:491-510.

6. Middleton, C. C., T. B. Clarkson, H. B. Lofland, and R. W. Prichard. 1967. Diet and atherosclerosis of squirrel monkeys. Arch. Pathol. 83:145-153.

7. Portman, O. W. and S. B. Andrus. 1965. Comparative evaluation of three species of New World monkeys for studies of dietary factors, tissue lipids, and atherogenesis. J. Nutr. 87:429-438.

8. Clarkson, T. B., H. B. Lofland, B. C. Bullock, N. D. M. Lehner, R. W. St. Clair, and R. W. Prichard. 1969. Atherosclerosis in some species of New World monkeys. Ann. N. Y. Acad. Sci. 162:102-109.

9. Wissler, R. W., L. E. Frazier, R. H. Hughes, and R. A. Rasmussen. 1962. Atherogenesis in the cebus monkey. Arch. Pathol. 74: 312-322.

10. Pucak, G. J., N. D. M. Lehner, T. B. Clarkson, B. C. Bullock, and H. B. Lofland. 1973. Spider monkeys (Ateles Sp.) as animal models for atherosclerosis research. Exp. Mol. Pathol. 18:32-49.

11. Srinivasan, S. R., A. Lopez-S, B. Radhakrishnamurthy, and G. S. Berenson. 1970. Complexing of serum pre-β- and β-lipoproteins and acid mucopolysaccharides. Atherosclerosis 12:321-334.

12. Berenson, G. S., S. R. Srinivasan, A. Lopez-S, B. Radhakrish-
     namurthy, P. S. Pargaonkar, and R. H. Deupree. 1972. Clinical
     application of an indirect method for quantitating serum lipo-
     proteins. Clin. Chim. Acta 36:175-183.

13. Srinivasan, S. R., A. Lopez-S, B. Radhakrishnamurthy, and G. S.
     Berenson. 1970. A simplified technique for semi-quantitative,
     clinical estimation of serum β- and pre-β-lipoproteins.
     Angiologica 7:344-350.

14. Srinivasan, S. R., R. R. Frerichs, and G. S. Berenson. 1975.
     Serum lipids and lipoprotein profile in school children from
     a rural community. Clin. Chim. Acta. 60:293-302.

15. Bowyer, D. E., J. S. Cridland, J. D. Pearson, J. P. King, and
     M. A. Reidy. 1974. A "Plasma cholesterol index" for the more
     precise prediction of atherosclerotic lesion formation in
     experimental animals. In Atherosclerosis III. Ed. by G.
     Schettler and A. Weizel, Springer-Verlag, New York, pp. 847-
     848.

16. Eggen, D. A., J. P. Strong, and W. P. Newman III. 1969.
     Experimental atherosclerosis in primates: a comparison of
     selected species. Ann. N. Y. Acad. Sci. 162:110-119.

17. Corey, J. E., K. C. Hayes, B. Dorr, and D. M. Hegsted. 1974.
     Comparative lipid response of four primate species to dietary
     changes in fat and carbohydrate. Atherosclerosis 19:119-134.

18. Manning, P. J., T. B. Clarkson, and H. B. Lofland. 1971.
     Cholesterol absorption turnover and excretion rates in hyper-
     cholesterolemic rhesus monkeys. Exp. Molec. Pathol. 14:75-89.

19. Dietschy, J. M. and J. D. Wilson. 1970. Regulation of choles-
     terol metabolism. Parts I-III. New Engl. J. Med. 282:1128-
     1138, 1179-1183, 1241-1249.

20. Kritchevsky, D. 1969. Experimental atherosclerosis in primates
     and other species. Ann. N. Y. Acad. Sci. 162:80-88.

21. Eggen, D. A. 1974. Cholesterol metabolism in rhesus monkey,
     squirrel monkey, and baboon. J. Lipid Res. 15:139-145.

22. Ho, K-J. and C. B. Taylor. 1970. Control mechanisms of cho-
     lesterol biosynthesis. Arch. Pathol. 90:83-92.

23. Gresham, G. A., A. N. Howard, J. McQueen, and D. E. Bowyer.
     1965. Atherosclerosis in primates. Brit. J. Exp. Pathol.
     46:94-103.

24. Armstrong, M. L., M. B. Megan, and E. D. Warner. 1974,
    Intimal thickening in normocholesterolemic rhesus monkeys
    fed low supplements of dietary cholesterol, Circ. Res. 34:
    447-454.

25. Kritchevsky, D. 1970. Cholesterol metabolism in the baboon.
    Trans. N. Y. Acad. Sci. 32:821-831.

26. Srinivasan, S. R., E. R. Dalferes, Jr., H. Ruiz, P. S. Par-
    gaonkar, B. Radhakrishnamurthy, and G. S. Berenson. 1972.
    Rapid serum lipoprotein changes in spider monkeys on short-
    term feeding of high cholesterol--high saturated fat diet.
    Proc. Soc. Exp. Biol. Med. 141:154-159.

27. Calvert, G. D. and P. J. Scott. 1974. Serum lipoproteins
    in pigs on high-cholesterol-high-triglyceride diets. Athero-
    sclerosis 19:485-492.

28. Morris, M. D. and W. E. Greer. 1972. Hyperalpha-lipoprotein-
    emia in cholesterol-fed rhesus monkeys. Fed Proc. 31:727.

29. Nichols, A. V. 1969. Functions and interrelationships of
    different classes of plasma lipoproteins. Proc. Nat. Acad.
    Sci. USA, 64:1128-1337.

THE BABOON IN ATHEROSCLEROSIS RESEARCH: COMPARISON WITH OTHER SPECIES AND USE IN TESTING DRUGS AFFECTING LIPID METABOLISM

A. N. Howard

Department of Medicine, University of Cambridge

England

USE OF NON-HUMAN PRIMATES

The use of monkeys in the production of hypercholes-terolaemia and atherosclerosis has many advantages. Firstly, the metabolism of cholesterol and the composition of the lipoproteins are similar to man. Then the arterial disease produced experimentally has a closer resemblance to human disease than that seen in other species, particularly the rabbit.

CHOLESTEROL CONTAINING DIETS

All non-human primates respond to cholesterol feeding, but there is a great variation in response. Table 1 lists the results obtained by several investigators using different species. By far the greatest response in serum cholesterol is given by the rhesus monkey, whilst the baboon gives rela-tively low values. Likewise, the extent of arterial disease seen in the baboon is small and is confined chiefly to sudano-philic streaks in the aorta, whereas in the rhesus monkey extensive coronary lesions have been reported.

One species of macaque - cynamolgus monkey (Maccaca iris) responds especially well to cholesterol feeding and the coronary lesions are so extensive that myocardial infarction is seen in 66% animals after two years (6).

Studies using baboon fed cholesterol diets are often

TABLE I

HYPERCHOLESTEROLAEMIA IN NON-HUMAN PRIMATES

Species	Ref.	Semi-synthetic diet	Dietary cholesterol	Weeks	Serum cholesterol mg/100ml
Baboon		control	-	-	120
	(1)	egg yolk (15%) butter (15%)	0.5	24	286
	(2)	cholesterol butter (15%)	2	24	383
Rhesus Monkey		control	-	-	131
	(3)	egg yolk (12%) butter (12%)	0.4	12	474
	(3)	cholesterol(2%) butter (25%)	2	4	688
Spider Monkey		control	-	-	169
	(3)	egg yolk (12%) butter (12%)	0.4	12	204
Chim-panzee		control	-	-	200
	(5)	cholesterol butter	2.5	24	450

disappointing. As shown in Fig. 1, baboons given a diet in which 2% cholesterol in corn oil was added to monkey chow gave a fairly large initial rise, and then a few weeks later the serum cholesterol fell to considerably lower values. Presumably, the animals have adapted to the increased cholesterol load by either greatly diminishing synthesis and/or decreasing absorption and/or increasing excretion of cholesterol and its metabolites such as the bile acids. The ability of the baboon to compensate appears to be much greater than some other non-human primates.

Following a ten week period on the diet, baboons were given either cholestyramine (400 mg/kg) or clofibrate (200 mg/kg) mixed in the diet. After four weeks no change in serum cholesterol was seen with clofibrate but the cholestyramine group had decreased 15%. The effect of cholestyramine is similar to that seen with anion exchange resins in the cholesterol fed chick and rabbit (7), although the magnitude of the effect is not so great in the baboon. Clofibrate has only been reported to lower cholesterol in animals fed normal diets (8).

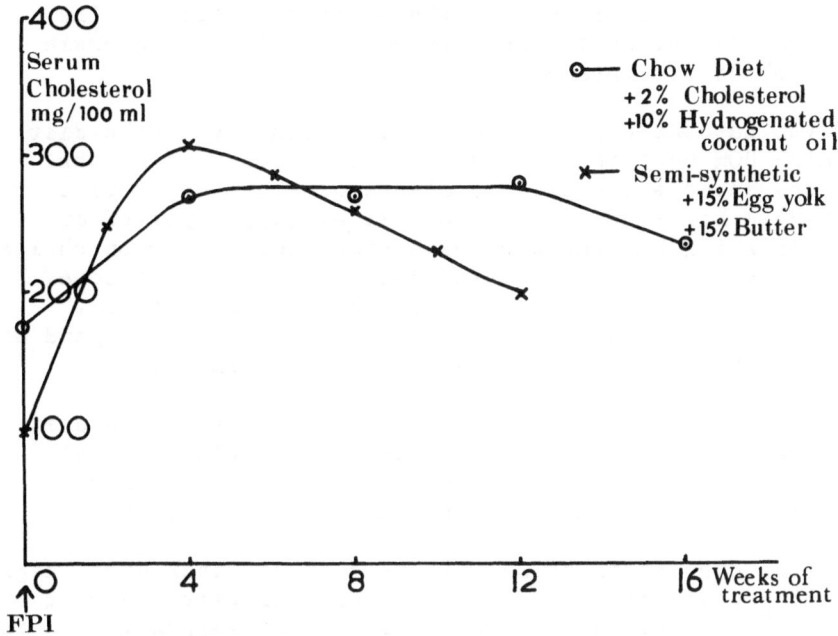

Fig. 1
Serum cholesterol in baboons given
hypocholesterolaemic diets

SEMI-SYNTHETIC DIETS

Rabbits, when given a semi-synthetic diet, develop hypercholesterolaemia and atherosclerosis. Although Malmros and
Wigand (9) claimed that the syndrome could be explained on the
basis of an essential fatty acid deficiency, this appeared not to
be the whole explanation. The situation has been clarified by
Carroll (10), who compared commercial and semi-synthetic diets
to which were added fat of different unsaturation. Saturated
fat only increased hypercholesterolaemia in a semi-synthetic
diet. Such an effect was also seen when casein was added to
the commercial diet. Thus, the hypercholesterolaemia is due
to a combination of factors: low polyunsaturated fatty acids
and a high animal protein content. It should also be noted
that vegetable protein(11) will also show the same potentiating
effect when in high concentration (25%).

The mechanism of the hypercholesterolaemia is not clear.
There is little cholesterol in the diet so the accumulation
must result from body synthesis. Liver cholesterol synthesis

is decreased but intestinal synthesis is unaffected. The
most likely defect is the ability of the animal to excrete
cholesterol or its metabolites.

      Seven baboons were maintained on a semi-synthetic diet
containing 20% beef tallow and 25% casein for nine months.
Two of the animals had serum cholesterol above the normal
range (12). Likewise, Kritchevsky et al (13) reported on
studies in which baboons were maintained for a year on cholesterol free semi-synthetic diets containing either glucose,
fructose, sucrose or starch as a source of carbohydrate.
Serum cholesterol rose approximately 35% in all groups, and at
autopsy fatty streaks were observed in all animals.

      Fig. 2 compares results of feeding semi-synthetic diets
in the baboon and four other primate species (14). In all
cases a significant rise in serum cholesterol is seen compared with similar animals fed a commercial chow diet.

      If the hypothesis of Carroll is correct, then diets high
in animal protein should be hypercholesterolaemic. Strong and
McGill (15) fed baboons for two years on semi-synthetic diets

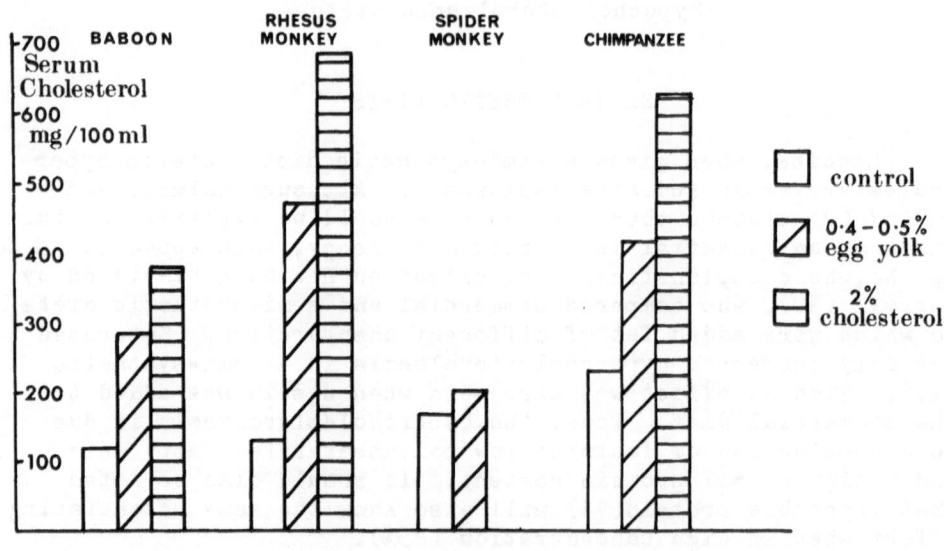

Fig. 2

Semi-synthetic diets in primates

containing different levels of casein (10 and 25%). Animals
on the high protein diets all showed increases in serum cholesterol of the order of 20 mg/100ml. Thus, the baboon does
respond to high protein semi-synthetic diets but very much
less than is seen in the rabbit.

In recent experiments a comparison was made between two
diets containing a moderate (A)or high (B)animal protein content
(Table II). After four weeks the serum cholesterol was
elevated by 31 mg/100ml (33%) in the high protein group.

TABLE II

EFFECT OF DIFFERENT COMMERCIAL DIETS IN BABOONS

Commercial diet	Protein Total	Protein Animal	Animal Fat	Fibre	Serum cholesterol* mg/100ml
A	15.9	12.0	2.4	4.8	95 (83 - 126)
B	23.5	20.0	7	3	126 (97 - 159)

* Mean and range

The above results provide substantial evidence of the
importance of animal protein in influencing the serum cholesterol levels of primates. At the present, the mechanism seems
obscure, but the problem represents a challenge which is not
insoluble using modern cholesterol-balance techniques.

Animals given the high protein commercial diet B were
given cholestyramine (400 mg/kg) or clofibrate (200 mg/kg)
for four weeks. The results were opposite to those obtained
using the high cholesterol diet. Cholestyramine had no effect
but clofibrate caused a drop of 25%.

The results closely parallel those seen in the rat given
a normal diet (16). Presumably, the baboon given a commercial
diet is able to completely compensate for the loss of cholesterol as bile acids when cholestyramine is fed.

COMBINATION OF HYPERCHOLESTEROLAEMIC AND IMMUNOLOGICAL INJURY

Because the extent of arterial disease is disappointing in baboons given hypercholesterolaemic diets, attempts were made to accelerate the disease by injuring the vessel wall by injecting protein antigens. This technique has been already employed successfully in the rabbit using bovine serum albumin or horse serum.

As shown in Table III, baboons given a diet of egg yolk and butter had an elevation of serum cholesterol to 280 mg/100ml and in the space of six months no aortic disease was evident. Likewise, the injection of bovine serum albumin (BSA), a substance which causes immunological injury, had no demonstrable effect on vascular pathology. However, the combination of hypercholesterolaemia and BSA produced extensive aortic sudanophilia and atherosclerosis. Neither the mild lipaemia nor injury alone were sufficient but both factors acted synergistically.

This method of producing atherosclerosis in baboons has been extensively useful in studying drugs which may be anti-atherogenic without affecting blood lipid levels, as discussed below.

DRUGS AFFECTING ARTERIAL ENZYMES

Prophylactic effect

The chief lipids which accumulate in the atherosclerotic lesion in man and animals are cholesterol and its esters and phospholipids. There is a relative increase in cholesterol esters compared with free cholesterol, much of the former being synthesised by esterification in situ. Fig. 3 shows the current status of our knowledge of the metabolism of lipoproteins in the arterial wall.

We have shown that in experimental atherosclerosis in rats and in rabbits, there is an increase in lipase and phospholipase activity and a decrease in cholesterol esterase activity in the arterial wall (17), and it is suggested that these might be contributing factors in the deposition of lipid (18). Injections of intravenous polyunsaturated phosphatidyl choline (EPL solution; 10% w/v in H_2O containing 4% sodium deoxycholate) in rabbits given atherogenic diets, reduced the extent of the aortic atherosclerotic lesions produced. This could not be explained on the basis of decreased hypercholesterolaemia but was probably due to change induced in aortic enzyme

TABLE III

MEAN PLASMA LIPIDS, AORTIC ATHEROSCLEROSIS AND LIPOLYTIC ENZYMES

Group	No. examined	Treatment* Diet	BSA	EPL solution	Plasma cholesterol mg%	Aortic atherosclerosis % area	Aortic Lipase	Aortic cholesterol esterase neq/min/mg
1	8	A	+	-	245	46.3	67	19
2	8	A	+	+	226	9.5	54	36
3	5	A	-	-	286	0		
4	5	C	+	-	118	0		
5	5	C	-	-	116	0	38	22

* A = atherogenic   C = control   BSA = bovine serum albumin

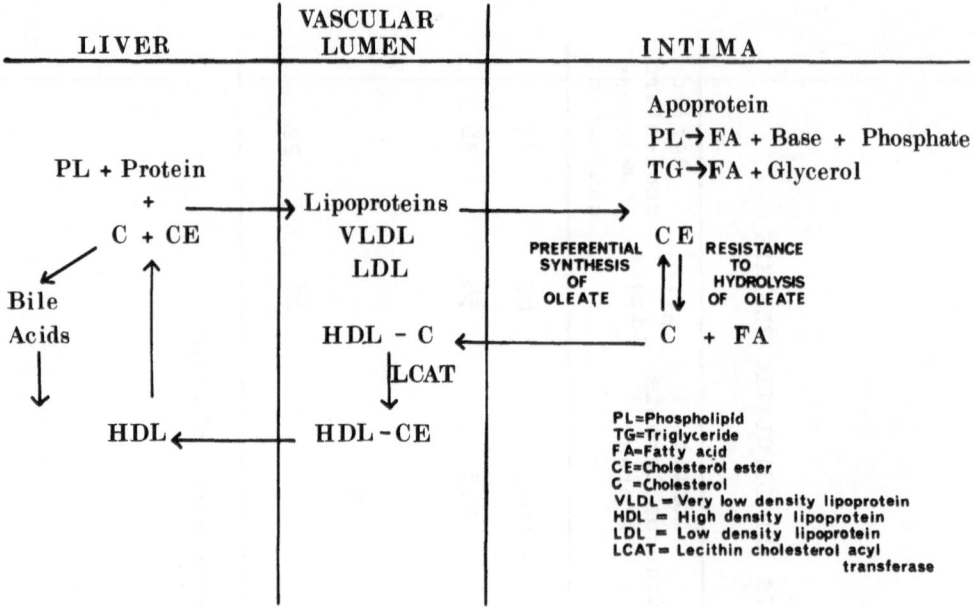

Fig. 3

Lipoprotein metabolism

activities. Of particular interest was the normalisation of
cholesterol ester hydrolase activity (19).

     A similar study was also made in hypercholesterolaemic
baboons given injections of bovine serum albumin (1). Groups
of 5 - 8 baboons were given either a control or hypercholesterolaemic diet for six months. During the last 90 days, each
group was given five i.v. injections of bovine serum albumin
(BSA) at 16 day intervals or control injections of saline.
Prophylactic injections of EPL solution caused a highly significant decrease in aortic atherosclerosis and a normalization
of aortic lipase. The activity of cholesterol esterase was
increased 50% above normal (Table IV).

                        Effect on regression

     Recent experiments have been concerned with the possible
effect of EPL solution on the regression of established
atherosclerotic lesions in the baboon (2). Animals were made

TABLE IV

SERUM CHOLESTEROL, AORTIC ATHEROSCLEROSIS AND ACAT IN BABOONS

			Serum cholesterol		Aortic	
Group	Injection		Initial diet	Control diet	athero-sclerosis (% disease)	ACAT activity (n equiv/min/ mg)
1	Saline	A	383	115	26.9	1.6
2	EPL soln.	A	388	114	26.8	0.1
3	None	C	104	112	0	0.6

A = atherogenic   C = control

to develop aortic atherosclerosis using a cholesterol containing diet and then injected with BSA as described above.
They were then changed to a control diet and treated with
saline or EPL solution (250 mg/kg EPL thrice weekly) for 16
weeks. As shown in Table IV, EPL solution had no demonstrable
effect on the regression of the lesions, as shown by analysis
of the aortic cholesterol content. However, it is recognised
that the cholesterol deposited in the aortic wall is extremely
immobile and a lack of effect may reflect a relatively short
period of treatment. It is obviously desirable to report such
critical experiments over a longer term.

However, one interesting result came to light in these
studies. EPL solution has a profound effect on the cholesterol ester synthetase enzyme acyl coA cholesterol acyl transferase (ACAT) in the aorta (Table IV). Compared with control
animals, enzyme activity was increased in atherosclerotic
aorta from saline injected animals. In atherosclerotic
animals injected with EPL solution the enzyme could not be
demonstrated. It is there concluded that the drug strongly
inhibits this enzyme, thus preventing the formation of cholesterol esters in the arterial wall.

CONCLUSIONS

Despite the demonstration of spontaneous atherosclerosis
in the wild state, the baboon is not the best species for
the production of atherosclerosis experimentally since it

develops only a mild hypercholesterolaemia when fed cholesterol.
Nevertheless, it is useful for the study of mild lipid deposition
in the aorta and the effect of drugs thereon, particularly if
protein antigens are also employed in addition. For studies of the
hypocholesterolaemic effect of potential therapeutic compounds in
man, the baboon fed a high protein commercial diet, with and without
cholesterol, is a useful second species to smaller laboratory
animals.

REFERENCES

1. Howard, A.N., J. Patelski, D.E. Bowyer and G.A. Gresham. 1971.
    Atherosclerosis induced in hypercholesterolaemic baboons by
    immunological injury; and the effects of intravenous polyun-
    saturated phosphatidyl choline. Atherosclerosis 14:17-29.

2. Howard, A.N. and J. Patelski. 1974. Hydrolysis and synthesis
    of aortic cholesterol esters in atherosclerotic baboons. Effect
    of polyunsaturated phosphatidyl choline on enzyme activities.
    Atherosclerosis 20:225-232.

3. Newman, W.P. III, D.A. Eggan and J.P. Strong. 1974. Comparison
    of arterial lesions and serum lipids in spider and rhesus
    monkeys on an egg and butter diet. Atherosclerosis 19:75-86.

4. Fraser, R., L. Dubien, F. Musil, E. Fosslien and R.W. Wissler.
    1972. Transport of cholesterol in thoracic duct lymph and
    serum of rhesus monkeys fed cholesterol with various food fats.
    Atherosclerosis 16:203-216.

5. Howard, A.N., V. Blaton, D. Vandamme, N. Van Landschoot and H.
    Peeters. 1972. Lipid changes in the plasma lipoproteins of
    baboons given an atherogenic diet. Part 3. A comparison between
    lipid changes in the plasma of the baboon and chimpanzee given
    atherogenic diets and those in human plasma lipoproteins of
    type II hyperlipoproteinaemia. Atherosclerosis 16:257-272.

6. Kramsch, D.M., A. Huvos and W. Hollander. 1970. A primate
    model for the study of coronary (atherosclerotic) heart disease.
    Circulation 42:III-9.

7. Parkinson, T.M. 1967. Hypolipidemic effects of orally admini-
    stered dextran and cellulose anion exchangers in cockerels and
    dogs. J. Lipid Res. 8:24-29.

8. Thorp, J.M. 1962. Experimental evaluation of an orally active
    combination of androsterone with ethyl chlorophenoxyisobutyrate.
    Lancet 1:1323-1326.

9. Malmros, H. and G. Wigand. 1959. Atherosclerosis and de-
    ficiency of essential fatty acids. Lancet 2:749-751.

10. Carrol, K.K. 1971. Plasma cholesterol levels and liver
    cholesterol biosynthesis in rabbits fed commercial or semi-
    synthetic diets with and without added fats or oils. Athero-
    sclerosis 13:67-76.

11. Howard, A.N., G.A. Gresham, D. Jones and I.W. Jennings. 1965.
    The prevention of rabbit atherosclerosis by soya bean meal.
    J. Atheroscler. Res. 5:330-337.

12. Howard, A.N., G.A. Gresham, C.N. Hales, F.T. Lindgren and A.A.
    Katzberg. 1965. Atherosclerosis in baboons: Pathological and
    biochemical studies. In: The Baboon In Medical Research Ed.
    by H. Vagtborg, Volume II, University of Texas Press, Austin,
    p. 333-350.

13. Kritchevsky, D., L.M. Davidson, I.L. Shapiro, H.K. Kim, M.
    Kitagawa, S. Malhotra, P.P. Nair, T.B. Clarkson, I. Bersohn
    and P.A.D. Winter. 1974. Lipid metabolism and experimental
    atherosclerosis in baboons: Influence of cholesterol-free
    semi-synthetic diets. Am. J. Clin. Nutr. 27:29-50.

14. Bullock, B.C., N.D.M. Lehner, T.B. Clarkson, M.A. Feldner,
    W.D. Wagner, and H.B. Lofland. 1975. Comparative primate
    atherosclerosis. I. Tissue cholesterol concentrations and
    pathologic anatomy. Exp. Molec. Path. 22:151-175.

15. Strong, J.P., and H.C. McGill. 1967. Diet and experimental
    atherosclerosis in baboons. Am. J. Path. 50:669-690.

16. Huff, J.W., J.L. Gilfillan and V.M. Hunt. 1963. Effect of
    cholestyramine, a bile acid binding polymer on plasma choles-
    terol and fecal bile acid excretion in the rat. Proc. Soc.
    Exp. Biol. Med. 114:252-255.

17. Patelski, J., D.E. Bowyer, A.N. Howard and G.A. Gresham. 1968.
    Changes in phospholipase A, lipase and cholesterol esterase
    activity in the aorta in experimental atherosclerosis in the
    rabbit and rat. J. Atheroscler. Res. 8:221-228.

18. Howard, A.N. In, C. Cowgill, D.L. Etrich and P.D. Wood. Edits.
    Proceedings of 1968 Deuel Conference, U.S. Dept. of Health,
    Educ. & Welfare, Washington, p. 171 (1968).

19. Patelski, J., D.E. Bowyer, A.N. Howard, I.W. Jennings, C.J.R.
    Thorne and G.A. Gresham. 1970. Modification of enzyme
    activities in experimental atherosclerosis in the rabbit.
    Atherosclerosis 12:41-53.

THE FINE STRUCTURE OF NONATHEROSCLEROTIC INTIMAL THICKENING,

OF DEVELOPING, AND OF REGRESSING ATHEROSCLEROTIC LESIONS

AT THE BIFURCATION OF THE LEFT CORONARY ARTERY

Herbert C. Stary and Jack P. Strong

Department of Pathology, Louisiana State University

School of Medicine, New Orleans, Louisiana 70112, U.S.A.

I.   INTRODUCTION

Ischemic heart disease is the major cause of death in the United States (1). Majority opinion holds that the underlying cause is obstruction of the coronary artery lumen by an atherosclerotic lesion with or without a superimposed thrombus (2). In coronary arteries, atherosclerotic lesions predominate at the bifurcation of the main stem of the left coronary artery and in the anterior descending branch just beyond (3,4). Stenosis by atherosclerotic plaques (5) and occlusion by plaques or thrombi (6-8) occur most frequently in the same areas.

Because of the obvious clinical importance of this highly susceptible coronary artery segment and because there is no information on its fine structure, we initiated studies of the segment under varying conditions. We began by studying normocholesterolemic animals and the fine structure of the nonatherosclerotic intimal thickening that is prominent at and about the left coronary artery bifurcation. Subsequently, we examined the evolution of atherosclerotic lesions in nonatherosclerotic intimal thickening at several time intervals after experimental induction of hypercholesterolemia. Most recently, we studied regression of the experimentally produced atherosclerotic lesions that follows when elevated serum cholesterol levels are returned to normal levels.

Experimental atherosclerotic lesions lose lipid and decrease in size when the serum cholesterol level is lowered (9), but

89

advanced lesions do not disappear completely (10-13). Therefore, in recent experiments on regression we studied the mechanism of regression since any attempt to bring about complete resolution of lesions must presuppose an understanding of the mechanism. Specifically, we explored the removal of foam cells, the mode by which intracellular lipid is removed from the cytoplasm of smooth muscle cells, and the mode by which extracellular lipid and cell debris is removed from the intima.

The purpose of this article is to review our earlier work on the structure of nonatherosclerotic intimal thickening and on the structure of atherosclerotic lesions that develop in nonatherosclerotic intimal thickening when hypercholesterolemia is induced experimentally, and to present new findings on the mechanism of regression of atherosclerotic lesions when high serum cholesterol levels are reduced.

II. DESIGN OF THE EXPERIMENTS

Nonatherosclerotic intimal thickening.-- Observations on the fine structure of nonatherosclerotic intimal thickening at and about the left coronary artery bifurcation (14) are of eight normocholesterolemic rhesus monkeys used as controls in several experiments.

Developing atherosclerotic lesions.-- The development of atherosclerotic lesions was studied in 12 hypercholesterolemic rhesus monkeys. Two animals were given a high-cholesterol diet for four weeks, four for 12 weeks, and six for 40 weeks. The animals were killed upon completion of the diet. The response of the serum cholesterol to the high-cholesterol diet and the extent of aortic lesions (15), and detailed observations on the fine structure of atherosclerotic lesions developing in the nonatherosclerotic intimal thickening of coronary arteries (16), have been reported

Regressing atherosclerotic lesions.-- Two regression experiments were combined for analysis of the fine structure of coronary arteries. The experimental design, the response of serum and aortic lipids, and gross and microscopic findings in the aorta have been reported for the first study (9). The two combined studies consisted of 11 dietary groups with a total of 43 rhesus monkeys. For 12 weeks, all animals initially received the same high-cholesterol diet used in the study on developing lesions. One group of animals was killed at the end of 12 weeks. Ten groups were changed to low-cholesterol food, and separate groups were killed after periods of 2, 3, 4, 8, 12, 16, 24, 32, 40, and 64 weeks.

III. MATERIALS AND METHODS

All animals were adolescent or young-adult, male, rhesus monkeys (<u>Macaca</u> <u>mulatta</u>). Age was estimated by body weight and by eruption of the third molar teeth. The animals were obtained from Shamrock Farms, Middleton, N.Y., and from Primate Imports, Port Washington, Long Island, N.Y. They had been conditioned for 6 to 8 weeks after arrival from India and Pakistan. During this period they were dewormed, tested for tuberculosis, and given low-fat, low-cholesterol food. From their arrival at the laboratory until the start of the experiment the animals received D & G research animal laboratory diet (Price Wilhoite Co., Frederick, Md.) which has a low content of fat and cholesterol. Control animals continued to receive this low-cholesterol food until they were killed.

The high-cholesterol diet consisted of D & G research animal laboratory diet supplemented with butter and beef tallow (3:1), casein, cholesterol, vitamin diet fortification mixture, and water. (We added unsweetened apple sauce to this diet recently in order to enhance palatability.) The diet contained 1 mg of cholesterol per calorie, or 0.37% cholesterol by weight. Food was offered once a day in a quantity just sufficient to maintain normal body growth.

Tissue taken for electron microscopy consisted of consecutive cross-sections of the main stem of the left coronary artery, of the bifurcation of the main stem into anterior descending and circumflex branches, and of the proximal left anterior descending branch. The tissue was fixed in two changes of buffered osmium tetroxide, dehydrated in graded alcohols and embedded in the epoxy resin Maraglas. Semithin sections of the complete cross-sections of the artery were prepared from several levels of each tissue block, stained with Paragon multiple stain and examined with the light microscope. Areas of special interest were fine sectioned with a diamond knife, stained with lead citrate and uranyl acetate, and examined and photographed in an RCA EMU 3F electron microscope.

Serum total cholesterol was quantitated for all animals by the method of Abell <u>et al</u>. (17). Serum samples were taken at one-week intervals initially, and less frequently later, from the time of the animals arrival at the laboratory until their death.

IV. ANATOMY OF THE LEFT CORONARY ARTERY

The left coronary artery originated from a single ostium and usually began as a distinct, single main stem of variable length which gave rise to the anterior descending and circumflex coronary arteries at the main bifurcation. In a few cases, the anterior descending and the circumflex artery both originated directly at

the left coronary ostium, and there was no distinct main stem. The
intermediate descending branch took its origin from either the
anterior descending or from the circumflex branch and sometimes
directly in between these two arteries, thus giving rise to a tri-
furcation.

V. NONATHEROSCLEROTIC INTIMAL THICKENING

The following observations on nonatherosclerotic intimal
thickening, made on eight animals receiving only low-cholesterol
food, provided a baseline for comparison of developing and regressing atherosclerotic lesions studied subsequently. The mean value
of all serum cholesterol determinations made in each animal ranged
from 110 to 180 mg/dl. The mean value for all eight animals was
142 mg/dl.

All animals had intimal thickening of some degree. The nature
of the intimal thickening varied characteristically with location
within the artery. Thickening occurred either as intimal cushions,
that is prominent but circumscribed thickenings at arterial forks,
or as less prominent diffuse intimal thickening away from, and
usually distal and lateral to, the mouth of branch vessels. The
highest degree of intimal thickening was a saddle-shaped cushion
at the apex of the bifurcation of the anterior descending and circumflex arteries (Fig. 1). The saddle-shaped cushion began on
opposite sides of the proximal segment of the main stem reaching a
thickness of up to six cells at the apex of the bifurcation. It
continued distally and laterally into the two branch vessels as
diffuse intimal thickening.

Intimal cushions differed from diffuse intimal thickening in
the number of cell layers, and in the nature of the cells and intercellular matrix. Cushions generally consisted of an upper loose
layer with a few randomly oriented cells in an abundant, finely
reticulated, intercellular matrix, and of deeper layers with a
higher cell density.

Intimal cushions contained two main cell types. Myofilament-
rich smooth muscle cells closely resembling medial smooth muscle
cells were the most frequent cell type. They were present throughout the cushions but tended to be the sole cell type at the base of
the cushions. The second, and less frequent, cell type were endoplasmic reticulum (ER)-rich smooth muscle cells which differed from
myofilament-rich cells by the presence of very abundant rough-surfaced ER. There was a scarcity of myofilament bundles, which were
frequently limited to the cell periphery, and a less prominent
basement membrane in this second type of cell. ER-rich cells were
scattered throughout cushions but tended to occur more frequently
in the luminal layer.

Diffuse intimal thickening was generally more homogeneous in character than intimal cushions, and similar in composition to the deeper layers of cushions (Fig. 2). The cell density was greater than that of cushions. The compactly arranged intimal cells consisted almost entirely of myofilament-rich smooth muscle cells (Fig. 2),although an isolated ER-rich cell was present now and then.

Degenerative changes were frequent in the elongated peripheral cell processes of intimal smooth muscle cells. Degenerative changes included swelling and loss of density of the cell cytoplasm, cystic dilatation of vesicles of endoplasmic reticulum,

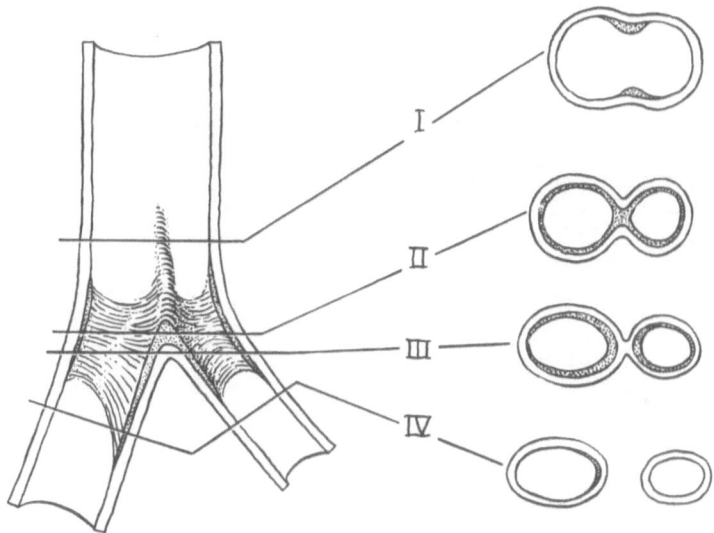

Figure 1. Schematic drawing of the most frequent type of left coronary artery bifurcation: The lumen, left; the corresponding arterial cross-sections, right. Intimal thickening is indicated by stippling. Level I: The main stem of the left coronary artery proximal to the bifurcation has paired, longitudinal intimal cushions. Level II: A thick saddle-shaped cushion forms at the apex of the bifurcation. Diffuse intimal thickening inconsistently extends to involve the circumference of the bifurcation. Level III: At the origin of the anterior descending and the circumflex branches, intimal thickening tends to involve the entire circumference of each branch diffusely. Level IV: Distal to the bifurcation, intimal thickening is progressively less extensive. (Reproduced from Stary and Strong, 1976, Primates in Medicine, vol. 9, pp. 321-358, Karger, Basel)

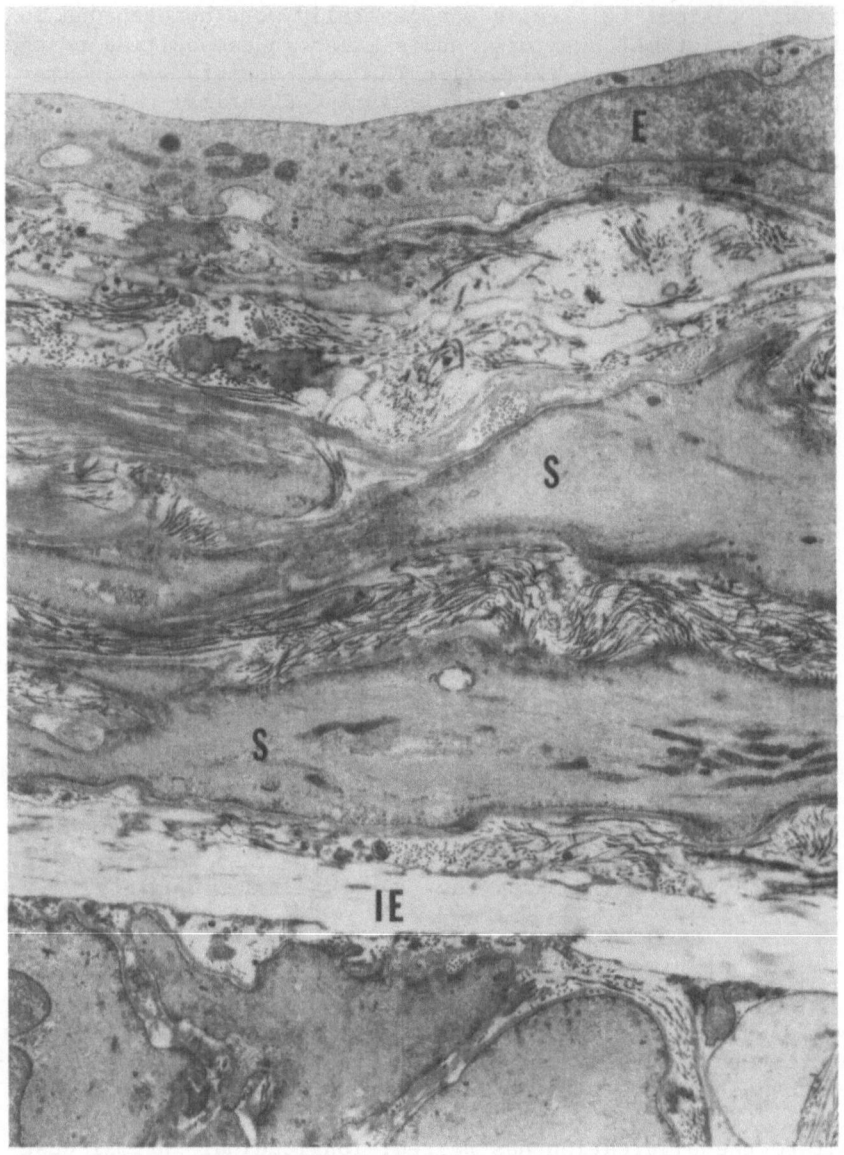

Figure 2. Diffuse intimal thickening in the proximal anterior descending branch, the continuation of a large intimal cushion at
the bifurcation. From a monkey receiving only low-cholesterol
food with a mean serum cholesterol level of 120 mg/dl. The intima
has two compact layers of myofilament-rich smooth muscle cells (S)
between endothelium (E) and internal elastic lamina (IE).
(Rhesus No. 20; X 12000) (Reduced 10% for reproduction.)

and, more often, loss of all organelles. Our observations indicate that degenerated cell processes separate from the main body of the cell and dissolve. Similar degenerative changes have been labeled "ghost bodies" in the aortas of rhesus monkeys fed either stock or atherogenic diets (18,19). Necrosis of whole intimal smooth muscle cells was not observed in these normocholesterolemic animals.

Some intimal smooth muscle cells had single or multiple intracytoplasmic lipid inclusions; however, inclusions were infrequent. Single, isolated foam cells of the macrophage type occurred rarely in the subendothelial portion of a few intimal cushions. Foam cells either showed degenerative change or were necrotic.

Endothelial cells on the surface of both cushions and diffuse thickening occasionally were richer in cell organelles than endothelial cells on intima that was not thickened. Vesicles of rough-surfaced ER sometimes were dilated and increased in number. One or several small lipid inclusions were infrequently present. Pinocytotic vesicles were abundant at the luminal surface and at the base of cells. Thin and thick filaments were prominent and sometimes formed filament bundles. Other cytoplasmic constituents such as mitochondria, Golgi apparatus, and Palade bodies were usually not prominent. A few endothelial cells showed degenerative change.

The internal elastic lamina usually was a prominent, compact membrane separating intima from media. Gaps in this membrane were frequent and extensive at the base of intimal cushions; gaps at the base of diffuse intimal thickening were less frequent and less extensive.

The media was composed of myofilament-rich smooth muscle cells which could be distinguished from intimal smooth muscle by their large size, regular arrangement, and greater prominence of the basement membrane. Intracytoplasmic lipid was infrequent; when present, it was different in appearance from that in intimal cells. It formed single, small droplets or grape-like clusters of small droplets, more osmiophilic than the lipid inclusions of intimal smooth muscle. The droplets were in close association with vesicles of smooth-surfaced ER at the center of the cells and probably represent lipofuscin. Adjacent to cushions and diffuse thickening, the space between internal elastic lamina and the first layer of medial smooth muscle cells sometimes contained the swollen and degenerated cell processes of medial smooth muscle cells.

VI. DEVELOPMENT OF ATHEROSCLEROTIC LESIONS

When the high-cholesterol diet was given to monkeys, the serum cholesterol level increased rapidly during the first four weeks, then more slowly, to reach an unsteady plateau after about 15 weeks. The degree of serum cholesterol elevation varied from animal to animal. The mean value was 440 mg/dl in the two animals given the high-cholesterol diet for four weeks; 470 mg/dl in four animals given the diet for 12 weeks; and 575 mg/dl in six animals given the diet for 40 weeks.

Four weeks after the high-cholesterol diet was started, intimal thickening was no greater than in control animals. The earliest changes were lipid inclusions in some of the smooth muscle cells of preexisting intimal cushions at the main bifurcation and the emergence of isolated foam cells just beneath the endothelium and occasionally at the periphery of cushions.

Twelve weeks after the start of the high-cholesterol diet there was a moderate increase in the thickness of intimal cushions and adjacent diffuse thickening as a result of the accumulation of foam cells, macrophages, and cell debris in the superficial portion of the intima near the endothelim. In the largest lesions cell debris formed pools in the interstitium of the intima. Eosinophil and neutrophil granulocytes were first seen in lesions at this time period, but they were rare. More intimal smooth muscle cells had single or multiple lipid inclusions.

Forty weeks after the start of the high-cholesterol diet, extensive atherosclerotic lesions blended into the preexisting intimal cushions at the main bifurcation. Smaller lesions were in the diffuse intimal thickening of the adjacent anterior descending and circumflex branches and in intimal cushions at the smaller distal bifurcations of branch vessels. The usual loose arrangement of cells in the superficial half of large intimal cushions and the finely reticulated ground substance between widely separated cells were replaced by a dence accumulation of cells. The largest lesions contained several layers of foam cells adjacent to the lumen. Other cells in lesions were macrophages and, less frequently, eosinophil and neutrophil granulocytes. The normally more densely arranged smooth muscle cells at the depth of cushions were widely separated by accumulations of coarsely grained cell debris and extracellular lipid derived from necrotic intimal smooth muscle cells and, more often, from necrotic foam cells. Cell debris and extracellular lipid tended to accumulate in pools adjacent to the internal elastic lamina. At gaps in the internal elastic lamina a few of the larger pools of extracellular material showed extension into the adjacent media.

The two types of intimal smooth muscle cells, myofilament-rich and ER-rich (Fig. 3), found in nonatherosclerotic intimal thickening were also present when atherosclerotic lesions were superimposed. ER-rich smooth muscle cells were more numerous in intimal cushions with superimposed atherosclerotic lesions than in cushions without lesions. Intimal smooth muscle cells of both types frequently contained intracytoplasmic lipid inclusions of the moderately electron dense type (Fig. 3). The borders of lipid inclusions were scalloped and usually not membrane bound. Laminated residual bodies thought to represent the degenerated end products of various cell constituents were sometimes present. Occassionally they filled the entire cytoplasm of a cell. Golgi stacks and vesicles of smooth-surfaced ER were more numerous in smooth muscle cells with lipid inclusions than in smooth muscle cells without and were more frequent in ER-rich than in myofilament-rich smooth muscle cells. Lysosomal activity, such as fusion of smooth-surfaced vesicles with lipid inclusions and formation of partial or complete membranes around lipid inclusions, occurred in both types of intimal smooth muscle cells, but more often in ER-rich smooth muscle cells. Lysosomal activity did not reach the same intensity in smooth muscle cells as in the macrophage derived foam cells in the same lesions. Degenerative changes occurred in the peripheral cell processes of intimal smooth muscle cells and resembled those seen in the smooth muscle cells of nonatherosclerotic intimal thickening of control animals. Degenerative changes were more frequent in atherosclerotic lesions. Necrotic smooth muscle cells of both types occurred in atherosclerotic lesions.

Foam cells were large spherical cells with numerous lipid inclusions within the cytoplasm (Fig. 4). Foam cells lacked the basement membrane and bundles of myofilaments characteristically associated with both types of smooth muscle cells. Filaments of a different type were, however, frequently present in the perinuclear region, and resembled the perinuclear filament bundles of macrophages. The perinuclear area of foam cells also contained a prominent Golgi apparatus and numerous vesicles of smooth-surfaced ER. Lipid inclusions were of several morphologically distinct types (Fig. 4). The majority usually were electron-lucent vacuoles. Less frequent were lipid inclusions of moderate electron density, similar to those in smooth muscle cells, and cholesterol crystals. Residual bodies, consisting of crinkled, coarsely laminated structures, almost always accompanied lipid inclusions. Although many lipid inclusions were not membrane bound, more inclusions were either completely or partially surrounded by a membrane in foam cells than in smooth muscle cells. Occasionally, smooth and delicate membranes formed several layers around lipid inclusions. Such coiled membranous structures associated with lipid inclusions are thought to represent phagolysosomes. Lipid droplets,

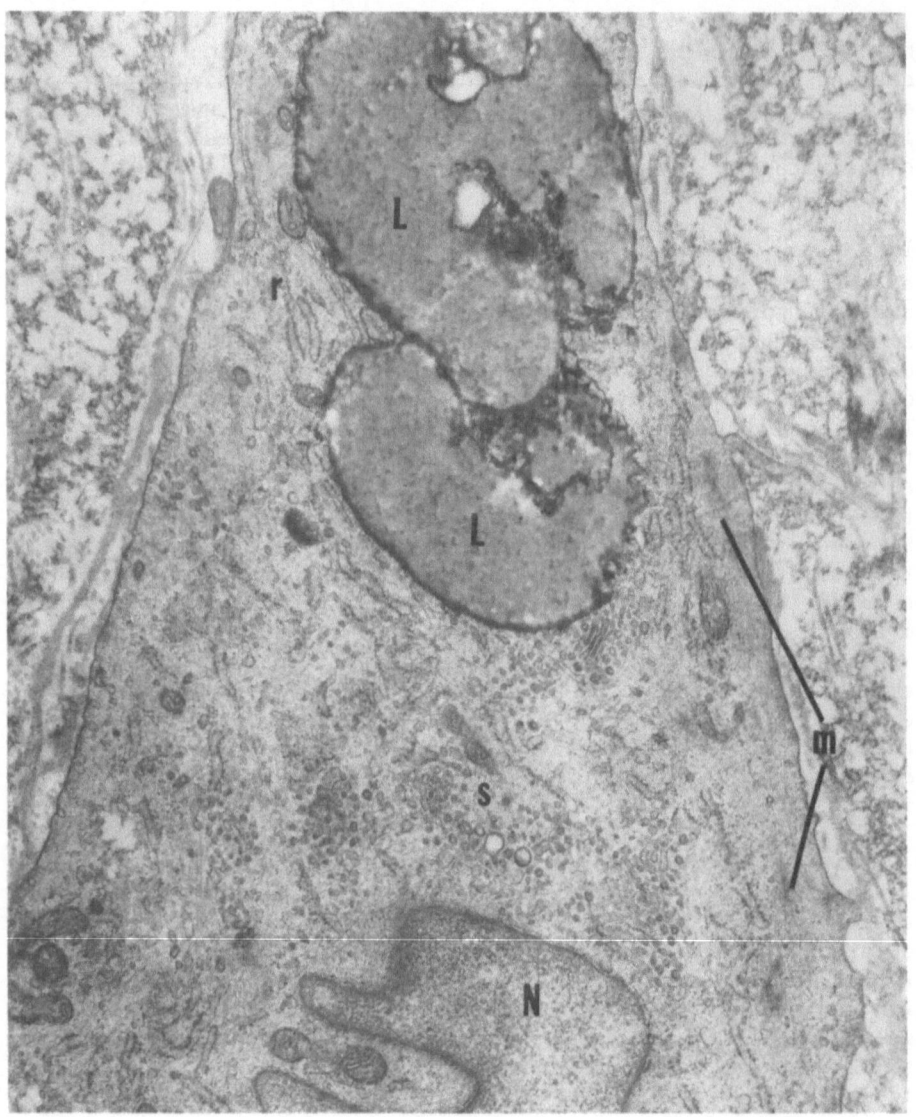

Figure 3. Detail of an ER-rich smooth muscle cell from the mid-
portion of an intimal cushion containing an atherosclerotic lesion.
From a monkey on the high-cholesterol diet for 40 weeks with a
mean serum cholesterol level of 850 mg/dl. ER is mainly rough-
surfaced (r), although smooth-surfaced ER (s) is prominent in the
perinuclear region of cells with lipid inclusions (L). Myofilament bundles with dense bodies (m) are at the periphery of the
cytoplasm. The basement membrane is less prominent than in
myofilament-rich smooth muscle cells. Nucleus (N). (Rhesus No.
31; X 24000) (Reduced 10% for reproduction.)

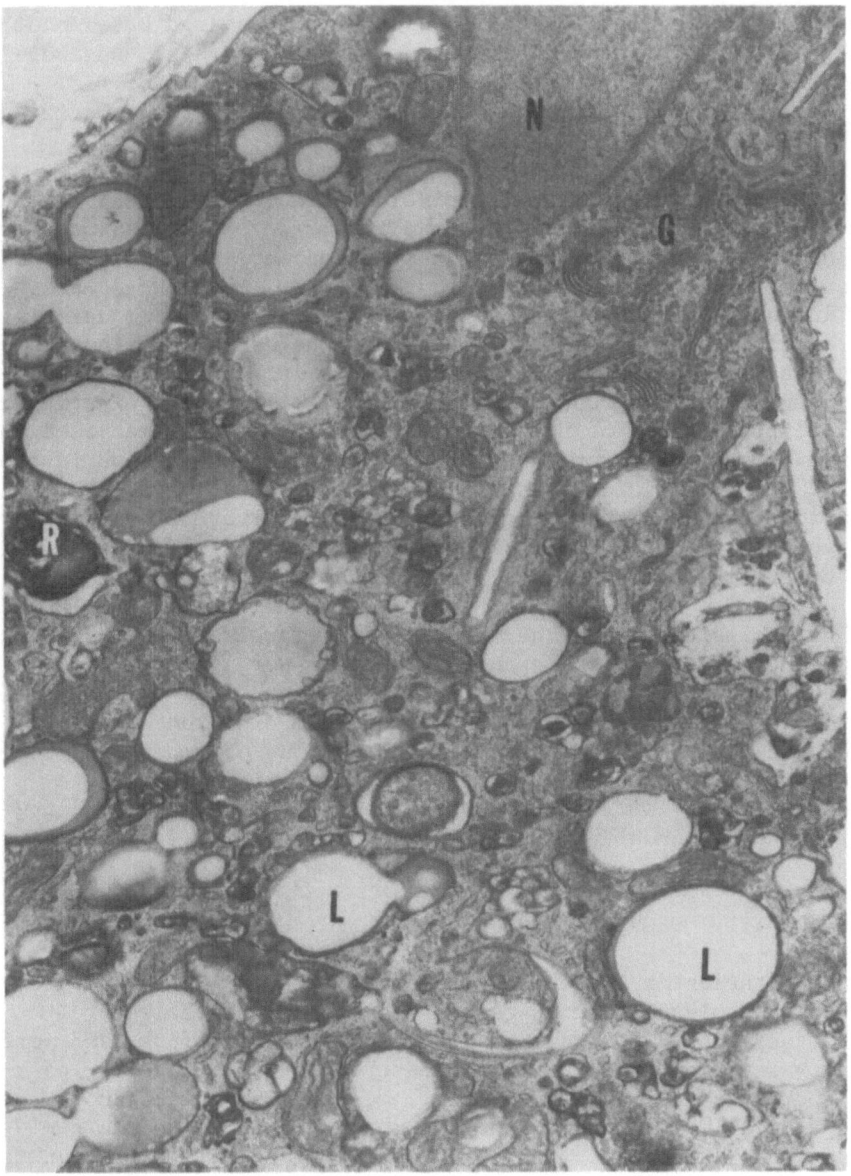

Figure 4. Detail of a macrophage derived foam cell from the
lesion shown in figure 3. Lipid inclusions are of several morphologically distinct types. Incompletely membrane-bound lipid
vacuoles (L) are usually more abundant than residual bodies (R).
Stilleto-shaped spaces are remnants of extracted cholesterol
crystals. The Golgi apparatus (G) and numerous vesicles of
smooth-surfaced ER are most abundant in the perinuclear area, the
"Hof" of the nucleus (N). (X 16875) (Reduced 10% for reproduction.)

cholesterol clefts, and residual bodies often appeared between or
at the center of the finely laminated membrane spirals. Degenerative changes in the foam cell cytoplasm and necrosis of foam
cells were frequent. More foam cells were necrotic than smooth
muscle cells.

Macrophages were either inactive or stimulated. The inactive
or immature cells contained few organelles, whereas the stimulated
cells had a prominent Golgi apparatus, lysosomes, and a plasma
membrane arranged as numerous microvilli. Some macrophages had
lipid inclusions and appeared to be in transition to foam cells.
Cells similar to those classified as macrophages in the present
study have been called monocytes (20) and undifferentiated cells
(21) in human fatty streaks, and primitive cells in the experimental aortic lesions of rhesus monkeys (18). Intimal macrophages
occurred in atherosclerotic lesions,although none were seen in the
nonatherosclerotic intimal thickening of control animals. The
derivation of intimal macrophages is unknown. There are indications that in experimental atherosclerotic lesions macrophages can
arise by proliferation of local intimal cells (22).

Endothelial cells on the surface of lesions sometimes had an
increased cytoplasmic volume and a prominent Golgi apparatus.
Pinocytotic vesicles were abundant. Some endothelial cells had
one or more large lipid inclusions of uniform electron density,
morphologically similar to the lipid inclusions of smooth muscle
cells. Grape-like clusters of small lipid droplets which have
been described as lipofuscin occurred rarely. Degenerative changes
occurred in some endothelial cells on the surface of lesions.

VII.   REGRESSION OF ATHEROSCLEROTIC LESIONS

Substitution of low-cholesterol food after a 12-week period
on the high-cholesterol diet caused elevated serum cholesterol
levels (range 260-830 mg/dl) to decrease rapidly at first and more
gradually later. Normal serum cholesterol levels (range 95-165
mg/dl) were regained within two to 12 weeks. The total time
varied from animal to animal and apparently depended on the response of each animal to the high-cholesterol diet, that is, on
the mean serum cholesterol elevation during the period of lesion
induction, and possibly on other as yet undetermined factors. Normal serum cholesterol levels were found within eight weeks after
diet change in the majority of animals.

In animals killed while serum cholesterol levels had not completely returned to normal, there was no apparent fine structural
evidence of lesion regression. On the contrary, the average size
of lesions increased during the period immediately after diet

reversal. Thus, in the majority of animals, the baseline atherosclerotic lesions from which regression had to be measured and
evaluated were the result of 14-20 weeks of hypercholesterolemia.
Although these lesions contained more lipid-laden cells than those
of animals killed immediately after 12 weeks on the high-cholesterol diet, they were, nevertheless, still largely limited to the
intimal thickening about the bifurcation.

The first signs of regression occurred about four weeks after
the serum cholesterol had returned to normal levels. Early changes
included a progressive decrease in the number of foam cells.
Within 16 weeks after return of the serum cholesterol level to
normal, most foam cells had disappeared from the intimal lesions.
Only infrequent and solitary foam cells were seen at this and at
later regression periods. While intact foam cells were decreasing
in number, necrotic foam cells were continually present (Fig. 5).
This suggests that the return to normal cellularity of the intima
was due to foam cell necrosis and not to emigration of foam cells
from the intima into the blood stream. The smooth muscle cells of
intimal lesions, either with or without lipid inclusions, ceased
to show morphologic features of necrosis as soon as the serum
cholesterol level returned to normal. A possible explanation for
the difference in susceptibility to necrosis between smooth
muscle cells and foam cells after reduction of the serum cholesterol level might be that after the immediate cause of cell
injury - hypercholesterolemia - had been removed, the difference
in cell survival came to depend on the difference in the overall
life span of two separate cell lines. Thus the accumulated macrophage-derived foam cells, having a limited life span, died over
a period of several months, while intimal smooth muscle cells with
a longer life span, survived and recuperated.

Studies of tritiated thymidine cell proliferation indicate
that the increased proliferation of intimal smooth muscle cells
seen during hypercholesterolemia returns to low normal levels
and that proliferation of foam cells stops after reduction of the
serum cholesterol level (23). The return to normal cell proliferation and the necrosis of the accumulated foam cells resulted in
a decrease in the number of intimal cells during the early phase
of lesion regression.

Certain changes in the organelles of intimal cells with lipid
inclusions occurred during lesion regression. In general, such
alterations in cell morphology occurred rapidly in foam cells and
gradually in intimal smooth muscle cells. Lipid inclusions became
associated with and enveloped by delicate smooth membranes. This
increase in intracellular membranous material was accompanied by
a decrease in the size of lipid inclusions. The membrane formation
around lipid inclusions in macrophage-derived foam cells was

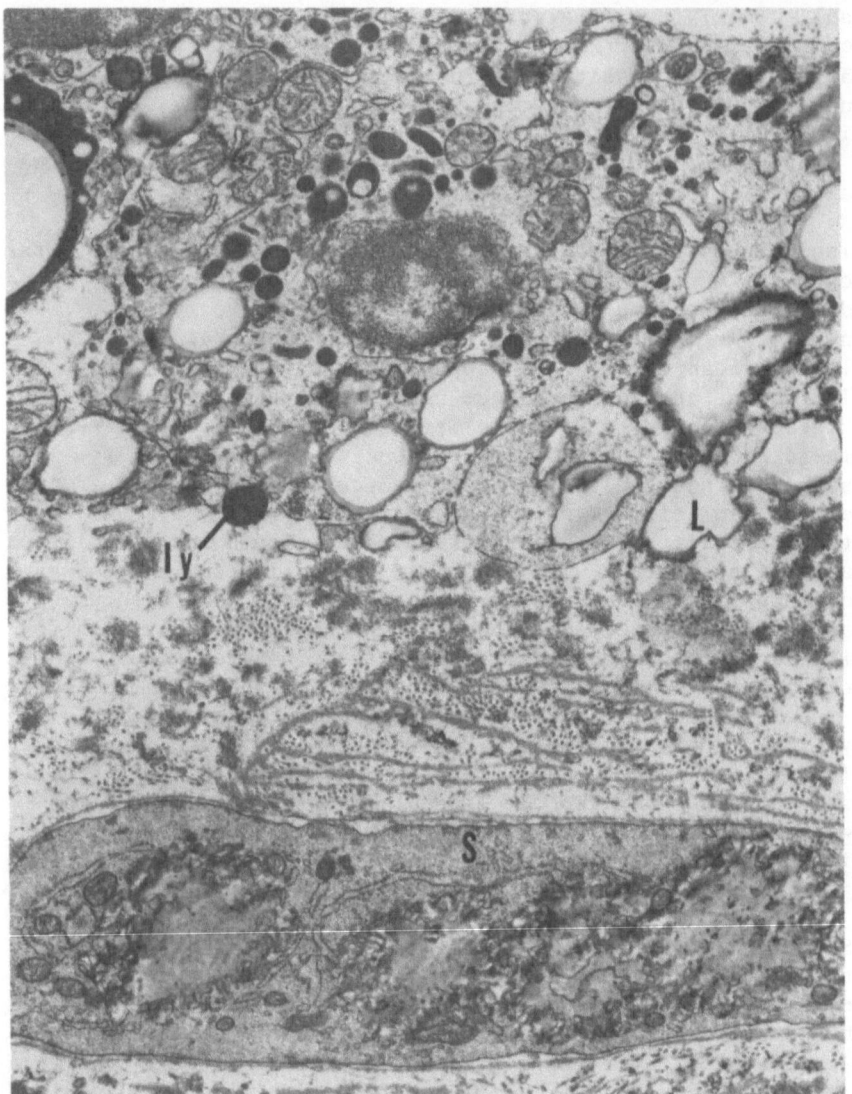

Figure 5. Upper part of an intimal cushion with an atherosclerotic lesion. From a monkey on the high-cholesterol diet for 12 weeks
and killed after an additional 8-week period on low-cholesterol
food. The mean serum cholesterol level over the 12-week period on
the high-cholesterol diet was 410 mg/dl; it had decreased to 190
mg/dl when the animal was killed. A necrotic foam cell shows
dissolution of the plasma membrane and release of lipid inclusions
(L), lysosomes (ly) and other cell components into the interstitial space of the intima. An adjacent ER-rich smooth muscle cell
(S) is intact and contains numerous lipid inclusions. (Rhesus
No. 122; X 14400) (Reduced 15% for reproduction.)

striking, and the cytoplasm frequently became entirely filled with
smooth multilamellated structures early in regression (Fig. 6).
These structures are thought to represent lysosome-lipid complexes,
that is, phagolysosomes or secondary lysosomes. Similar structures, although smaller and less frequent, occurred in the foam
cells of developing atherosclerotic lesions during hypercholesterolemia.

During hypercholesterolemia, lipid inclusions in smooth
muscle cells consisted of homogeneous droplets with scalloped
borders without a limiting membrane. In regressing lesions,
membranes progressively enclosed lipid inclusions at least
partially in most smooth muscle cells. These membranes occasionally were multilamellated, and lipid-membrane complexes resembled
the phagolysosomes of foam cells. The phagolysosomes of smooth
muscle cells, however, reached neither the size nor the number of
those in foam cells. Some smooth muscle cells did not contain
lipid inclusions with distinct membranes, although lipid inclusions decreased in size in all smooth muscle cells. At late
stages of regression and after foam cells had disappeared from the
intima, the few residual inclusions of smooth muscle cells appeared
as small clusters of lipid-membrane complexes in the perinuclear
area (Fig. 7). The progressive decrease in the size of lipid inclusions in smooth muscle cells indicates that exocytosis of
metabolized inclusions from smooth muscle cells into the interstitial space might occur.

Intracellular lipid and cell debris released into the
interstitial space of the intima from necrotic foam cells accumulated and formed pools in deep portions of the intima. While
necrosis of foam cells continued during regression, interstitial
debris and lipid decreased slowly. Pools were still present after
foam cells had disappeared from the regressing lesions. Debris
and lipid derived from necrotic cells were probably cleared from
the intima through the media and adventitial lymphatics. The
clearing process was slow, and removal of debris and lipid occurred more slowly during regression than lipid accumulation during
development of lesions.

Interstitial lipid and debris, and lipid inclusions in intimal
smooth muscle cells, persisted longest in the intimal thickening of
animals with the highest serum cholesterol levels during lesion
induction and, thus, presumably in those with the largest lesions.
Sixty-four weeks after diet change even these animals had only a
small amount of interstitial debris in the intima and only small,
infrequent inclusions in some intimal smooth muscle cells. The
normal structure of intimal cushions about the main coronary artery
bifurcation was largely restored.

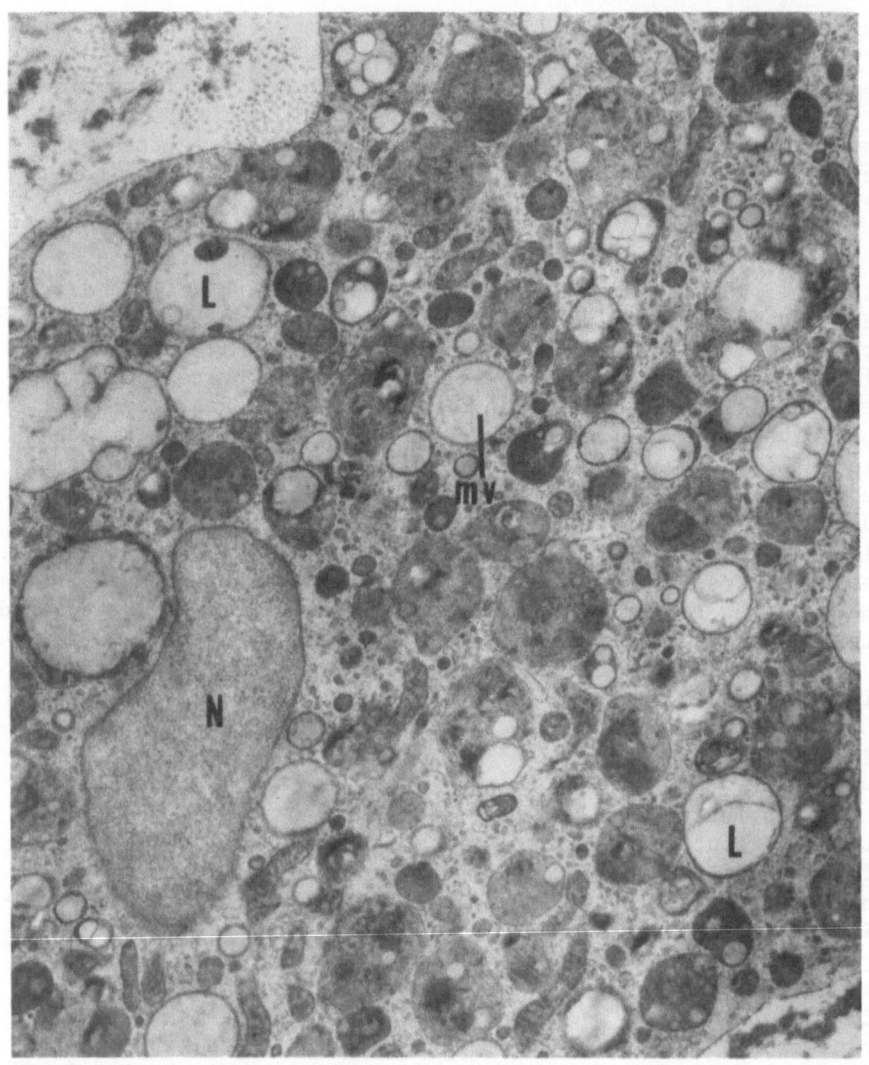

Figure 6. Detail of a foam cell from a regressing atherosclerotic
lesion in an intimal cushion. From a monkey killed after a 12-week
period on high-cholesterol and an additional 32-week period on
low-cholesterol food. The mean serum cholesterol level over the
12-week period on the high-cholesterol diet was 520 mg/dl. Normo-
cholesterolemia (145 mg/dl) returned eight weeks after diet reversal. Foam cells in regressing lesions differ from those in
developing lesions. (Compare with foam cell in figure 4.) Lipid
inclusions (L) are numerous but generally small. All are enveloped
by single or multiple membranes to form phagolysosomes. Some inclusions are multivesicular (mv), with vesicles of variable size.
Nucleus (N). (Rhesus No. 91: X 16875)(Reduced 10% for reproduction.)

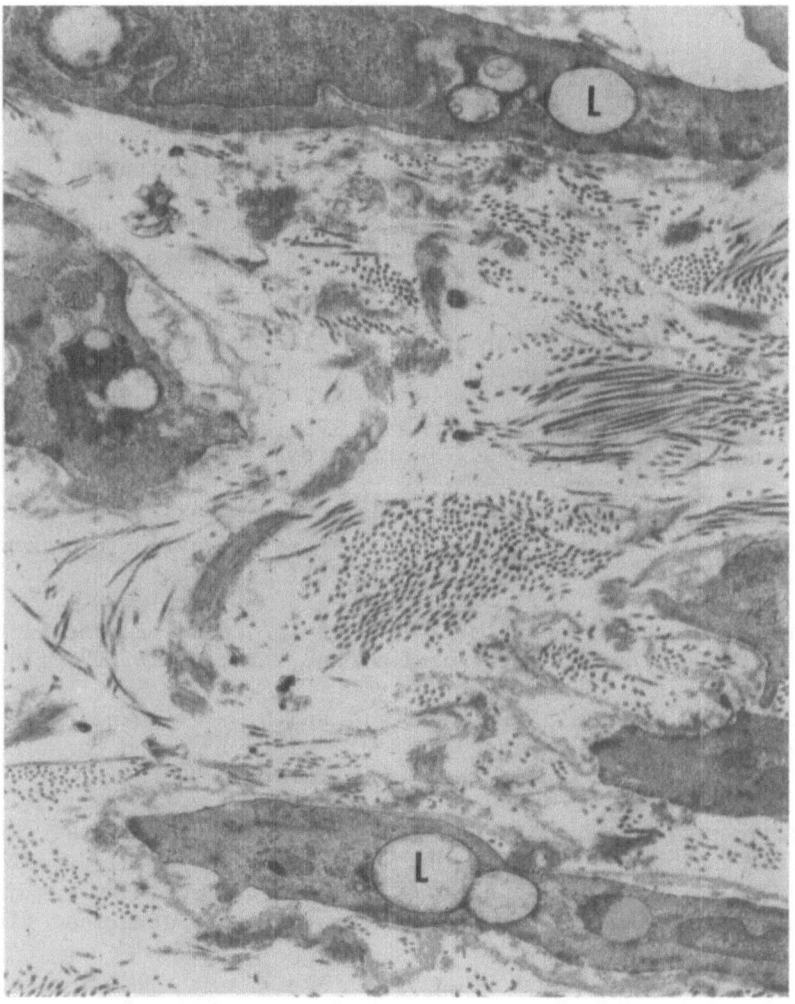

Figure 7. Upper part of a large intimal cushion at the bifurcation
with evidence of residual regression. From a monkey killed after a
12-week period on high-cholesterol and an additional 64-week period
on low-cholesterol food. Mean serum cholesterol level, 520 mg/dl
during the 12-week period on the high-cholesterol diet, returned
to normocholesterolemic levels (150 mg/dl) four weeks after diet
reversal. Neither foam cells nor extracellular debris remain, but
lipid inclusions (L) in several smooth muscle cells indicate that
a lesion had previously been present. In the late phase of regression, the lipid inclusions of smooth muscle cells differ from
those seen in developing lesions. (Compare with smooth muscle cell
in figure 3). Lipid inclusions are smaller and surrounded by smooth
membranes to form phagolysosomes. (Rhesus No. 60; X 14400)
(Reduced 15% for reproduction.)

REFERENCES

1. National Center for Health Statistics. 1969. Vital statistics
    of the United States, 1967: Volume II -- Mortality, Part A.
    US Department of Health, Education and Welfare, Public Health
    Service. US Government Printing Office, Washington, D.C.

2. Strong, J.P., L.A. Solberg, and C. Restrepo. 1968. Athero-
    sclerosis in persons with coronary heart disease. Lab. Invest.
    18: 527-537.

3. Wolkoff, K. 1929. Ueber die Atherosklerose der Coronarar-
    terien des Herzens. Beitr. Path. Anat. 82: 555-596.

4. Montenegro, M.R., and D.A. Eggen. 1968. Topography of athero-
    sclerosis in the coronary arteries. Lab. Invest. 18: 586-593.

5. Berger, R.L., and H.C. Stary. 1971. Anatomic assessment of
    operability by the saphenous vein bypass operation in coronary
    artery disease. New Engl. J. Med. 285: 248-252.

6. Schlesinger, M.J., and P.M. Zoll. 1941. Incidence and local-
    ization of coronary artery occlusions. Arch. Path. 32: 178-188.

7. Pitt, B., P.M. Zoll, H.L. Blumgart, and D.G. Freiman.
    1963. Location of coronary arterial occlusions and their re-
    lation to the arterial pattern. Circulation 28: 35-41.

8. Rodriguez, F.L., S.L. Robbins, and M. Banasiewicz. 1964. Post-
    mortem angiographic studies on the coronary arterial circula-
    tion. Incidence and topography of occlusive coronary lesions;
    relation to anatomic pattern of large coronary arteries. Amer.
    Heart J. 68: 490-499.

9. Strong, J.P., D.E. Eggen, and H.C. Stary. 1976. Reversibility
    of fatty streaks in rhesus monkeys. Primates in Medicine, vol.
    9, pp. 300-320, Karger, Basel.

10. Anitschkow, N.N. 1928. Ueber die Rueckbildungsvorgaenge bei
    der experimentellen Atherosklerose. Verh. dtsch. Path. Ges.
    23: 473-478. Zentralbl. Allg. Path. path. Anat., Suppl. to
    vol. 43.

11. Anitschkow, N.N. 1967. A history of experimentation on ar-
    terial atherosclerosis in animals. In: Cowdry's Arterio-
    sclerosis: A Survey of the Problem. Ed. by H.T. Blumenthal,
    Charles C. Thomas, Springfield, p. 32.

12. Armstrong, M.L., E.D. Warner, and W.E. Connor. 1970. Regression of coronary atheromatosis in rhesus monkeys. Circ. Res. 27:59-67.

13. Vesselinovitch, D., R.W. Wissler, K. Fisher-Dzoga, R. Hughes, and L. Dubien. 1974. Regression of atherosclerosis in rabbits Part 1. Treatment with low-fat diet, hyperoxia and hypolipidemic agents. Atherosclerosis 19: 259-275.

14. Stary, H.C., and J.P. Strong. 1976. Coronary artery fine structure in rhesus monkeys: Nonatherosclerotic intimal thickening. Primates in Medicine, vol. 9, pp. 321-358, Karger, Basel.

15. Stary, H.C. 1972. Progression and regression of experimental atherosclerosis in rhesus monkeys. In: Medical Primatology 1972, part III. Ed. by E.I. Goldsmith and J. Moor-Jankowski, Karger, Basel, pp. 356-367.

16. Stary, H.C. 1976. Coronary artery fine structure in rhesus monkeys: The early atherosclerotic lesion and its progression. Primates in Medicine, vol. 9, pp. 359-395, Karger, Basel.

17. Abell, L.L., B.B. Levy, B.B. Brodie, and F.E. Kendall. 1952. A simplified method for the estimation of total cholesterol in serum and demonstration of its specificity. J. Biol. Chem. 195: 357-366.

18. Scott, R.F., R. Jones, A.S. Daoud, O. Zumbo, F. Coulston, and W.A. Thomas. 1967. Experimental atherosclerosis in rhesus monkeys II. Cellular elements of proliferative lesions and possible role of cytoplasmic degeneration in pathogenesis as studied by electron microscopy. Exp. Molec. Path. 7: 34-57.

19. Tucker, C.F., C. Catsulis, J.P. Strong, and D.A. Eggen. 1971. Regression of early cholesterol-induced aortic lesions in rhesus monkeys. Amer. J. Path. 65: 493-514.

20. Geer, J.C. 1965. Fine structure of human aortic intimal thickening and fatty streaks. Lab. Invest. 14: 1764-1783.

21. Geer, J.C., and W.S. Webster. 1974. Morphology of mesenchymal elements of normal artery, fatty streaks, and plaques. Adv. Exp. Med. Biol., vol. 43, pp. 9-33, Plenum Press, New York.

22. Stary, H.C. 1974. Proliferation of arterial cells in athero-
     sclerosis. Adv. Exp. Med. Biol., vol. 43, pp. 59-81,
     Plenum Press, New York.

23. Stary, H.C. 1974. Cell proliferation and ultrastructural
     changes in regressing atherosclerotic lesions after reduction
     of serum cholesterol. In: Atherosclerosis III. Ed. by G.
     Schettler and A. Weizel, Springer-Verlag, Berlin, pp. 187-190.

APO-LIPOPROTEIN LOCALIZATION IN HUMAN ATHEROSCLEROTIC ARTERIES

H.F.Hoff, R.L. Jackson, and A.M. Gotto, Jr.

Departments of Neurology and Medicine
Baylor College of Medicine and The Methodist Hospital
Houston, Texas 77025

ABSTRACT

A study documenting the localization in human arteries of apoproteins from human plasma high density (HDL), low density (LDL), and very low density (VLDL) lipoproteins was undertaken in light of their possible roles in the pathogenesis and regression of the atherosclerotic process in man. Apo A-I from HDL, apo B from LDL, apo C-III from VLDL were all·localized by immunohisto-chemical techniques to generally the same areas of atherosclerotic lesions. These consisted of certain bands of collagen and elastic fibers in fatty streaks and fibrous plaques, and extracellular pools of neutral lipid in fibrous plaques. Apoproteins were also occasionally present in areas of diffuse intimal thickening in coronary arteries. Extensiveness and frequency of appearance of apo B in atherosclerotic lesions was greatest in type II hyperlipo-proteinemics, thus correlating with the plasma apo B levels. Employing an immuno-peroxidase procedure, apo B was localized ultra-structurally in atherosclerotic lesions to the outer surface of spheres ranging in diameter between 250 and 700 A. These spheres, localized predominantly in lipid cores and between collagen bands, were also seen in negatively-stained preparations of arterial extracts which also reacted positively against anti-apo B, suggest-ing that the spheres may represent native LDL and VLDL. The super-imposed localization of apo A-I, apo B, and apo C-III in athero-sclerotic lesions suggests that a specific interaction exists between certain lesion components and these apoproteins.

INTRODUCTION

Epidemiological studies in man suggest that elevations of both
plasma low (LDL) and very low (VLDL) density lipoproteins are risk
factors for atherosclerosis (1-4). In particular the cholesterol-
rich LDL has been linked to the atherosclerotic process by virtue
of its accumulation in arterial lesions (5). Elevation of plasma
LDL in experimental animals leads to enhanced atherosclerosis (6).
Results from recent reports suggest that apo B, the major apoprotein
from LDL, may be directly involved in atherogenesis (7-9) while
apo A-I, the major protein in high density lipoproteins (HDL) may
be involved in regression of the atherosclerotic lesion (10, 11).
Since HDL, LDL, and VLDL share common apoproteins that result in
immunological cross-reactivity (12), their identification in human
lesions can best be approximated by the presence of antigens primarily specific for their individual lipoprotein fraction, namely apo A-I
for HDL, apo B for LDL, and apo C-III for VLDL. We have, therefore,
undertaken a study to localize these three apoproteins in uninvolved
and atherosclerotic human arteries employing immunohistochemical
techniques.

METHODS

Antibodies raised against purified human apo A-I, apo B, and
apo C-III were conjugated to fluorescein isothiocyanate (FITC) for
light microscopic observations (13, 14) and to horseradish peroxidase
(for apo B) (15) for electron microscopic observations. The conjugated antibodies were further purified by affinity chromatography
on a column of Sepharose 4B to which the individual apoproteins or
lipoproteins had been covalently coupled (13). Cryostat sections of
normal and involved segments from the aortic, carotid, cerebral
and coronary arterial beds obtained at autopsy or surgery were incubated with the appropriate fluorescein-conjugated antibodies as described previously (13, 14). Paraformaldehyde-fixed arterial segments
were incubated with peroxidase-conjugated anti-apo B (15), treated
with the peroxidase localization medium, and embedded in epoxy for
electron microscopic observations.

RESULTS

The initial study undertaken was the localization on the light
microscopic level of apo B in arteries from normo- and hyperlipidemics
(16). The localization pattern for apo B was found to be about the
same in each lipemic group. Apo B was localized only to atherosclerotic arteries and occasionally to areas of diffuse intimal
thickening, usually in the coronary arteries. The localization
pattern consisted of localization to certain collagen bands (fig. 1c),

fragmented and reduplicated elastica (fig.1d), and extracellular
pools of neutral lipid in fibrous plaques (fig.1a,b). Although this
pattern was essentially the same in each lipemic group (with the
exception of some positive localization in intimal cells of plaques
in the type II group), extensiveness and frequency in appearance of
positive localization was greatest in the type II cases and about
equal in the type IV and normolipemic cases (14). This correlates
with the levels of apo B in the patient's plasma and may indicate
greater accumulations of apo B due to the larger original concentration gradient.

When employing an immunoperoxidase technique in conjunction
with the electron microscope, apoB was localized to the surface
of spheres ranging in diameter from 250 to 700 A$^{\circ}$ and found predominantly in lipid cores, but also between collagen bands in atherosclerotic lesions (fig. 2a,b). The reaction product for peroxidase
can be seen distinctly because of its electron density often filling
the spaces between spheres. Such spheres are also seen without the
immunoperoxidase technique, and in abundance in lesions from type II
hyperlipoproteinemics. Spheres of the same size range were also
found in negatively-stained preparations of saline extracts from
unfixed segments of atherosclerotic lesions from neighboring (fig 2d)
areas. These extracts also gave a precipitin line against anti-apoB
in double gel diffusion plates (fig. 2c). The results suggest that
apoB resides on the surface of these spheres which are presumed to
represent intact LDL and VLDL.

In preliminary studies determining the localization of apo A-I,
apo B, and apo C-III in the same artery with immunofluorescence
techniques, there was a tendency of the three apoproteins and neutral
lipid to have superimposed localizations (fig. 3). In order to semi-
quantitate the degree of superposition, each arterial segment was
graded from 0 to 4 according to the maximum number of the three
apoproteins and neutral lipid that were found together in one major
area of the artery (18). In the first study (Series I) separate
slides containing six cryostat sections each were utilized for the
localizations of the four factors (Table I). Results from the
different arterial beds were pooled in this series of experiments.
It can be seen that 46% of the fibrous plaques and 39% of the fatty
streaks demonstrated the superposition of all four factors in at least
one major area of the lesion. These values rose to 80% and 84%,
respectively, when analyzing the frequency of at least three out of
four together. By contrast 50% of the uninvolved areas, defined as
lipid free but containing areas of diffuse intimal thickening, failed
to demonstrate the presence of any of these factors (18).

Using immunofluorescence techniques fibrinogen was found in 52%
of fibrous plaques, 70% of fatty streaks, but only 26% of uninvolved
arteries, usually on the lumen surface, but also in deeper areas of

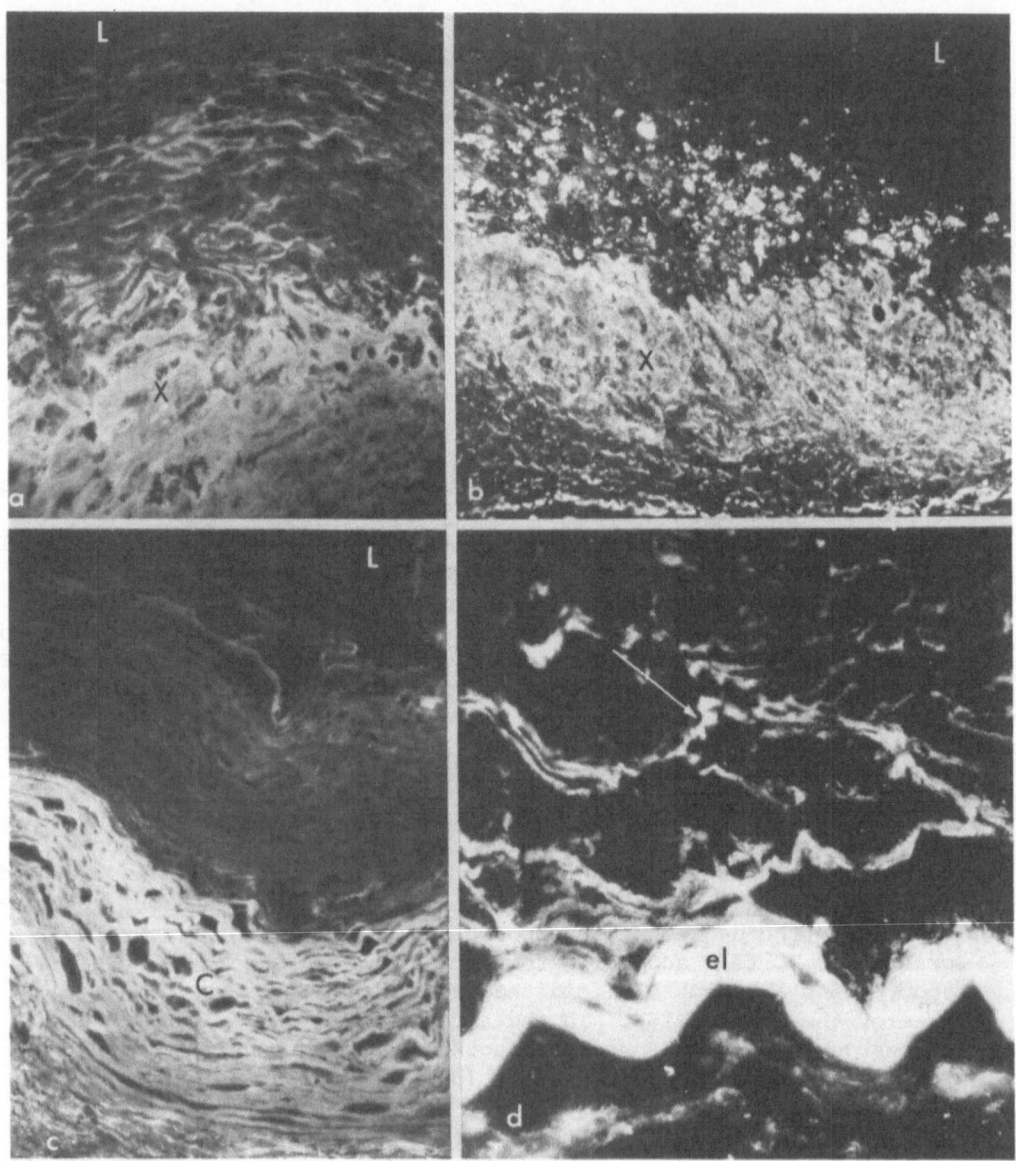

Fig. 1. Localization of apoB in cryostat sections of arterial lesions
using immunofluorescence techniques L = lumen Fig. 1a. ApoB is
seen as white areas in the lipid core (X) and along collagen fibers
of a coronary artery fibrous plaque X 100. Fig. 1b. Large apoB-posi-
tive area in a lipid core from a coronary artery fibrous plaque X 80.
Fig. 1c. Localization of apoB to collagen bands (c) in the deeper
layers of a carotid artery plaque X 100. Fig. 1d. Localization of
apoB to fragmented or reduplicated elastic fibrils (arrow) on the
intimal side of the internal elastic membrane (e 1) which auto-
fluoresces X 300. (Reduced 10% for reproduction.)

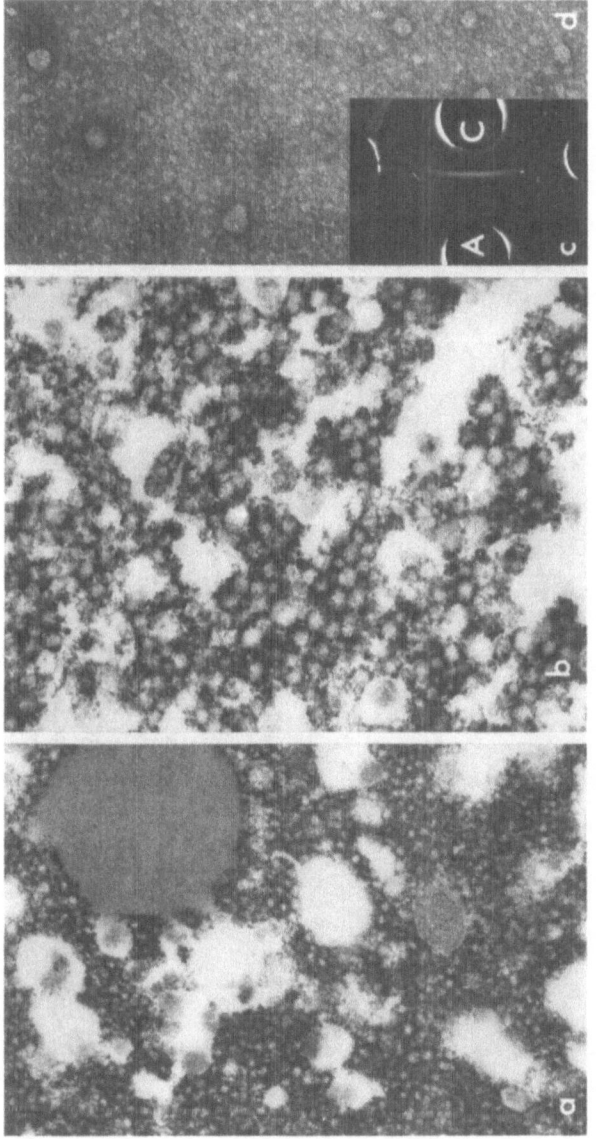

Fig. 2a. Electron micrograph of human intracranial artery with atherosclerotic involvement. ApoB depicted by electron-dense reaction product for peroxidase is localized on the outer surface of spheres in the plaque lipid core x 20,000. Fig. 2b. Same as Fig. 2a. but at higher magnification x 40,000. Fig. 2c. Double gel diffusion plate illustrating single precipitin line formed between anti-apoB (A) and a plaque saline extract (C). Fig. 3d. Negatively stained electron micrograph of a plaque saline extract illustrating particles of the same size as those seen in sections and as native LDL and VLDL. x 75,000.

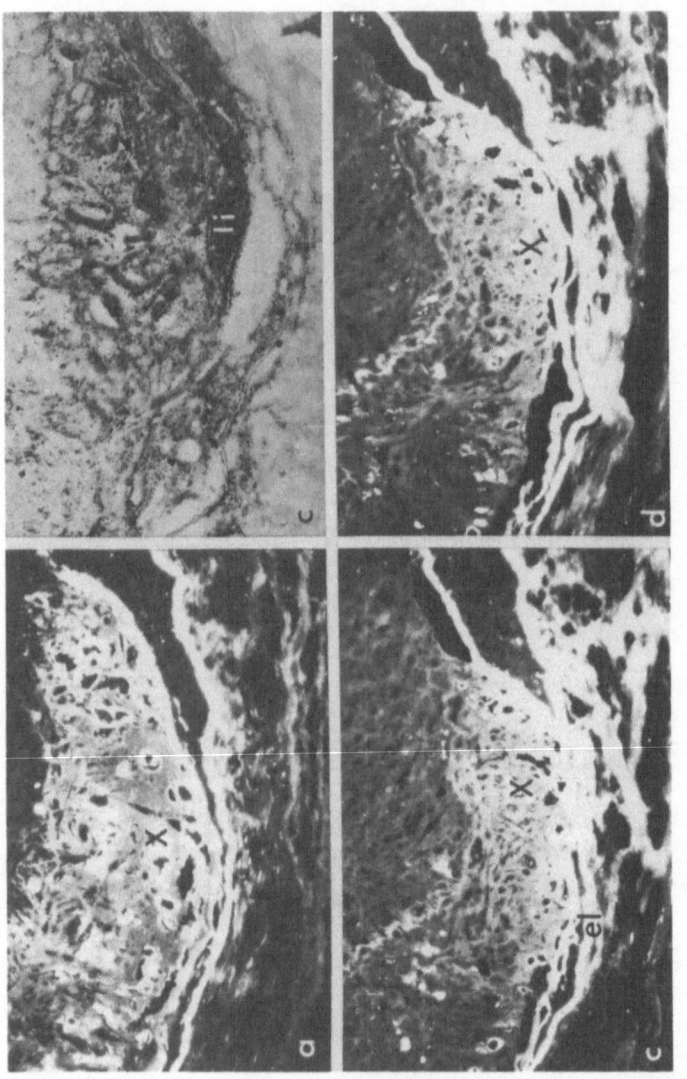

Fig. 3. Serial cryostat sections of human intracranial arterial plaque illustrating the superimposed localization in the lipid core of apoB (Fig. 3a), neutral lipid (Fig. 3b) stained with oil red 0, apo A-I (Fig. 3c), and apo C-III (Fig. 3d). X = apoprotein localization (light areas using immunofluorescence techniques), li = neutral lipid (dark areas).

TABLE I

Frequency of Maximum Superposition of Localizations of Lipid
and Apoproteins in Human Atherosclerotic Lesions

Category	Total no. blocks	Classification+					F	F'	A	A'
		0	1	2	3	4				
Series 1										
Fibrous plaques	101	0 0%	5 5%	16 16%	34 34%	46 46%	52%	37%	10%	4%
Fatty streaks	31	0 0%	4 13%	1 3%	14 45%	12 39%	70%	64%	10%	5%
Uninvolved	30	15 50%	9 30%	2 7%	4 13%	0 0%	26%	0%	0%	0%
Series 2										
Fibrous plaques	83	0 0%	2 2%	4 5%	10 12%	67 81%				
Fatty streaks	25	0 0%	4 16%	1 4%	5 20%	15 60%				
Uninvolved	10	9 90%	1 10%	0 0%	0 0%	0 0%				
*Carotid plaques	65	0 0%	4 6%	4 6%	23 35%	34 53%				

+ = Classification. Each block was classified from 0 to 4 according to the maximum number of apoproteins (apoA-I, apoB, and apoC-III) and neutral lipid localized in any one area of tissue.

F = Percentage of blocks with demonstrable fibrinogen

F'= Percentage of blocks showing fibrinogen in area of maximum superposition of localizations of lipid and apoproteins.

A = Percentage of blocks with demonstrable albumin

A'= Percentage of blocks showing albumin in area of maximum superposition of localizations of lipid and apoproteins.

* = Blocks of carotid plaques were taken from both Series 1 and 2

TABLE II

Frequency of Apolipoprotein
Localization in Human Arteries

		Total number blocks	apoA	apoB	apoC	apoB +apoC	apoC +apoA	apoB +apoA	apoA +apoB +apoC
EXTRA- AND INTRACRANIAL ARTERIES	plaque	62	37 60%	54 87%	49 79%	40 65%	37 60%	38 61%	30 48%
	fatty streak	24	16 67%	14 58%	15 63%	11 46%	15 63%	16 67%	11 46%
	uninvolved	25	3 12%	1 4%	0 0%	0 0%	0 0%	0 0%	0 0%
CORONARY ARTERIES	plaque	52	45 87%	46 88%	46 88%	41 79%	44 85%	43 83%	39 75%
	fatty streak	12	8 67%	7 58%	10 83%	9 75%	10 83%	9 75%	9 75%
	uninvolved	10	4 40%	7 70%	4 40%	4 40%	4 40%	4 40%	4 40%
AORTA	plaque	24	19 79%	21 88%	20 83%	15 63%	18 75%	14 58%	13 54%
	fatty streak	16	13 81%	11 69%	11 69%	5 31%	8 50%	8 50%	5 30%
	uninvolved	4	2 50%	2 50%	2 50%	0 0%	2 50%	1 25%	0 0%

advanced lesions (Table I). Fibrinogen was also localized together with the three apoproteins and neutral lipid in areas of maximum superposition of localizations in 37% of the fibrous plaques, 64% of the fatty streaks, but none of the normal arteries. Albumin, another plasma protein, was localized in only 10% of both fatty streaks and fibrous plaques and in not more than 5% of the areas of lesions showing a maximum superposition of localizations.

In another study, the degree of superposition of localization of apoproteins and neutral lipid in carotid artery bifurcations obtained from endarterectomies was determined (Table I). In this study 53% of the advanced lesions showed the presence of all four factors together, and 88% at least three out of the four factors together.

During the course of this study it was observed that due to the focal nature of the changes in arterial structure resulting from the atherosclerotic process, the topography of sections used for the different incubations varied resulting in an appreciable error in maximum superposition of factors (18). In a second series of experiments (Series 2) apo A-I and apo C-III were localized in three sections each on one slide, and apo B on a second slide, which was subsequently also stained with oil red 0 to stain neutral lipid. We had hoped to minimize this error by utilizing as close to serial sections as was technically possible. By this procedure 81% of fibrous plaques and 60% of fatty streaks showed the presence of all four factors together. By contrast 90% of the uninvolved arteries failed to demonstrate the presence of any of the three apoproteins or neutral lipid.

The frequencies of individual and superimposed localizations of the three apoproteins in arteries from different vascular beds as obtained from the pooled results of both series of experiments have also been tabulated (Table II). The individual apoproteins were found in 60 to 88% of the fibrous plaques, and 58 to 81% of the fatty streaks. Seven out of ten uninvolved coronary arteries and two out of four uninvolved aortas demonstrated the presence of apo B, but always in areas of diffuse intimal thickening. The frequency of superimposed localization of apoproteins in lesions ranged between 30 and 85%. The highest frequencies of superposition of all three apoproteins was found in the group of extra- and intracranial arteries, the lowest in the aorta. However, this may merely reflect the smaller number of specimens studied in the latter (44 blocks) relative to the former (111 blocks).

DISCUSSION

These results suggest that there exist some tissue components indigenous to the atherosclerotic lesion which have a specific

affinity for the three apoproteins. These components are comprised
of essentially connective tissue and extracellular pools of neutral
lipid. Association of apo B (19, 20) and apo C-III (21) to such
areas has been documented previously and may represent an interaction
of LDL and VLDL (or breakdown products thereof) with these components.
These results may also explain the correlation in man of elevated
plasma LDL and VLDL and the atherosclerotic process, assuming that
the accumulation of these lipoproteins or their apoproteins is
atherogenic (7-9, 22). The specificity of this interaction is
suggested by the fact that two other plasma proteins, fibrinogen
and albumin have, in part, different localizations or are present in
nominal amounts. Moreover, uninvolved arteries devoid of the plaque
components rarely accumulate any apoproteins. It is also possible
that the lipid moiety of lipoproteins interact with plaque components
rather than apoproteins. The superimposed localizations of neutral
lipid and apoproteins in this study may suggest the presence of native
lipoproteins in lesions.

   The presence of apo A-I in generally the same areas as apo B
and apo C-III could represent a trapping of HDL as well as LDL and
VLDL as they perfuse from the lumen through the artery to the lymphatics. It could also represent a mechanism for cholesterol removal
from involved arteries in which free apo A-I together with phospholipid might bind and remove free cholesterol as was demonstrated in
tissue culture cells (10, 11).

   Although these studies have demonstrated the existence and
localization of plasma lipoproteins or their apoproteins in human
atherosclerotic lesions, quantitation of this accumulation still
needs to be done. Moreover, it is still unclear whether this
accumulation is the cause or the result of the initial structural
changes in the atherosclerotic process. Morphologic and quantitative
procedures are presently in progress on experimental animal model
systems of atherogenesis to elucidate this question.

ACKNOWLEDGEMENTS

   We are indebted to members of the Departments of Pathology and
Surgery at The Methodist Hospital and Ben Taub General Hospital in
assisting in the procurement of arterial specimens; to Dr. H.K.
Thompson of the Department of Medicine for performing the statistical
evaluations; and to Dr. J.S. Meyer, Chairman, Department of Neurology,
and Dr. J.L. Titus, Chairman, Department of Pathology for their
continual support. This investigation was supported in part by H.E.W.
grants HL-14194 and HL-05434/34 and USPH 09287. R.L.J. is an Established Investigator of the American Heart Association.

REFERENCES

1. Dawber, T.R., F.E. More, and J.V. Mann. 1957. Coronary heart disease in the Framingham Study. Am. J. Public Health 47 (Suppl. 4):4-24.

2. Kannel, W.B., T.R. Dawber, and G.D. Friedman. 1964. Risk factors in coronary heart disease: An evaluation of several serum lipids as predictors of coronary heart disease. The Framingham Study. Am. Intern. Med. 61:888-899.

3. Kannel, W.B., T. Gordon, and T.R. Dawber. 1974. Role of lipids in the development of brain infarction. The Framingham Study. Stroke 5:679-685.

4. Goldstein, J.L., W.R. Hazzard, H.G. Schrodt, E.L. Bierman, and A.F. Motulsky. 1973. Hyperlipidemia in coronary heart disease: I. Lipid levels in 500 survivors of myocardial infarction. J. Clin. Invest. 52:1533-1577.

5. Smith, E.B. 1974. Relationship between plasma and tissue lipids in human atherosclerosis. Adv. Lipid Res. 12:1-49.

6. Adams, C.W.M. 1971. Lipids, lipoproteins and atherosclerotic lesions. Proc. Roy. Soc. Med. 64:902-905.

7. Goldstein, J.L., and M.D. Brown. 1975. Lipoprotein receptors, cholesterol metabolism, and atherosclerosis. Arch. Pathol. 99: 181-184.

8. Fischer-Dzoga, K., R.M. Jones, D. Vesselinovitch, and R.W. Wissler. 1974. Increased mitotic activity in primary cultures of aortic medial smooth muscle cells after exposure to hyperlipemic serum. In: Atherosclerosis, III, Proc. Third Inter. Symposium on Atherosclerosis Ed. by G. Schettler and A. Weizel, Springer-Verlag, New York, pp. 193-195.

9. Ross, R. and J.A. Glomset. 1973. Atherosclerosis and the arterial smooth muscle cell. Science 180:1332-1339.

10. Stein, Y., M.C. Glangeaud, M. Fainaru, and O. Stein. 1975. The removal of cholesterol from aortic smooth muscle cells in culture and Landschutz ascites cells by fractions of human high density apolipoproteins. Biochim. Biophys. Acta. 380:106-118.

11. Jackson, R.L., O. Stein, A.M. Gotto, and Y. Stein. 1975. A comparative study on the removal of cellular lipids from Landschutz ascites cells by human plasma apolipoproteins. J. Biol. Chem. 250:7204-7209.

12. Pearlstein, E., P. Eggena, and F. Aladjem. 1971. Human serum high density lipoproteins and chylomicrons. Immunochemistry 8:865-87.

13. Hoff, H.F., R.L. Jackson, J.T. Mao, and A.M. Gotto. 1974. Localization of low density lipoproteins in arterial lesions from normolipemics employing a purified fluorescent-labeled antibody. Biochim. Biophys. Acta. 351:407-415.

14. Hoff, H.F., J.T. Lie, J.L. Titus, R.L. Jackson, R. Bayardo, M.E. DeBakey, and A.M. Gotto. 1975. Localization of apo-low density lipoproteins (apo LDL) in atherosclerotic lesions of human normo- and hyperlipemics. Arch. Pathol. 99:253-258.

15. Modesto, R.R., and A.J. Pesce. 1973. Use of tolylene diisocy-anate for the preparation of a peroxidase-labelled antibody con-jugate: Quantitation of the amount of diisocyanate bound. Bio-chim. Biophys. Acta. 295:283-295.

16. Frederickson, D.S., and R.I. Levy. 1972. Familial hyperlipo-proteinemia. In: Metabolic Basis of Inherited Diseases. Ed. by J.B. Standburg, J.B. Wyngaarden, and D.S. Frederickson, Mc-Graw-Hill Book Company, New York, p. 545.

17. Hoff, H.F., and J.W. Gaubatz. 1976. Ultrastructural localization of plasma lipoproteins in human intracranial arteries. Virchows Archiv (in press).

18. Hoff, H.F., C.L. Heideman, R.L. Jackson, R.J. Bayardo, H.S. Kim, and A.M. Gotto. 1975. Localization patterns of plasma apolipo-proteins in human atherosclerotic lesions. Circ. Res. 37:72-79.

19. Kao, V.C., and R.W. Wissler. 1965. A study of the immunohisto-chemical localization of serum lipoproteins and other plasma proteins in human atherosclerotic lesions. Exp. Mol. Path. 4:465-479.

20. Walton, K.W., and N. Williamson. 1968. Histological and immuno-fluorescent studies on the human atheromatous plaque. J. Athero-scler. Res. 8:599-624.

21. Walton, K.W. 1974. Identification of lipoproteins involved in human atherosclerosis. In: Atherosclerosis III, Proc. Third Inter. Symposium on Atherosclerosis. Ed. by G. Schettler and A. Weizel, Springer-Verlag, Berlin, Heidelberg, New York, pp. 93-95.

22. Zilversmit, D. 1973. A proposal linking atherogenesis to the interaction of endothelial lipoprotein lipase with triglyceride-rich lipoproteins. Circ. Res. 33:633-638.

SECTION 2

RABBIT MODELS

RABBITS AS A MODEL FOR THE STUDY OF HYPERLIPOPROTEINEMIA AND ATHEROSCLEROSIS

B. Shore and V. Shore

Biomedical Division, Lawrence Livermore Laboratory

University of California, Livermore, California 94550

ABSTRACT

Lipoproteins of normal and cholesteremic plasma were compared in New Zealand White (hyperresponder) and Dutch Belt (hyporesponder) rabbits. Three major differences were observed between the strains: (1) New Zealand White rabbits developed much higher plasma levels of very low, intermediate, and low density lipoproteins after cholesterol feeding; (2) Dutch Belt rabbits, normal and cholesteremic, had higher ratios of the more dense high density lipoproteins HDL_3 (d 1.125-1.20 g/ml) to the less dense HDL_2 (d 1.081-1.125 g/ml); (3) cholesteremic Dutch Belt rabbits had higher plasma levels of the more dense HDL_3 subfraction than did cholesteremic New Zealand White rabbits.

Cholesteremic very low density lipoproteins of both strains are large particles of beta electrophoretic mobility that are rich in cholesteryl esters and an arginine-rich apolipoprotein(s). The intermediate and low density lipoprotein fractions were similarly altered in composition, although the proportion of arginine-rich protein to total protein was less than in the very low density fraction. Although the high density lipoproteins were greatly decreased in concentration in cholesteremic plasma, no major changes in their apolipoproteins were seen in either strain of rabbits. The major high density apolipoprotein of rabbits occurs in two electrophoretically separable forms and is similar to human apo A-I. Six minor apolipoproteins were isolated from the high density lipoproteins; some of these occur also in other density fractions.

Erythrocyte membranes of both strains of rabbits before and after cholesteremia were quantitatively similar in their Na^+-K^+-ATPase, Mg^{++}-ATPase, and Ca^{++}-ATPase activities.

INTRODUCTION

Cholesteremia, hyperlipoproteinemia, and atherosclerosis can be induced experimentally in a variety of animals by feeding diets rich in cholesterol or cholesterol plus fat (1,2). There is considerable variation among animal species in the degree of cholesteremic and atherogenic responses (1,2) and in the plasma lipoproteins that are elevated in association with the cholesteremia (3-7). Within a given species, considerable variation in the susceptibility to induction of cholesteremia and atherosclerosis is related to genetic differences (1,8). Genetically determined differences are a major determinant of hyperresponders and hyporesponders within a species, including man.

The rabbit has been used quite extensively for many years in studies of atherosclerosis and is a useful animal for investigating lipoprotein metabolism and the molecular and biochemical bases determining the "hyper" or "hypo" response to the induction of cholesteremia and atherogenesis. The normal rabbit has plasma lipoprotein classes, although at lower concentrations, comparable to those of man (9). The present investigation and earlier work (5) indicate that the rabbit apolipoproteins are also comparable to those of man. Since apolipoproteins are major determinants of the metabolism of lipoproteins and lipids and of lipoprotein structure and properties, it can be expected that many biological processes for synthesis and catabolism of the lipoproteins and for lipoprotein-lipoprotein and lipoprotein-cell interactions will be essentially similar in the rabbit and man. Furthermore, rabbits respond rapidly to changes in dietary cholesterol, provide adequate blood and tissue samples for molecular and biochemical studies, and are relatively inexpensive and easy to maintain. Finally, strains of hyperresponders and hyporesponders among rabbits have been identified (10).

New Zealand White rabbits are hyperresponders with respect to cholesteremia and atherosclerosis and develop atheroma after a few weeks of cholesterol-enriched diet (3,10). Within a few days on the diet there is a marked elevation in plasma cholesterol, particularly in cholesteryl esters, that is associated with beta-migrating lipoproteins in the very low and low density fractions (3,5). These lipoproteins contain little triglycerides (3,5) and relatively little of certain of the apolipoproteins found in the fractions of corresponding density in the normal New Zealand White rabbit (5). The cholesteremic lipoproteins are specifically

enriched in an arginine-rich apolipoprotein and contain counterparts to the human apoVLDLserine (C-I) and to the B proteins (5).
Accumulation of these lipoproteins in the plasma increases over a
period of several weeks so that after four to six weeks a plasma
total cholesterol level of 3000 mg per 100 ml is common in rabbits
of this strain. The plasma high density lipoproteins decrease in
concentration on cholesterol feeding (5). On the other hand, the
cholesterol levels are elevated in Dutch Belt rabbits, which are
hyporesponders, to a much less extent than in hyperresponder
rabbits (10).

In this investigation, we compared Dutch Belt and New Zealand
White rabbits with respect to changes following cholesterol feeding
in plasma concentrations of lipoproteins in the various density
classes and in the apolipoprotein and lipid compositions of the
isolated lipoproteins. Previous work (5) on the isolation and
characterization of the rabbit apolipoproteins was extended to the
high density lipoproteins of normal and cholesteremic rabbits. In
addition, we compared erythrocyte membranes before and after cholesteremia with respect to Na^+-K^+-ATPase, Mg^{++}-ATPase, and Ca^{++}-
ATPase activities.

MATERIALS AND METHODS

Material Isolation

Animals, Plasma, and Erythrocyte Membranes. Twelve female New
Zealand White and eight female Dutch Belt rabbits were matched
according to age (10 weeks in age in most cases at the start of
the experiment) and placed on a diet consisting of Purina[1] rabbit
pellets plus 1% cholesterol. Control animals of the same age received no cholesterol supplement. A solution of cholesterol in
peroxide-free ether was slowly added to the pellets and the solvent
was allowed to evaporate. The animals were bled at 10 days and
again at 32 days. About 15 ml of blood per animal (unfasted) was
taken from the ear vein at each interval. Each of the plasma and
lipoprotein samples was analyzed individually except as noted, e.g.,
for isolation of proteins by ion exchange chromatography. Hemoglo-
bin-free erythrocyte membranes were prepared from the freshly drawn
heparinized blood by lysis in tris-HCl buffer (11).

---

[1]Reference to a company or product name does not imply approval or
recommendation of the product by the U.S. ERDA or the University
of California to the exclusion of others that may be suitable.

Plasma Lipoproteins. Isolation of the lipoproteins was begun on the same day as the bleeding. The very low density lipoproteins (VLDL, d less than 1.006 g/ml), intermediate density lipoproteins (IDL, d=1.006-1.019 g/ml), low density lipoproteins (LDL, d=1.019-1.065 g/ml), high density lipoprotein$_2$ (HDL$_2$, d=1.081-1.125 g/ml), and the high density lipoprotein$_3$ (HDL$_3$, d=1.125-1.200 g/ml) fractions were isolated sequentially by centrifugation in solutions adjusted with NaCl and NaNO$_3$ plus D$_2$O to the appropriate densities (12,13). Prior to the initial centrifugation, the cholesteremic plasma was diluted 8-10 fold with a NaCl solution of density 1.006 g/ml. EDTA at 0.0008 M and 0.01 M tris-HCl buffer at pH 7.5 were present throughout. Protein concentration of lipoprotein and apolipoprotein solutions was determined colorimetrically (14) and/or from amino acid analysis. In the colorimetric analysis of turbid lipoproteins, the samples were extracted one or two times with diethyl ether. The concentrations of the various lipoprotein fractions in plasma were estimated from the quantity of lipoprotein (total lipid plus apolipoproteins) isolated from a known volume of plasma, or in some cases from analysis of the schlieren pattern of the lipoprotein in the analytical ultracentrifuge (15).

Analytical Methods

Lipid Analysis. The total plasma cholesterol levels were determined by the method of Mann (16). Total lipids of the isolated lipoproteins were determined gravimetrically. Lipid composition of lipoproteins was determined by one-dimensional thin layer chromatography (17), cholesterol (16), and phosphorus (18) analyses.

Delipidation of Lipoproteins. The lipids were extracted from the lipoproteins with combinations of ethyl ether and ethanol as described previously (5,12). Precautions were taken to recover small amounts of protein carried over in the lipid extract. The delipidated, dialyzed protein was water soluble; amino acid analyses indicated that it was the same in composition and quantity as the protein moiety of the undialyzed ether-extracted material.

Disc Electrophoresis. The delipidated protein moieties so obtained were subjected to electrophoresis in 10% polyacrylamide gels at pH 8.3 in the presence of 8M urea (19) or sodium dodecyl sulfate (20). The urea gels were fixed in cold 12.5% trichloroacetic acid and stained at room temperature with 0.05% Coomassie Blue in trichloroacetic acid solution. The detergent gels were fixed and stained with 25% isopropanol-10% acetic acid containing 0.05% Coomassie Blue.

Fractionation of Apolipoproteins. The entire protein moiety (i.e., no losses as insoluble protein, etc.) of the high density lipoproteins was taken for ion exchange chromatography. The procedure was that used for fractionation of human high density lipoproteins (13).

Amino Acid Analysis. Amino acid analysis was by the 4 hour methodology described in Beckman Instruments' (Palo Alto, Calif.) technical bulletin A-TB-033. Measured aliquots of the protein solutions were lyophilized. The protein was then hydrolyzed at 110°C for 30 hours essentially by the method of Liu and Chang (21) except that the 3N p-toluenesulfonic acid was replaced by 4N methanesulfonic acid. This method permitted estimation of tryptophan content.

Enzyme Assays. Assays of the Na^+-K^+-activated, ouabain-sensitive ATPase and Mg^{++}-activated, ouabain-insensitive ATPase activities were carried out as described by Gibbs et al.(22). Ca^{++}-ATPase was assayed as described by Coleman and Bromley (23). Reaction times were 20 and 40 minutes with controls at zero time and, in the absence of either membranes or ATP, at 20 and 40 minutes; the hydrolysis of ATP was essentially linear with time.

RESULTS

Plasma Lipoproteins of Hyperresponder and Hyporesponder Strains of Rabbits

Dutch Belt (hyporesponder) and New Zealand White (hyperresponder) rabbits developed qualitatively similar hyperlipoproteinemias on feeding commercial rabbit food supplemented with 1% cholesterol. In both strains, there were marked elevations in the very low density and intermediate density lipoproteins and, to a lesser extent, in the low density lipoproteins (Table I). Unlike certain other species after cholesterol feeding, such as swine or the dog (6,7), neither strain of cholesteremic rabbits developed a marked elevation in plasma lipoprotein species resembling high density lipoproteins and containing the arginine-rich apolipoprotein and the major high density apolipoprotein apo A-I.

The major differences in the hyperlipoproteinemias of hyporesponder and hyperresponder strains of rabbits were found at both 10 day and one month periods of investigation. The differences were quantitative rather than qualitative ones in lipoprotein composition and were observed in all density classes, including the high density lipoproteins (Table I). The total plasma cholesterol values were consistently less in Dutch Belt rabbits than in New Zealand White rabbits, and this was manifest in significantly lower levels of the cholesteremic very low, intermediate, and low density lipoproteins, particularly the latter, in Dutch Belt rabbits.

TABLE I

Rabbit Plasma Lipoproteins and Total Cholesterol

Rabbits	Cholesterol	Plasma Concentrations, mg/100 ml			
		VLDL	IDL	LDL	HDL
New Zealand White:					
Normal	80 (70–100)*	25 ± 5	100 ± 7	115 ± 8	130 ± 9
Cholesteremic, 10 day	1640 (1260–2200)	1880 ± 335	820 ± 175	380 ± 60	75 ± 11
Dutch Belt:					
Normal	75 (65–90)	25 ± 5	85 ± 8	105 ± 9	140 ± 8
Cholesteremic, 10 day	880 (675–1200)	1110 ± 140	270 ± 58	170 ± 36	95 ± 9

*Range among individual animals.

Other differences between the Dutch Belt and New Zealand rabbits, both normal and cholesteremic, were seen in the quantitative distribution of plasma high density lipoproteins. In the Dutch Belt rabbits (hyporesponders), the ratio of the more dense HDL_3 subfraction to the less dense HDL_2 subfraction in plasma was on the average considerably higher than in New Zealand White rabbits. Based on protein concentrations and the total volume of the fractions, the average ratios of apoHDL$_3$ to apoHDL$_2$ in Dutch Belt rabbit plasma were 1.6 (range 1.2-2.4) and 1.6 (range 1.1-2.3) for normal and cholesteremic animals, respectively. For New Zealand White rabbits, on the other hand, the corresponding ratios were 0.9 (range 0.4-1.6) and 1.0 (0.6-1.6), respectively.

Agarose electrophoretic patterns, not presented, of normal and cholesteremic sera indicated in general a greater decrease in concentration in alpha-migrating (high density) lipoproteins in New Zealand White rabbits than in Dutch Belt rabbits. This was supported by data on the amount of high density lipoproteins isolated centrifugally from the plasma, with the exception of 2 of the 12 New Zealand animals. The agarose electrophoresis patterns of sera

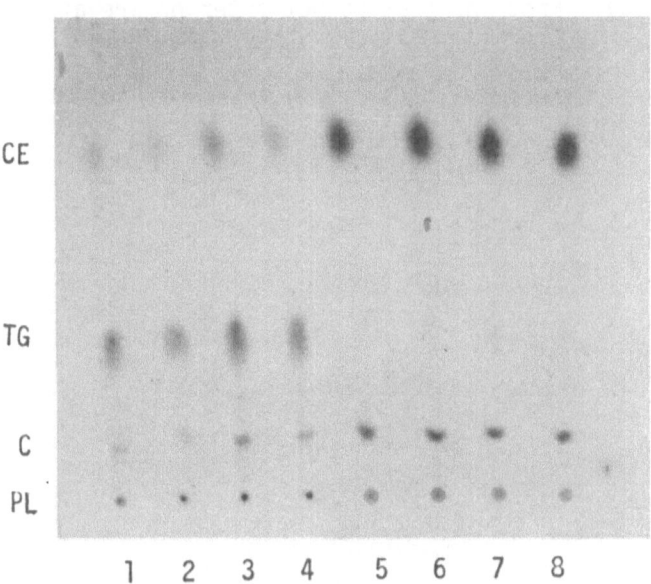

Figure 1. Thin-layer chromatography on silica gel of the lipids of very low density lipoproteins isolated from normal (1,2) and cholesteremic (7,8) Dutch Belt rabbits and from normal (3,4) and cholesteremic (5,6) New Zealand White rabbits. Solvent was petroleum ether-diethyl ether-acetic acid, 85:15:2. CE=cholesteryl esters, TG=triglycerides; C=cholesterol; PL=phospholipids.

and isolated lipoproteins of both strains resembled those published
earlier (5) for New Zealand White rabbits in that the lipoprotein
elevation was in beta-migrating species, including beta-migrating
very low density lipoproteins. These beta-migrating very low density lipoproteins were cholesteryl ester rich and triglyceride poor
lipoproteins in both strains of rabbits (Figure 1).

Apolipoproteins of Hyperresponder and Hyporesponder Strains of Rabbits

There were no major or consistant differences in the apolipoproteins of the very low density and high density lipoproteins isolated from the plasma of both strains of rabbits; the low density
lipoprotein apolipoproteins have not yet been studied. The cholesteremic very low density lipoproteins of both strains were very
similar and differed from the normal, as shown in urea (Figure 2)
and sodium dodecyl sulfate (Figure 3) polyacrylamide gel electrophoretic patterns in which equal amounts (70 micrograms) of apolipoprotein samples were compared. The major components seen in the
cholesteremic patterns correspond to the arginine-rich apolipoprotein isolated previously from cholesteremic rabbit very low density
lipoproteins (5). Proteins that do not enter or are at the top of

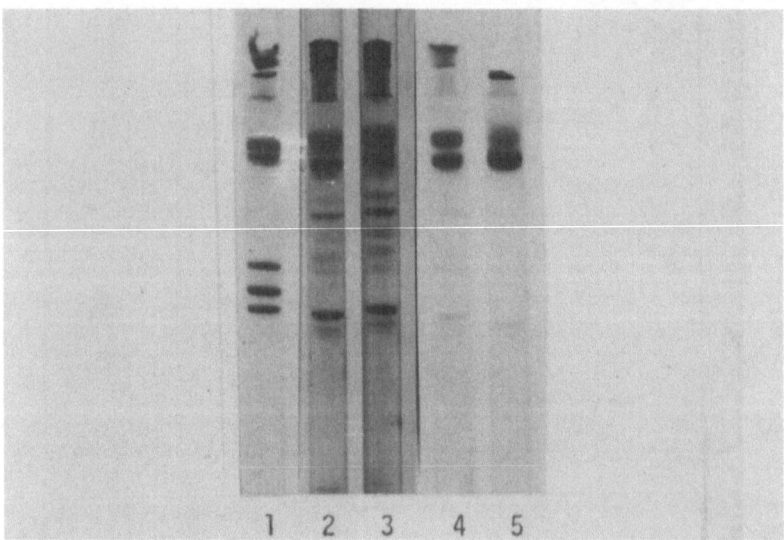

Figure 2. Electrophoretic patterns of very low density apolipoproteins (70 micrograms/ml) at pH 8.3 in 8% polyacrylamide gels containing 8M urea. 1, normal human; 2, normal New Zealand White
rabbit; 3, normal Dutch Belt rabbit; 4, cholesteremic Dutch Belt
rabbit; 5, cholesteremic New Zealand White rabbit.

the separating gels (presumably B or low density apolipoproteins) and an apolipoprotein that appears to correspond to human apoVLDL-serine (C-I) (5) and to the fast-migrating protein in the presence of sodium dodecyl sulfate (Figure 3) are also present. Similarly, electrophoretic patterns show that the proportion of arginine-rich apolipoprotein in cholesteremic intermediate density and low density lipoproteins is greater than normal, although the relative amount of this apolipoprotein to total protein (or to B protein) decreases as the density of the fraction increases and is much less in low density lipoproteins than in the very low density fraction.

In contrast, there are at most very minor changes from the normal pattern in the high density apolipoproteins on induction of cholesteremia, even though their concentration in plasma decreases. Two major protein bands, whose proteins have been isolated chromato-graphically, are seen in the electrophoretic patterns of apoHDL$_3$ and apoHDL$_2$ in polyacrylamide gels containing urea (Figure 4).

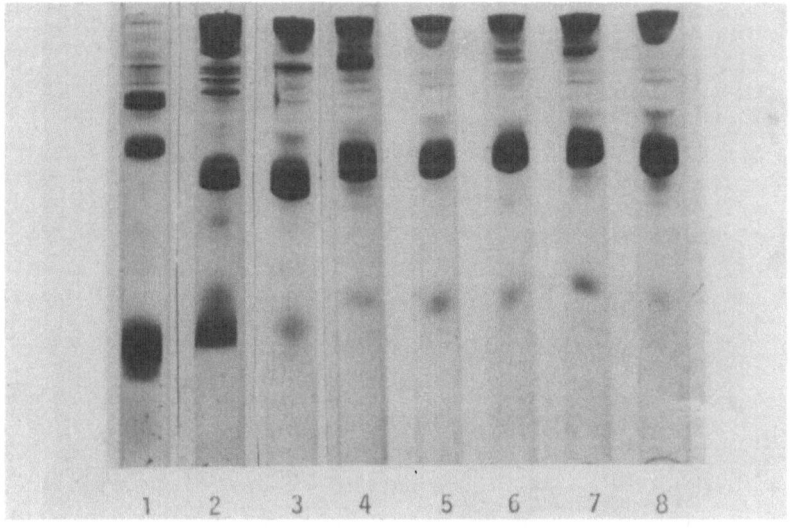

Figure 3. Polyacrylamide gel electrophoretic patterns of rabbit very low density apolipoproteins in the presence of sodium dodecyl sulfate. 1, bovine serum albumin + ovalbumin + cytochrome c; 2, normal very low density lipoproteins; 3-5, cholesteremic Dutch Belt very low density lipoproteins; 6-8, cholesteremic New Zealand White very low density lipoproteins.

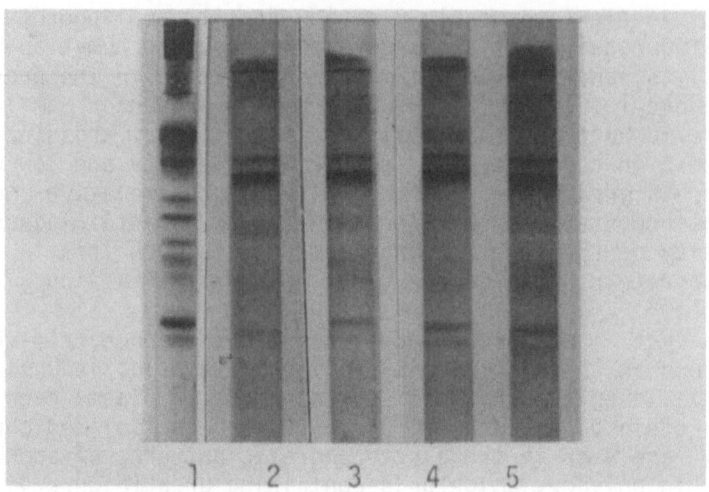

Figure 4. Electrophoretic patterns of rabbit apolipoproteins at pH 8.3 in polyacrylamide gels containing 8M urea. 1, normal very low density lipoproteins; 2,4, normal high density lipoprotein subfractions HDL_3 and HDL_2, respectively; 3,5, cholesteremic high density lipoprotein subfractions HDL_3 and HDL_2, respectively.

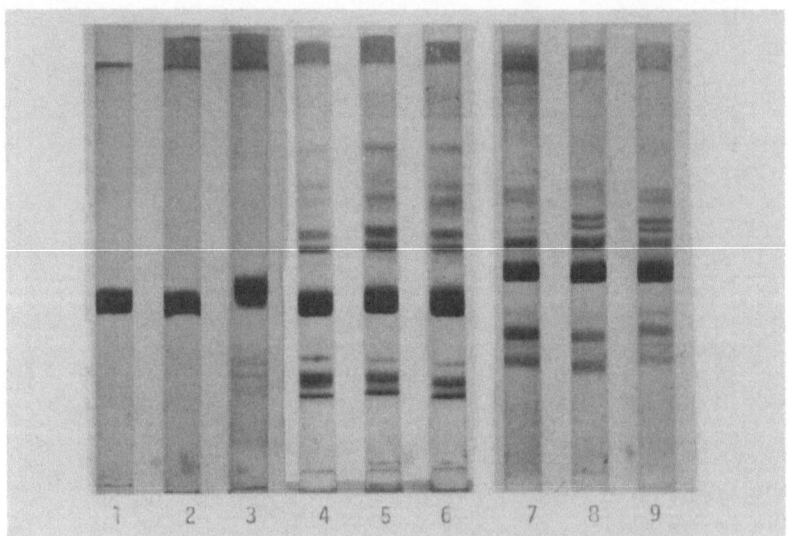

Figure 5. Electrophoretic patterns of human and rabbit high density apolipoproteins in 10% polyacrylamide gels containing 0.1% sodium dodecyl sulfate. 1, human apo A-I; 2, rabbit apo A-I or fraction (1) of Table II; 3, fraction (2) of Table II; 4,5, normal Dutch Belt HDL_3 and HDL_2, respectively; 6, cholesteremic Dutch Belt HDL_2; 7,8, normal New Zealand White HDL_3 and HDL_2, respectively; 9, cholesteremic New Zealand White HDL_2.

These two isolated peptides resemble human apo A-I in electrophoretic mobility in sodium dodecyl sulfate polyacrylamide gels
(Figure 5). Normal and cholesteremic high density apolipoprotein
patterns of Dutch Belt rabbits were indistinguishable from those
of the New Zealand White strain. The arginine-rich apolipoprotein,
a major component of very low density lipoproteins, is one of
several minor components in high density lipoproteins and occurs to
a greater extent in the HDL_2 than in the HDL_3 subfraction (Figure 5).
Small amounts of proteins of low molecular weight are also present
(Figure 5).

The rabbit high density apolipoproteins were isolated from
normal and cholesteremic lipoproteins (pooled HDL_2 and HDL_3 subfractions) by ion exchange chromatography, as used previously for
human high density apolipoproteins (13). Amino acid compositions
of fractions 1 and 2 in Table II as well as the polyacrylamide gel
electrophoresis patterns suggest that the two major proteins correspond closely to human apo A-I (24). The composition of the arginine-
rich apolipoprotein (fraction 4 in Table II) is also very similar
to its human counterpart (25). Rabbit high density lipoproteins,
like human very low density and high density lipoproteins (25),
contain a protein (fraction 5 in Table II) that is rich in hydro-
philic or polar amino acids. Possibly this protein accounts for
the relatively high glycine content of normal rabbit very low density lipoproteins (5). Fraction 3, found previously in cholesteremic rabbit very low density lipoproteins (5), appears to correspond to human apoVLDLserine (C-I), and it is possible that fraction
8 corresponds to human apoVLDLalanine (C-III).

Erythrocyte ATPase Activities

Membranes isolated from Dutch Belt and New Zealand White
rabbits, normal and cholesteremic, were compared with respect to
their Na^+-K^+-ATPase, Mg^{++}-ATPase, and Ca^{++}-ATPase activities
(Table III). This preliminary comparison involving eight rabbits
did not reveal a major difference among the cells. Possibly the
Ca^{++}-ATPase activity is lower than normal in erythrocytes of cholesteremic New Zealand White rabbits,but further experiments are
necessary to establish this point. Rabbit erythrocyte membranes
have less Na^+-K^+-ATPase and more Mg^{++}-ATPase activities than do
human erythrocyte membranes prepared and assayed under the same
conditions (26).

DISCUSSION

The cholesterol-induced, highly atherogenic hyperlipoproteinemia in the rabbit brings to mind certain hyperlipoproteinemias in

TABLE II

Amino Acid Composition of Apolipoproteins of Rabbit High Density Lipoproteins

| | HDL$_2$ | | Isolated Apolipoproteins | | | | | | | |
| | Normal | Cholesteremic | Major | | | | Minor | | | |
			(1)	(2)	(3)	(4)	(5)	(6)	(7)	(8)
Lys	80	82	83	79	149	43	24	58	58	55
His	10	10	8	11	16	9	13	7	14	21
Arg	59	54	67	68	33	102	18	28	29	21
Asp	88	86	88	90	63	48	67	111	93	89
Thr	47	50	43	45	114	30	58	70	62	52
Ser	79	78	74	81	102	57	170	114	75	109
Glu	194	195	209	200	161	229	176	147	157	151
Pro	38	38	35	36	23	33	38	38	58	44
Gly	48	46	41	41	23	59	216	66	67	81
Ala	79	87	78	80	42	120	64	104	80	102
Cys			0	0	0	0		0		
Val	57	55	61	55	16	62	36	39	56	58
Met	13	11	5	6	16	30	17	19	24	30
Ile	10	11	7	7	81	9	20	14	28	20
Leu	124	124	132	127	70	112	44	114	107	90
Tyr	25	26	25	27	0	15	15	48	36	26
Phe	33	31	26	27	81	15	24	13	43	35
Trp	19	19	20	20				12	14	19

TABLE III

Erythrocyte ATPase Activities of Normal and Cholesteremic Rabbits

Erythrocytes	μ moles Pi/mg protein/hr		
	Na^+-K^+-ATPase	Mg^{++}-ATPase	Ca^{++}-ATPase
Dutch Belt:			
Normal	0.18	1.16	0.86
Cholesteremic	0.20	1.19	0.82
New Zealand White:			
Normal	0.18	1.01	1.03
Cholesteremic	0.18	1.01	0.68

man in which elevated very low density and intermediate density lipoproteins are enriched in cholesteryl esters (27-30) and in the arginine-rich apolipoprotein (29-31). The genetic disorder dysbetalipoproteinemia (xanthoma tuberosum, type III hyperlipoproteinemia) and hypothyroidism are associated with changes in lipoprotein composition qualitatively similar to those observed in the cholesteremic rabbit very low density lipoproteins. However, these human fractions contain considerably more triglycerides and both beta- and prebeta-migrating lipoproteins, in contrast to the cholesteremic rabbit fractions which contain predominantly beta-migrating species and very little triglycerides. The cholesteremic rabbit possibly also differs from man in that much of the cholesteryl esters of its lipoproteins is derived from the liver (32), whereas in man the plasma lecithin-cholesterol acyl transferase system is the major source of plasma cholesteryl esters (33). However, observations in both man and rabbits and in other species (4,6,7,34) suggest that the arginine-rich apolipoprotein or its phospholipid complex is associated primarily with cholesterol and/or cholesteryl esters. Since the arginine-rich apolipoprotein is preferentially enriched in certain cholesteryl ester-rich particles, it could be associated with specific metabolic pathways for the utilization of cholesterol as well as with the synthesis of lipoprotein particles.

It has been postulated that high density lipoproteins protect against atherogenesis (35,36); lipoproteins that are rich in cholesteryl esters and the arginine-rich apolipoprotein are atherogenic (5-7). Hence, elucidation of mechanisms that determine plasma levels of these lipoproteins is of great interest for elucidation of atherogenesis. For example, it is not clear why excess dietary cholesterol in rabbits leads primarily to high plasma levels of the beta-migrating very low density lipoproteins and intermediate density lipoproteins rather than in low density lipoproteins.

In addition, the mechanism by which the plasma high density lipoproteins are decreased concomitantly with the increase in the very low density and intermediate density lipoproteins in the cholesteremic rabbit is also not evident. In humans as well, low levels of plasma high density lipoproteins have not infrequently been observed in association with elevated plasma very low density lipoproteins (27; Shore, B. and V. Shore, unpublished observations). The HDL_2 subfraction contains more than does the HDL_3 subfraction of the minor apolipoproteins that cycle between the very low density and high density lipoproteins. High density components containing the minor apolipoproteins could be transferred to the very low density fraction (the major apolipoproteins are not similarly transferred), thus depleting the high density fractions to some extent. However, the proportion of the less dense high density subfraction HDL_2 to the more dense HDL_3 subfraction was not changed in rabbits on cholesterol feeding as one would expect were the mechanism so simple.

The mechanisms for regulation of the ratio of the high density subfractions HDL_3 to HDL_2 are not well understood, but a sex difference in humans is known (27), and plasma lecithin-cholesterol acyl transferase may be involved. Whether the ratio is of significance for atherogenesis is not known. However, it was noted that the (female) hyporesponder Dutch Belt strain of rabbits, both normal and cholesteremic, had a higher ratio than the (female) hyper-responder New Zealand White rabbits.

The atherogenecity of plasma lipoproteins is no doubt related to their composition with respect to specific apolipoproteins and lipids as well as to their concentration in plasma. For example, very low density lipoproteins that are enriched in cholesteryl esters, the arginine-rich apolipoprotein, and B proteins, may be more atherogenic than the normal triglyceride-rich very low density lipoproteins. The apolipoproteins probably contain specific sites for interaction with specific cell membrane receptors; hence the composition of proteins as well as lipids can determine the kind of lipoprotein-cell interaction and subsequent effects upon membrane properties and cell function. However, it is probable that other determinants of the atherogenic response are to be found at the cell membrane and intracellular sites. In addition to synthetic, catabolic, and exchange processes that regulate plasma concentration and composition of the lipoproteins, possibly there are membrane differences, normal variations as well as the abnormal genetic defects, that determine the effects of lipoproteins on cells. Thus, metabolic processes account for the differences in plasma lipoproteins in Dutch Belt and New Zealand White rabbits that have been given the same cholesterol-rich diet. But are there also differences at the membrane level that determine a hyper- or hypo- response of arterial walls with respect to atherosclerosis?

Erythrocytes loosely interact with plasma lipoproteins and the very low density lipoproteins and some of their apolipoproteins can markedly stimulate the Mg^{++}-ATPase of isolated membranes (26). The precise function of this enzyme in cells has not yet been elucidated completely, but it is thought to play an important role in the cellular transport of small molecular weight substances and in cell-cell interactions; thus it may play a role in the growth of cells. Hence, it seemed possible that membrane changes due to the cholesterol-rich diet or due to altered cell-lipoprotein interactions in the cholesteremic animal could result in changes in membrane ATPase activity. It was also possible that hyper- and hypo-responder strains could differ quantitatively in membrane enzyme activities. However, the comparison of ATPase activities of erythrocyte membranes isolated from normal and cholesteremic rabbits, both Dutch Belt and New Zealand White strains, indicated that the erythrocyte ATPase activities of the different strains were very similar if not identical. Further studies comparing the interactions of the erythrocytes and cells from atherosclerotic tissues with normal and cholesteremic lipoproteins and apolipoproteins derived from them might reveal effects of cholesteremia on cells.

In summary, the results of the studies on the rabbit lipoproteins and particularly the evidence that several of the rabbit apolipoproteins are very similar to their human counterparts further establish the value of the rabbit as a model for study of hyperlipoproteinemia and atherogenesis. The rabbit is an abundant source of cholesteremic very low density and intermediate density lipoproteins for structural and biochemical studies. The rabbit should be valuable also for studies of the mechanisms that regulate plasma levels of these lipoproteins and the high density lipoproteins. It should also be valuable for elucidation of the role of the arginine-rich apolipoprotein in lipoprotein metabolism and in the atherogenic process associated with cholesteremia characterized by plasma elevations in beta-migrating very low density and intermediate density lipoproteins that are enriched in this apolipoprotein. Finally, the availability of hyperresponder and hyporesponder strains of this animal should greatly facilitate all of these kinds of studies.

ACKNOWLEDGMENTS

This research was supported by United States Public Health Service Grants HL-17463 and HL-16559 from the National Heart and Lung Institute and carried out under the auspices of the United States Energy Research and Development Administration. We wish to express our appreciation to Mr. Stanley Krotz and Miss Marie Laskaris for their technical assistance.

REFERENCES

1. Kritchevsky, D. 1963. Experimental atherosclerosis. In: Lipid Pharmacology. Ed. by R. Paoletti, Academic Press, New York, pp. 63-130.

2. Clarkson, T.B. 1971. Animal models for atherosclerosis. North Carolina Med. J. 32:88-98.

3. Schumaker, V.N. 1956. Cholesteremic rabbit lipoproteins: serum lipoproteins of the cholesteremic rabbit. Am. J. Physiol. 184:35-42.

4. Lasser, N.L., P.S. Roheim, D. Edelstein, and H.A. Eder. 1973. Serum lipoproteins of normal and cholesterol-fed rats. J. Lipid Res. 14:1-8.

5. Shore, V.G., B. Shore, and R.G. Hart. 1974. Changes in apolipoproteins and properties of rabbit very low density lipoproteins on induction of cholesteremia. Biochemistry 13:1579-1584.

6. Mahley, R.W., K.H. Weisgraber, T. Innerarity, H.B. Brewer, Jr., and G. Assmann. 1975. Swine lipoproteins and atherosclerosis. Changes in the plasma lipoproteins and apoproteins induced by cholesterol feeding. Biochemistry 14:2817-2823.

7. Mahley, R.W., K.H. Weisgraber, and T. Innerarity. 1974. Canine lipoproteins and atherosclerosis. II. Characterization of the plasma lipoproteins associated with atherogenic and non-atherogenic hyperlipidemia. Circ. Res. 35:722-733.

8. Clarkson, T.B., H.B. Lofland, Jr., B.C. Bullock, and H.O. Goodman. 1971. Genetic control of plasma cholesterol: studies in squirrel monkeys. Arch. Pathol. 92:37-45.

9. Mills, G.L. and C.E. Taylaur. 1971. The distribution and composition of serum lipoproteins in eighteen animals. Comp. Biochem. Physiol. 40B:489-501.

10. Adams, W.C., E.M. Gaman, and A.S. Feigenbaum. 1972. Breed differences in the responses of rabbits to atherogenic diets. Atherosclerosis 16:405-411.

11. Israel, Y., H. Kalant, E. LeBlanc, J.C. Bernstein, and I. Salazar. 1970. Changes in cation transport and (Na + K)-activated adenosine triphosphatase produced by chronic administration of ethanol. J. Pharmacol. Exp. Ther. 174:330-336.

12. Shore, V. and B. Shore. 1967. Some physical and chemical studies on the protein moiety of a high-density (1.126-1.195 g/ml) lipoprotein fraction of human serum. Biochemistry 6: 1962-1969.

13. Shore, B. and V. Shore. 1969. Isolation and characterization of polypeptides of human serum lipoproteins. Biochemistry 8: 4510-4516.

14. Lowry, O.H., N.J. Rosebrough, A.L. Farr, and R.J. Randall. 1951. Protein measurement with the folin phenol reagent. J. Biol. Chem. 193:265-275.

15. Lindgren, F.T., L.C. Jensen, and F.T. Hatch. 1972. The isolation and quantitative analysis of serum lipoproteins. In: Blood Lipids and Lipoproteins: Quantitation, Composition and Metabolism. Ed. by G.J. Nelson, Wiley-Interscience, New York, pp. 182-274.

16. Mann, G.   1961.   A method for measurement of cholesterol in blood serum.   Clin. Chem. 7:275-284.

17. Nelson, G.   1967.   Composition of neutral lipids from erythrocytes of common mammals.   J. Lipid Res. 8:374-379.

18. Chen, P.S., Jr., T.Y. Toribara, and H. Warner.   1956.   Microdetermination of phosphorus.   Anal. Chem. 28:1756-1758.

19. B.J. Davis.   1964.   Disc electrophoresis: method and application to human serum proteins.   In: Gel Electrophoresis, Ann. N.Y. Acad. Sci. 121. Ed. by H.E. Whipple, pp. 404-427.

20. U.K. Laemmli.   1970.   Cleavage of structural proteins during the assembly of the head of bacteriophage T4.   Nature 227: 680-685.

21. Liu, T.Y. and Y.H. Chang.   1971.   Hydrolysis of proteins with p-toluenesulfonic acid.   J. Biol. Chem. 246:2842-2848.

22. Gibbs, R., P.M. Roddy, and E. Titus.   1965.   Preparation, assay and properties of an Na^+ and K^+-requiring adenosine triphosphatase from beef brain.   J. Biol. Chem. 240:2181-2187.

23. Coleman, R. and T.A. Bromley.   1975.   Hydrolysis of erythrocyte membrane phospholipid by a preparation of phospholipase C from Clostridium Welchii: deactivation of (Ca^{++}, Mg^{++})-ATPase and its reactivation by added lipids.   Biochim. Biophys. Acta 382: 565-575.

24. Morrisett, J.D., R.L. Jackson, and A.M. Gotto, Jr.   1975. Lipoproteins: structure and function.   In: Annual Review of Biochemistry.   Ed. by E.E. Snell, Annual Reviews, Inc., Palo Alto, Calif., pp. 184-207.

25. Shore, B. and V. Shore.   1970.   Apoproteins and substructure of human serum lipoproteins.   In: Atherosclerosis: Proceedings of the Second International Symposium.   Ed. by R.J. Jones, Springer-Verlag, New York, pp. 144-150.

26. Shore, V. and B. Shore.   1975.   Stimulation of human erythrocyte Mg^{++}-ATPase by plasma lipoproteins.   Biochem. Biophys. Res. Comm. 65: 1250-1256.

27. Gofman, J.W., O. DeLalla, F. Glazier, N.K. Freeman, F.T. Lindgren, A.V. Nichols, B. Strisower, and A.R. Tamplin.   1954.   The serum lipoprotein transport system in health, metabolic disorders, atherosclerosis and coronary heart disease.   Plasma (Milan) 2:413-484.

28. Hazzard, W.R., F.T. Lindgren, and E.L. Bierman. 1970. Very
     low density lipoprotein subfractions in a subject with broad-
     beta disease (type III hyperlipoproteinemia) and a subject with
     endogenous lipemia (type IV hyperlipoproteinemia). Chemical
     composition and electrophoretic mobility. Biochim. Biophys.
     Acta 202:517-525.

29. Havel, R.J. and J.P. Kane. 1973. Primary dysbetalipoprotein-
     emia: predominance of a specific apoprotein species in tri-
     glyceride rich lipoproteins. Proc. Nat. Acad. Sci. (Washington)
     70:2015-2019.

30. Shore, B., V. Shore, A. Salel, D. Mason, and R. Zelis. 1974.
     An apolipoprotein preferentially enriched in cholesteryl ester-
     rich very low density lipoproteins. Biochem. Biophys. Res.
     Comm. 58:1-7.

31. Shore, V.G. and B. Shore. 1973. Heterogeneity of human plasma
     very low density lipoproteins. Separation of species differing
     in protein components. Biochemistry 12:502-507.

32. Rose, H. 1972. Origin of cholesteryl esters in the blood of
     cholesterol fed rabbits: relative contributions of serum leci-
     thin-cholesterol acyl transferase and hepatic ester synthesis.
     Biochim. Biophys. Acta 260:312-326.

33. Glomset, J.A. 1972. Plasma lecithin:cholesterol acyl trans-
     ferase. In: Blood Lipids and Lipoproteins: Quantitation,
     Composition and Metabolism. Ed. by G.J. Nelson, Wiley-
     Interscience, New York, pp. 745-787.

34. Ostwald, R. and L.S.S. Guo. 1975. Changes in the high density
     lipoprotein apoproteins of guinea pigs in response to dietary
     cholesterol. Fed. Proc. 34:499.

35. Bondjers, G. and S. Bjorkerud. 1974. Cholesterol transfer
     between arterial smooth muscle tissue and serum lipoproteins
     in vitro. Artery 1:3-9.

36. Miller, G.J. and N.E. Miller. 1975. Plasma high density
     lipoprotein concentration and development of ischaemic heart
     disease. Lancet (January 4):16-19.

SEASONAL VARIATIONS IN SEVERITY OF EXPERIMENTAL ATHEROSCLEROSIS IN RABBITS

David Kritchevsky, Shirley A. Tepper and Jon A. Story

Wistar Institute of Anatomy and Biology

Philadelphia, Pennsylvania 19104

For fifteen years, we have been conducting numerous experiments on the induction of atherosclerosis in male Dutch belted rabbits, testing a variety of dietary fats and several hypolipidemic drugs. In all of these experiments, the standard atherogenic regimen that provided the basis for comparison of treatments was 2% cholesterol and 6% corn oil added to laboratory ration. Although each experiment contained its own control, we noted that the atheromata in the control rabbits varied from experiment to experiment. In an effort to ascertain a possible seasonal variation in atherosclerosis we have collated by month of autopsy data from 74 experimental identical 2-month feeding periods.

EXPERIMENTAL

The experimental groups consisted of 8 to 15 rabbits with starting weights of approximately 1.5-2.0 kg. The diet was fed ad libitum although these rabbits ate from 75-100 g daily. After two months the rabbits were killed (by intracardial injection of barbiturate) and the aortas graded in the manner of Duff and McMillan (1). Serum cholesterol levels were always determined; the methods varied but usually involved direct determination on the serum (2-4).

RESULTS AND DISCUSSION

Our findings are presented in Table I and Figure 1. The average values for arch and thoracic atheromata for the reporting period were 2.0 and 1.3, respectively. The range of arch athero-

TABLE I

Monthly Variation in Atherosclerosis in Rabbits Fed 2% Cholesterol

and 6% Corn Oil for 2 Months

Month*	Number of Experiments	Average Atheromata $\pm$ S.E.M.**	
		Arch	Thoracic
January	2	2.4 ± 1.1	1.6 ± 0.7
February	7	$2.2 \pm 0.2_{ab}$	1.4 ± 0.2
March	9	$1.6 \pm 0.1_{acd}$***	$1.2 \pm 0.1_{k}$
April	5	$1.7 \pm 0.2_{e}$	1.1 ± 0.2
May	7	$1.6 \pm 0.1_{bfg}$***	$1.0 \pm 0.1_{lm}$***
June	4	$2.4 \pm 0.4_{cf}$	$1.7 \pm 0.3_{l}$
July	7	$1.9 \pm 0.2_{h}$	$1.2 \pm 0.1_{n}$
August	6	$1.9 \pm 0.2_{i}$	1.4 ± 0.1
September	8	$2.5 \pm 0.2_{deghij}$***	$1.7 \pm 0.2_{kmno}$
October	6	2.0 ± 0.2	1.3 ± 0.2
November	1	2.2	1.5
December	12	$1.9 \pm 0.2_{j}$	$1.1 \pm 0.1_{o}$
TOTAL	74	2.0 ± 0.1	1.3 ± 0.1

*Month in which rabbits were autopsied.

**Values bearing same subscript are significantly different.

***Significantly different from average for all 74 experiments.

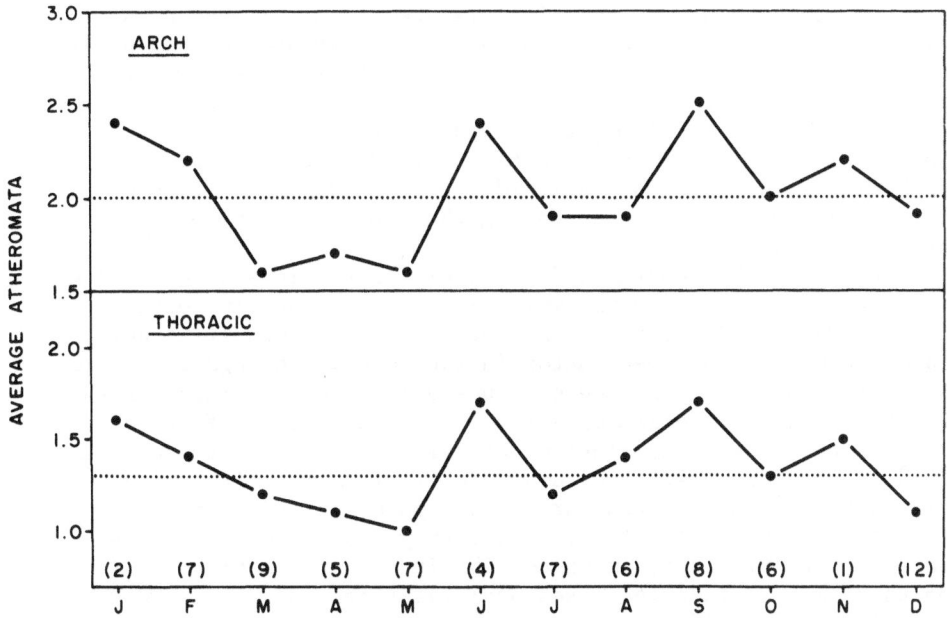

Figure 1. Variation of severity of experimentally induced atherosclerosis in rabbits.

sclerosis was 1.6-2.5, and for the thoracic aorta was 1.0-1.7.

The seasonal variations of the severity of atherosclerosis in the two sections of aorta were similar. Thus the highest levels of aortic arch atherosclerosis were observed in January, June and September, and thoracic atherosclerosis peaked in the same months. The lowest levels of atherosclerotic involvement occurred in March and May in the arch and April, May and December in the thoracic aorta.

We could not relate the levels of atherosclerosis to average serum cholesterol levels. The highest average level was 2431 mg/dl in August and the lowest was 1468 mg/dl in January. This finding is not unexpected since even the lowest cholesterol level is about 20 times normal for this breed of rabbit. Temporal variations in serum cholesterol levels have been reported in man (5-7), baboon (8-10), monkeys (11,12) and the rat (13).

The observed variation in average atheromata in this report may, in part, reflect differences in the composition of the stock

diet to which the atherogenic factors are added. It has been
pointed out (14) that stock diets are less atherogenic than semipurified diets. Since little is known about the fine composition
of the stock diet, it is possible that some variation in mineral,
carbohydrate or fiber (amount or type) content may affect the
atherogenicity of the added cholesterol. However, if only the
stock diet were involved, we would expect a completely random
distribution of results considering the number of experiments and
the time span.

Thorp (13) has correlated seasonal fluctuations in endocrine
function in both rat and man which fluctuate either in concert
with, or in opposition to serum cholesterol levels. It is possible, then, that another factor in the observed swings in atherogenic effects of diet may be some phase of endocrine function that
affects aortic metabolism directly. We presume the effect is
directly upon the aorta since no correlation exists between serum
lipid levels and severity of atherosclerosis. The effect may be
related to thyroid function or to the synthesis and hydrolysis
of aortic cholesteryl esters. Cholesteryl esterase activity appears to vary with species susceptibility to atherosclerosis (15)
and there may be individual seasonal variations as well. We are
examining several of these possibilities.

ACKNOWLEDGEMENTS

This work was supported, in part, by a grant (HL 03299) and
a Research Career Award (HL-0734) from the National Heart and Lung
Institute, USPHS.

REFERENCES

1.   G.L. Duff and G.C. McMillan. The effect of alloxan diabetes
     on experimental cholesterol atherosclerosis in the rabbit.
     J. Exp. Med. 89:611-630 (1949).

2.   P. Trinder. Determination of cholesterol in serum. Analyst
     77:321-326 (1952).

3.   G.V. Mann. A method for measurement of cholesterol in blood
     serum. Clin. Chem. 7:275-284 (1961).

4.   S. Pearson, S. Stern and T.H. McGavack. A rapid, accurate
     method for the determination of total cholesterol in serum.
     Analyt. Chem. 25:813-814 (1953).

5. C.B. Thomas, H.W.D. Holljes and F.F. Eisenberg. Observations on seasonal variations in total serum cholesterol levels among healthy young prisoners. Ann. Int. Med. 54:413-430 (1961).

6. J. Paloheimo. Seasonal variations of serum lipids in healthy young men. Ann. Med. Exp. Biol. Fenn. 39:Suppl. 8 (1961).

7. J. Kocemba, L. Szopinska-Ciba, T. Ciba and L. Tochowicz. Seasonal variations of serum cholesterol levels in healthy and in atherosclerotic subjects. Bull. Polish Med. Sci. History 6:10-13 (1963).

8. J.P. Strong, P.B. Radelat, M.H. Guidry and C.A. McMahon. Variability of serum cholesterol levels in baboons. Circ. Res. 14:367-372 (1964).

9. D. Kritchevsky, E.S. Kritchevsky, P.P. Nair, J.A. Jastremsky and I.L. Shapiro. Effect of free fatty acids on cholesterol metabolism in the baboon. Nutr. Dieta 9:283-299 (1967).

10. D. Kritchevsky, L.M. Davidson, I.L. Shapiro, H.K. Kim, M. Kitagawa, S. Malhotra, P.P. Nair, T.B. Clarkson, I. Bersohn and P.A.D. Winter. Lipid metabolism and experimental atherosclerosis in baboons: influence of cholesterol-free, semisynthetic diets. Am. J. Clin. Nutr. 27:29-50 (1974).

11. D. Kritchevsky and R.F.J. McCandless. Weekly variations in serum cholesterol levels of monkeys. Proc. Soc. Exp. Biol. Med. 95:152-154 (1957).

12. G.E. Cox, C.B. Taylor, L.G. Cox and M.A. Counts. Atherosclerosis in rhesus monkeys. I. Hypercholesteremia induced by dietary fat and cholesterol. Arch. Pathol. 66:32-52 (1958).

13. J.M. Thorp. Effects of seasonal variation on lipid metabolism in animals and man. In "The Control of Lipid Metabolism", ed. J.K. Grant, Academic Press, N.Y., 1963, pp. 163-168.

14. D. Kritchevsky. Experimental atherosclerosis in rabbits fed cholesterol-free diets. J. Atheroscler. Res. 4:103-105 (1964).

15. D. Kritchevsky and H.V. Kothari. Aortic cholesterol esterase in species resistant or susceptible to atherosclerosis. Steroids and Lipids Res. 5:23-27 (1974).

STUDY OF DRUGS AFFECTING CHOLESTEROL-INDUCED ATHEROSCLEROSIS IN

RABBITS

Y.S.Kwak, K.T.Lee and D.N.Kim

Clinical Chemistry Section, Laboratory Service, VA
Hospital, Albany, N.Y. 12208 (Y.S.K.) and Department
of Pathology, Albany Medical College, Albany,N.Y.12208

INTRODUCTION

Studies in man and animal models reveal that the major events
involved in early atherogenesis include lipid deposition and
degeneration and proliferation of smooth muscle cells or mesenchymal cells in the intima of aortae (1-4). An atherogenic insult
such as hypercholesterolemia may have a direct effect on the endothelial and/or smooth muscle cells of arteries, or an indirect
effect on these cells mediated through plasma or tissue factors
including platelets, lipoprotein and vasoactive amines including
histamine, serotonin and angiotensin (5).

Mustard and Packham (6) have recently shown that many factors
which lead to vascular injury and atherosclerosis may also injure
platelets and cause them to aggregate and release substances,
many of which may be potentially inflammatory and atherogenic.
These substances are histamine, epinephrine, prostaglandin, adenosine diphosphate, permeability factors, elastase and other proteo-
lytic enzymes.

Recent studies of Peters, Takano and de Duve (7) and from our
laboratory (8,9) lend support to the view that lysosomes in arterial
smooth muscle cells play a role in the early atherogenesis. An
inherent deficiency in the amount of cholesterol metabolizing
enzymes in the arterial wall probably leads to an accumulation of
cholesteryl esters and eventually to atherosclerosis. Our earlier
studies in vitro on interaction of lipids and the stability of
lysosomes seemed to indicate that increased concentration of
phospholipids and esterified cholesterol in incubation media
labilized incubated aortic and hepatic lysosomes of swine.

ATHEROGENESIS AND TREATMENT OF ATHEROSCLEROSIS

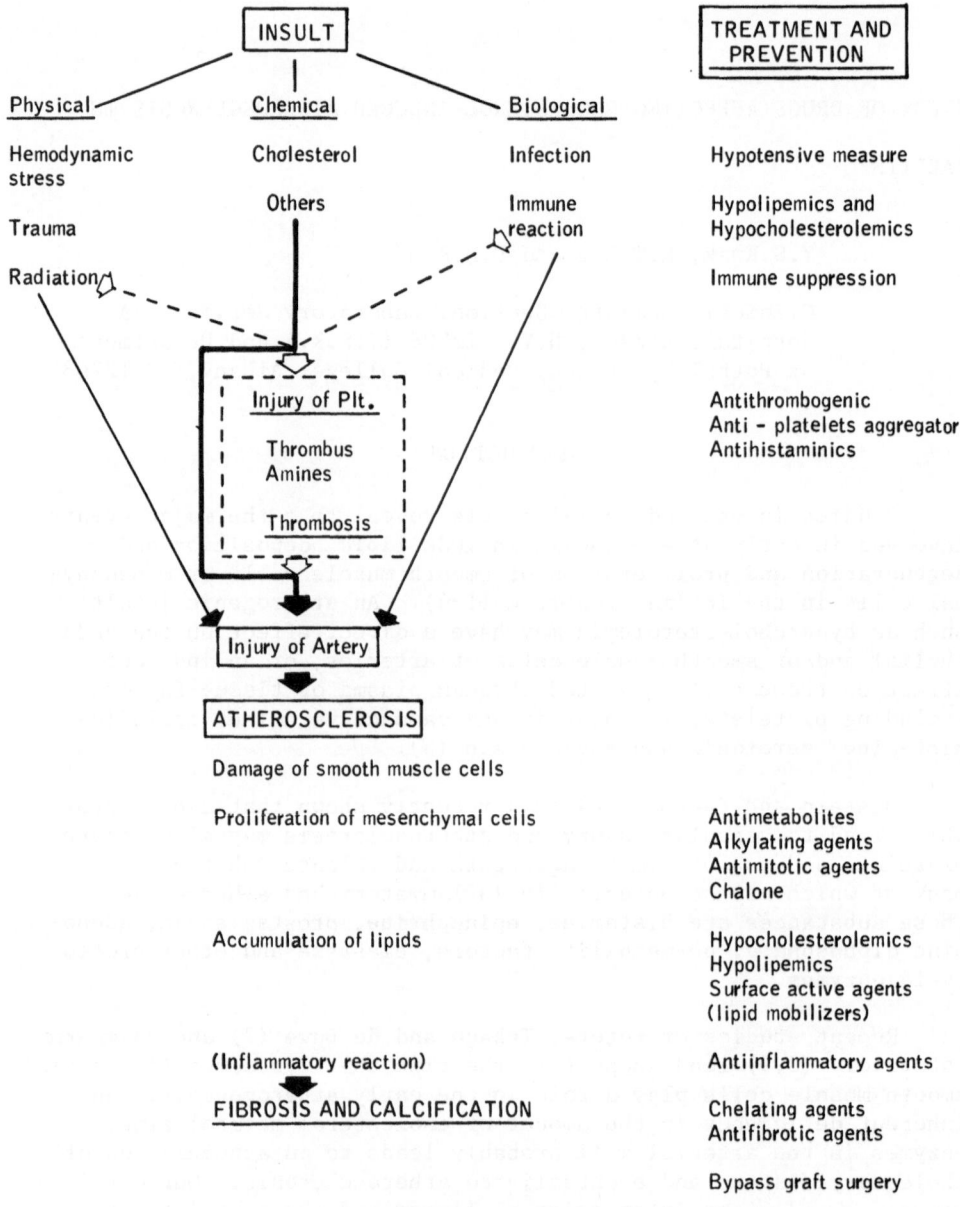

Figure 1

Therefore, an increased concentration of lipids in the mesenchymal cells of aorta during early atherogenesis might result in a labilization of lysosomes and the triggering of cells into mitoses or degeneration.

In addition, there is ample evidence indicating that various types of injuries to the arterial wall may cause atherosclerosis. These injuries include physical, chemical and biological forms (10-13). A hypothetical scheme of atherogenesis is summarized in Figure 1. Various insults (physical, chemical and biological) act individually or synergistically on arterial wall or through mural thrombosis. Then the injured artery further progresses toward accumulation of lipids and degeneration and proliferation of mesenchymal cells. Finally, the diseased arteries become fibrous, necrotic and calcified.

For the treatment and prevention of atherosclerosis, obviously a reasonable approach would be removal of causative factors or blockade of the disease process by using therapeutic agents and other means. The commonly used therapeutic measures to promote regression of atherosclerosis are lipid lowering drugs and low-fat diets. The effect of these measures appears to be promising in both human and experimental animal models(14-30). During the past several years, we have primarily focused our study on drugs affecting atherosclerotic processes. We are not concerned principally with altering the levels of serum and tissue lipids but with interfering with metabolic events which lead to the development of atherosclerotic lesions. The drugs studied were chosen according to our scheme and included lysosome stabilizers, antihistaminics, anti-platelet aggregators, inhibitors of steroid hormone synthesis by adrenal cortex, cholesterol binders (polyenoic antibiotics), surface active agents and antimetabolites.

We have studied the effects of various drugs on both the progression and regression phases of cholesterol-induced atherosclerosis in rabbits. In this communication, however, we have summarized findings of the effects of these drugs only on the progression phase.

MATERIALS AND METHODS

One hundred and fifty male, New Zealand white rabbits weighing 2.5 $\pm$ 0.3 kg were divided into 17 experimental groups, each group consisting of 7 to 10 animals (Table I). The normal control diet group was fed 100 g daily of rabbit pellets (Agway, Inc., Syracuse, N.Y.). The experimental groups were given 100 g of rabbit pellets mixed with 1% cholesterol and 6% peanut oil or corn oil by weight with or without drugs. The drugs studied were chloroquine, acetylsalicyclic acid + chlorpheniramine, pyridinolcarbamate, 1,1-dichloro-2-(o-chlorophenyl)-2-(P-chlorophenyl)-ethane

TABLE I. EXPERIMENTAL GROUPS AND NUMBER OF ANIMALS

GROUP	DIETS[a]			NUMBER OF
	Cholesterol	Corn Oil	Peanut Oil	ANIMALS
Untreated	+	+		10
Chloroquine	+	+		10
Acetylsalicylic Acid + chlorpheniramine	+	+		10
Pyridinolcarbamate[b]	+	+		10
Untreated	+	+		13
Nystatin	+	+		7
o, p' –DDD	+	+		8
Untreated	+	+		9
Mercaptopurine	+	+		9
Hydroxyurea	+	+		8
Untreated	+		+	8
Sodiumdodecyl sulfate	+		+	8
Pellet[c]	–		–	8
Untreated	+		+	8
Mercaptopurine	+		+	8
Hydroxyurea	+		+	8
Pyridinolcarbamate[d]	+		+	8

a: 100 g of commercial rabbit pellets was mixed with 1% cholesterol
   and 6% oil by weight;
b: mixed with diet;
c: commercial pellets only;
d: given at fasting in one dose prior to the meal

TABLE II. MODE OF ACTION AND DOSES OF DRUGS

DRUGS	MODE OF ACTION	DAILY DOSE[a]
Mercaptopurine	Purine and DNA syntheses inhibitor	2.5 mg/kg
Hydroxyurea	DNA synthesis inhibitor	25 mg/kg
o,p'-DDD	Adreno-cortical steroid synthesis inhibitor	150 mg/kg
Nystatin	Cholesterol binder, polyenoic antibiotic	10^4U
Acetylsalicylic acid	Lysosome stabilizer Anti-platelet aggregator	75 mg/kg
+ Chlorpheniramine	Antihistaminic	2 mg/kg
Chloroquine	Lysosome stabilizer	5 mg/kg[b]
Pyridinolcarbamate	Endothelial cell relaxant Anti-platelet aggregator	25 mg/kg[c] 12.5 mg/kg[d]
Sodiumdodecyl sulfate	Surface active agent (detergent)	250 mg/kg

a: all drugs were mixed with diet except for chloroquine and pyridinolcarbamate in second experiment.

b: given once a day between the meals.

c: mixed with diet in the first experiment.

d: given at fasting in one dose prior to the meal.

(o, p'-DDD), nystatin,sodiumdodecyl sulfate, mercaptopurine and
hydroxyurea. The drugs were administered orally in doses comparable to those used in human on the body weight basis, except for
nystatin. A high dose of nystatin was used because the rate
of absorption of this drug is very low. Table II illustrates
the mode of action and doses.

At the end of 2 months of the experiment, all animals were
killed; the aorta was removed,and blood samples were taken for
cholesterol measurement. The aorta was opened,and the adventitia
was cleaned. A thin transparent vinyl sheet was placed over the
aorta,and the atherosclerotic lesions were traced. The percent
of aortic surface area involved by atherosclerosis was calculated
via planimetry.

The serum and tissue cholesterol was measured by the method
of Leffler (31). The aorta was saponified with alcoholic KOH and
the non-saponifiable lipids were extracted.

Representative sections from the thoracic aorta was processed
routinely for light microscopy. Hematoxylin-eosin, Weigert-Von
Giesson and Alcian blue stains were used.

RESULTS

The results are summarized in Table III. The most significant
finding was obtained from the groups treated with antimetabolites,
mercaptopurine and hydroxyurea. These drugs significantly reduced
the area of the aorta involved in atherosclerotic lesions. In the
hydroxyurea-treated group, both the aortic cholesterol concentration and the lesion area were reduced with no reduction in serum
cholesterol levels. On the other hand, the mercaptopurine group
showed more drastic reductions in both the aortic cholesterol
concentration and the lesion area,and the serum cholesterol level
was also lower in this group than the control group. This portion
of the study was performed twice; the first with the diet containing 1% cholesterol and 6% corn oil, and the second with 1%
cholesterol and 6% peanut oil. The effect of the drugs was reproducible,but the effect of peanut oil on atherogenesis was more
severe than that of corn oil. Although antimetabolites were
known to be toxic, the rabbits tolerated the drugs well and gained
weight as the controls.

Pyridinolcarbamate showed little effect on both aortic
cholesterol concentrations and the extent of aortic atherosclerosis
when it was mixed with the diet. But when it was given orally
once a day prior to the meal, the extent of atherosclerosis was
reduced slightly.

TABLE III. SUMMARY OF THE EFFECTS OF DRUGS ON CHOLESTEROL-INDUCED
ATHEROSCLEROSIS IN RABBITS
(Relative ratios against untreated controls)

| DRUG | CHOLESTEROL | | ATHEROSCLEROTIC |
	SERUM	AORTA	LESION
Untreated control	1.00 (2,100 mg/dl) [a]	1.00 (18 mg/g) [a]	1.00 (72%) [a]
Mercaptopurine (CO) [b]	0.53[s]	0.27[s]	0.06[s]
(PO) [c]	0.62[s]	0.11[s]	0.06[s]
Hydroxyurea (CO)	0.86[s]	0.38[s]	0.25[s]
(PO)	0.90[s]	0.46[s]	0.39[s]
o, p' -DDD	1.14	0.57	0.50
Nystatin	1.14	0.71	0.69
Acetylsalicylic acid + Chlorpheniramine	1.05	1.43	1.82
Chloroquine	1.06	1.24	1.26
Pyridinolcarbamate (1) [d]	0.92	0.95	1.00
(2) [e]	0.86	0.66	0.63
Sodiumdodecyl sulfate	1.43	0.69	0.44

a: mean values for the untreated control group.
b: CO: the diet mixed with 1% cholesterol and 6% corn oil.
c: PO: the diet mixed with 1% cholesterol and 6% peanut oil.
d: Pyridinolcarbamate was given 25 mg/kg/day mixed with diet.
e: Pyridinolcarbamate was given 12.5 mg/kg/day orally one dose
   a day prior to the meal.
s: significantly different from the untreated control group
   ($P < 0.05$).

An inhibitor of adreno-cortical steroid synthesis, o,p'-DDD seemed to reduce the extent of the lesions as well as aortic cholesterol concentrations, but the differences were not statistically significant.

A surface active agent, sodiumdodecyl sulfate, increased serum cholesterol levels when rabbits were fed a high cholesterol diet but it did not alter the serum cholesterol levels when rabbits were on pellets. The extent of atherosclerotic lesions in the aorta was reduced by this agent. The dosage utilized in this study did not affect the growth of the animals.

A cholesterol binder, nystatin did not show significant effect in the tissue cholesterol concentrations nor the extent of atherosclerosis.

On the other hand, lysosome stabilizers with or without an antihistaminic, chloroquine or acetylsalicyclic acid + chlorpheniramine, seemed to increase both the extent of aortic lesions and aortic cholesterol concentrations, but these were not statistically significant.

Histologically, there was no difference in the type of aortic lesions among the various drug-treated groups. All lesions consisted of foam cells. The thickness of intimal lesions of the aorta was closely correlated with the concentration of aortic cholesterol.

DISCUSSION

There have been numerous studies utilizing various drugs in experimental animal models to learn if the course of experimental atherosclerosis can be modifed by these therapeutic agents (28-68). Corticosteroids (32-39), estrogen (40-44), pyridinolcarbamate (45,46), colchicine (39,47), penicillamine (47), acetylsalicylic acid (38,47-49) and heparin (50) have been most widely tested aside from the hypocholesterolemics. Their effects appear to be species-specific and the summary of a review on the effects of non-hypocholesterolemic drugs on the experimental atherosclerosis from the literature is tabulated in Table IV.

Cortisone (32-34,37,38), estrogen (40-44), pyridinolcarbamate (45,46) and colchicine (47) are reported to be inhibitory on the development of atherosclerosis in hypercholesterolemic rabbits. However, cortisone enhances the development of atherosclerosis in rats (35), chickens (36) and swine (39). Colchicine is not effective on swine atherosclerosis which is produced by combination of endothelial denudation injury and a high-cholesterol diet (39). The effect of pyridinolcarbamate on the experimental atherosclerosis

TABLE IV. EFFECTS OF DRUGS ON EXPERIMENTAL[a]
ATHEROSCLEROSIS, A REVIEW

DRUGS	EFFECTS	
	Serum Cholesterol	Atherosclerotic lesion
Immune Suppressive Agents		
Antimetabolites (53)[b]	D or N.C.	D
Corticosteroid (32-39)	I	D or I
Chloroquine (64)[b]	N.C.	N.C. or ? I
Anti-platelet Aggregator		
Pyridinolcarbamate (45,46)[b]	N.C.	D or N.C.
Acetylsalicyclic acid (38,47-49)	N.C.	N.C. or ? D
Antithrombogenic agents		
Heparin (50)	N.C.	N.C.
Antihistaminic		
Chlorpheniramine (51,52)	N.C.	D or N.C.
Antimetabolites		
Mercaptopurine (53)[b]	D	D
Hydroxyurea (53)[b]	N.C.	D
Actinomycin D (54)	N.C.	D
O,P'-DDD	N.C.	D
Antimitotic Agents		
Colchicine (39,47)	N.C.	D or I
Chalone (aortic) (55)	N.C.	D
Surface Active Agents		
Tween 80 (56-60)	I	D
Surfactant (61)	I	D
Sodiumdodecyl sulfate[b]	I	D
Lecithin (62, 63)	N.C.	D
Cholesterol Binder		
Nystatin[b]	N.C.	N.C.

TABLE IV. (continued)

DRUGS	EFFECTS	
	Serum Cholesterol	Atherosclerotic lesion
Anti-inflammatory Agents		
Corticosteroids (32-39)	I	D or I
Salicylates (38,47-49)	N.C.	N.C.
Chloroquine (64)	N.C.	N.C. or I
Antifibrotic Agents		
Estrogen (40-44)	N.C. or ?D	D
Penicillamine (47)	N.C.	N.C. or ? D
Decalcifying Agent		
Ethane-1-hydroxy-1,1- diphosphonate (65)	N.C.	D
Combination of Drugs		
Acetylsalicylic acid (64)[b] + chlorpheniramine	N.C.	N.C. or ? I
Cholestyramine + O_2 (26) + Estrogen	N.C.	D
Others		
Reserpine (? decalcification)(66)	?	D
Acorus Calamus (herb) (54,67)	N.C.	D
Chondroitin sulfate A (68)	N.C.	D

a: This review excludes hypolipemic or hypocholesterolemic agents
b: Results from the current study:
I: increase; D: decrease; N.C.: no change;
Numbers in parenthesis represent references.

of the progression phase is also controversial at present (46).

In the current study, the most effective agents for the inhibition of progression of cholesterol-induced atherosclerosis in rabbits appear to be antimetabolites, mercaptopurine and hydroxyurea. The next effective agents are surface active agent, sodiumdodecyl sulfate, and an inhibitor of adreno-cortical steroid synthesis, o,p'-DDD. Pyridinolcarbamate showed a slight beneficial effect on the prevention of atherosclerosis, only when it was administered prior to the meal. Nystatin does not appear to be beneficial. On the other hand, chloroquine and acetylsalicyclic acid + chlorpheniramine seem to enhance the atherosclerotic process. The mode of action of most of these drugs on the arterial wall metabolism is not clear at present.

Antimetabolites probably inhibit the smooth muscle cell proliferation in the intima of arteries and perhaps block the syntheses of key cellular proteins and lipids, leading to an inhibition of the development of atherosclerosis. However, there was a notable difference between mercaptopurine and hydroxyurea; a significant reduction in the serum cholesterol levels in the mercaptopurine-treated groups was seen.

An analogue of sodiumdodecyl sulfate, sodiumdecyl sulfate, and other surface active agents such as Tween 20 and Tween 80 are reported to inhibit aortic microsomal cholesterol esterifying system (69). Therefore, these agents might reduce the accumulation of cholesteryl esters in the aortic tissue.

Of particular interest was the effects of lysosome stabilizers, chloroquine and acetylsalicylic acid + chlorpheniramine (an antihistaminic) on atherogenesis. We found that usual therapeutic doses of these drugs caused enhancement of atherogenesis in rabbits, Peters, Takano and de Duve (7) have recently observed that there is less increase in lysosomal cholesteryl ester hydrolase activity in the atherosclerotic rabbit aorta than the other lysosomal enzymes. Therefore, they suggested that a relative deficiency of cholesterol metabolizing enzymes may lead to an accumulation of cholesteryl esters in the aorta. If these drugs stabilize the lysosomal membranes to segregate cholesteryl ester hydrolase from its substrate (cholesteryl ester), the esters may accumulate more rapidly in the aortic tissue. This might enhance the disease process.

A study of effects of various drugs on the regression of experimental rabbit atherosclerosis is in progress.

SUMMARY

1. Effects of various drugs on cholesterol-induced atherosclerosis in rabbits during the progression phase have been studied.
The drugs tested are antimetabolites (mercaptopurine, hydroxyurea),
endothelial cell relaxant and platelet aggregate inhibitor
(pyridinolcarbamate), surface active agents (sodiumdodecyl sulfate), inhibitor of adrenocoritcal steroid synthesis (o,p'-DDD),
lysosome stabilizers (chloroquine, acetylsalicylic acid) with
antihistaminic (chlorpheniramine) and cholesterol binder (nystatin).

2. Mercaptopurine treatment showed marked reduction in both
atherosclerotic lesions and cholesterol concentrations of the
serum and aorta.

3.   Hydroxyurea reduced both the aortic cholesterol concentration and the lesions, but the serum cholesterol concentration
remained high.

4. Sodiumdodecyl sulfate and o,p'-DDD showed slight inhibition
of the development of atherosclerosis.

5. Pyridinolcarbamate showed a slight beneficial effect on the
prevention of atherosclerosis only when it was administered prior
to the meal.

6. Nystatin, chloroquine and acetylsalicylic acid + chlorpheniramine showed little effect.

ACKNOWLEDGEMENTS

This study was supported by USPHS Grant HL-14177. We would
like to thank Drs. T. Shimamoto and F. Numano, Department of
Internal Medicine, Tokyo Dental and Medical University, Tokyo,
Japan for their generous supply of pyridinolcarbamate. We are
also grateful to Burroughs Wellcome Co., Research Triangle Park,
North Carolina for the supply of mercaptopurine.

REFERENCES

1. Florentin, R.A., S.C. Nam, A.S.Daoud, R. Jones, R.F.Scott,
    E.S. Morrison, D.N.Kim, K.T.Lee, W.A.Thomas, W.J.Dodds and
    K.D. Miller. 1968. Dietary-induced atherosclerosis in minia-
    ture swine. Exptl. Mol. Pathol. 8: 263-301.

2. Adams, C.W.M. 1967. Vascular Histochemistry in Relation to
    the Chemical and Structural Pathology of Cardiovascular
    Disease. Year Book Medical Publishers, Inc., Chicago, p.35.

3. Imai, H., K.T.Lee, S. Pastori, E.Panlilio, R. Florentin and
    W.A.Thomas. 1966. Atherosclerosis in rabbits. Architectural
    and subcellular alterations of smooth muscle cells of aortas
    in response to hyperlipemias. Exptl. Mol. Pathol. 5: 273-310.

4. Geer, J.C. and M.D.Haust. 1972. Smooth Muscle Cells in
    Atherosclerosis. S. Karger, Basel, München, Paris, London,
    New York, Sydney.

5. Hollander, W. 1973. Hypertension, antihypertensive drugs and
    atherosclerosis. Circulation 48: 1112-1127.

6. Mustard, J.F. and M.A. Packham. 1970. Thromboembolism, A
    manifestation of the response of blood to injury. Circulation
    42: 1-21.

7. Peters, T.J., T. Takano and C. de Duve. 1973. Subcellular
    fractionation studies on the cells isolated from normal and
    atherosclerotic aorta. In: Atherogenesis: Initiating Factors
    Ciba Foundation Symposium 12, Elsevier, Excerpta Medica.
    North-Holland, Associated Scientific Publishers, Amsterdam,
    London, New York, pp. 197-214.

8. Kwak, Y.S., D.N.Kim, and K.T.Lee.1975. Effects of lipids on
    the stability of lysosomes in vitro. I. Effects of egg-
    lecithin, lysolecithin, sphingomyelin and cholesterol on the
    stability of isolated aortic and hepatic lysosomes of swine.
    Exptl. Mol. Pathol. 23: 266-275.

9. Kwak, Y.S., D.N. Kim and K.T.Lee, 1976. Effects of lipids
    on the stability of lysosomes in vitro. II. Exchange of
    lecithin and cholesterol between lysosomal membrane and incu-
    bating medium and its effect on the functional integrity of
    the membrane. Exptl. Mol. Pathol. in press.

10. Taylor, C.B. 1954. The reaction of arteries to injury by
    physical agents. With a discussion of factors influencing
    arterial repair. In: Symposium on Atherosclerosis, National

Academy of Sciences–National Research Council Publication
338, Washington, D.C., pp. 74–90.

11. Waters, L.L. 1954. The reaction of the artery wall to injury
     by chemicals or infection. In: Symposium on Atherosclerosis,
     National Academy of Sciences–National Research Council
     Publication 338, Washington, D.C. pp. 91–98.

12. Haust, M.D. 1970. Injury and repair in the pathogenesis of
     atherosclerotic lesions. In: Atherosclerosis, Proceedings
     of the Second International Symposium. Ed. by R.J.Jones,
     Springer–Verlag, New York, pp. 12–20.

13. Lamberson, H.V., Jr. and K.E.Fritz. 1974. Immunological
     enhancement of atherosclerosis in rabbits. Persistent
     susceptibility to atherogenic diet following experimentally
     induced serum sickness. Arch. Path. 98: 9–16.

14. Armstrong, M.L., E.D.Warner and W.E.Connor, 1970. Regression
     of coronary atheromatosis in rhesus monkeys. Circ. Res.
     27: 59–67.

15. Armstrong, M.L. and M.B.Megan. 1972. Lipid depletion in
     atheromatous coronary arteries in rhesus monkeys after
     regression diets. Circ. Res. 30: 675–680.

16. Tucker, C.F., C. Catsulis, J.P. Strong and D.A.Eggen. 1971.
     Regression of early cholesterol–induced aortic lesions in
     rhesus monkeys. Am. J. Pathol. 65: 493–502.

17. Eggen, D.A., J.P.Strong, W.P.Newman,III. C. Catsulis, G.T.
     Malcom and M.G.Kokatnur. 1974. Regression of diet–induced
     fatty streaks in rhesus monkeys. Lab. Invest. 31. 294–301.

18. Depalma, R.G., W.Insull, Jr., E.M.Bellon, W.T.Roth and A.V.
     Robinson. 1972. Animal models for the progression and
     regression of atherosclerosis. Surgery 72: 268–278.

19. Vesselinovitch, D., R. Hughes, L. Frazier and R.W.Wissler.
     1973. Studies of the reversal of advanced atherosclerosis
     in the rhesus monkey. Am. J. Pathol. 70: 41a.

20. Horlick, L. and L.N.Katz. 1949. Retrogression of atheroscl–
     erotic lesions on cessation of cholesterol feeding in the
     chick. J.Lab.Clin.Med. 34: 1427–1442.

21. Bevans, M., J.D.Davidson and F.E.Kendall. 1951. Regression

of lesions in canine arteriosclerosis. Arch. Pathol. 51: 288-292.

22. DePalma, R.G., C.A.Hubay, W. Insull, Jr., A.V.Robinson and P.H.Hartman. 1970. Progression and regression of experimental atherosclerosis. Surg. Gynecol. Obstet. 131: 633-647.

23. Bortz, W.M. 1968. Reversibility of atherosclerosis in cholesterol-fed rabbits. Circ. Res. 22: 135-139.

24. St. Clair, R.W., T.B.Clarkson and H.B.Lofland. 1972. Effects of regression of atherosclerotic lesions on the content and esterification of cholesterol by cell-free preparations of pigeon aorta. Circ. Res. 31: 664-671.

25. Clarkson, T.B., J.S.King, H.B.Lofland and M.A.Feldner. 1971. Changes in pathologic characteristics and composition of plaques during regression. Circulation 44:II-48.

26. Vesselinovitch, D., R.W.Wissler, K.Fisher-Dzoga, R. Hughes and L. Dubien. 1974. Regression of atherosclerosis in rabbits. Part I. Treatment with low-fat diet, hyperoxia and hypolipidemic agents. Atherosclerosis 19: 259-275.

27. Daoud, A.S., J. Jarmolych, J.M.Augustyn, K.E.Fritz, J.K.Singh and K.T.Lee. 1975. Regression of advanced swine athero- sclerosis. Arch. Path. in press.

28. Dayton, S., M.L.Pearce, S. Hashimoto, W.J.Dixon and U.Tomoyasu. 1969. A controlled clinical trial of a diet high in unsatu- rated fat in preventing complication of atherosclerosis. Circulation 39/40 Suppl. II: 1-63.

29. Bierenbaum, M.L., A.J.Fleishman, D.P.Green, R.I.Raichelson, T.Hayton, P.B.Watson and A.B.Caldwell, 1970. The 5-year experience of modified fat diets on younger men with coronary heart disease. Circulation 42: 943-952.

30. Miettinen, M., O.Turpeinen, M.J.Karvonen, R.Elosuo and E. Paavilainen. 1972. Effect of cholesterol-lowering diet on mortality from coronary heart-disease and other causes. A twelve-year clinical trial in men and women. Lancet II:835-838.

31. Leffler, H.H. 1959. Estimation of cholesterol in serum. Am. J. Clin. Path. 31:310-313.

32. Gordon, D., S.D.Kobernick, G.C.McMillan and G.L.Duff. 1954.
     The effect of cortisone on the serum lipids and on the
     development of experimental cholesterol atheroslcerosis in
     the rabbit. J. Exp. Med. 99: 371-386.

33. Dury, A. 1959. Influence of cortisone on lipid distribution
     and atherosclerosis. Ann. N.Y. Acad. Sci. 72: 870-884.

34. Friedman, M., S. Byers and S. St. George, 1964. Cortisone
     and experimental atherosclerosis: effects upon administration.
     Arch. Pathol. 77: 142-158.

35. Stamler, J., R. Pick and L.N.Katz. 1951. Intensification of
     cholesterol-induced atherogenesis by cortisone in the chick.
     Circulation 4: 461-462.

36. Wexler, B.C. 1969. Exacerbation of spontaneously occuring
     arteriosclerosis in breeder rats following chronic treatment
     with cortisone. J. Atheroscler. Res. 9:267-277.

37. Bailey, J.M. and J. Butler. 1966. Influence of anti-inflam-
     matory agents on experimental atherosclerosis. Nature 212:
     731-732.

38. Bailey, J.M. and J. Butler, 1973. Anti-inflammatory drugs in
     experimental atherosclerosis. Part I. Relative potencies
     for inhibiting plaque formation. Atherosclerosis 17:515-522.

39. Lee, W.M., R.F.Scott, and E.S. Morrison. 1976. Effects of
     prednisolone and colchicine on the swine atherosclerosis.
     submitted for publication.

40. Moses, C. 1963. Atherosclerosis, Mechanisms as a Guide to
     Prevention. Lea and Febiger, Philadelphia, pp. 128-130.

41. Pick, R., J. Stamler, S. Rodbard and L.N.Katz. 1952. Estrogen-
     induced regression of coronary atherosclerosis in cholesterol-
     fed chicks. Circulation 6: 858-861.

42. Wolinsky, H. 1972. Effects of estrogen and progesterone
     treatment on the response of the aorta of male rats to
     hypertension. Cir. Res. 30: 341-349.

43. Numano, F., M. Takenobu, A. Sagara, M. Kobayashi, K.Moriya,
     T. Kuroiwa, S. Yamazawa, T. Shimamoto, H.Hidaka and K.Mohri.
     1972. The search for antiatherosclerotic agents. Histologi-
     cal and biochemical analysis of the preventive effect of

estrogen, progesterone and pyridinolcarbamate on experiment-
ally inudced atherosclerosis. In: Atherogenesis II. Ed. by
T. Shimamoto, F. Numano and G.M.Addison, Excerpta Medica,
Amsterdam, pp. 98-112.

44. Rhee, C.Y., T.H. Spaet, E. Gaynor, F. Lajam, H.H.Shiang, E.
     Karuso and R.S. Litwak. 1974. Suppression of surgically
     induced vascular intimal hypertrophy by estrogen. Circulation
     50: III-92.

45. Shimamoto, T. and F. Numano. 1969. Atherogenesis I. Proceed-
     ings of the First International Symposium on Atherogenesis
     Thrombosis and Pyridinolcarbamate Treatment. Excerpta Medica,
     Amsterdam.

46. Shimamoto, T., F. Numano and G.M.Addison. 1972. Atherogenesis
     II, Proceedings of the Second International Symposium on
     Atherogenesis, Thrombosis and Pyridinolcarbamate Treatment.
     Excerpta Medica, Amsterdam.

47. Hollander, W., D.M.Kramsch, C. Franzblau, J. Paddock and M.A.
     Columbo. 1974. Suppression of atheromatous fibrous plaque
     formation by antiploriferative and anti-inflammatory drugs.
     Circ. Res. Suppl. 34/35. I: 131-141.

48. Elwood, P.C., A.L. Cochrane, M.L.Burr, P.M.Sweetnam, G.
     Williams, E. Welsby, S.J. Hughes and R. Renton. 1974. A
     randomized controlled trial of acetylsalicyclic acid in
     the secondary prevention of mortality from myocardial infarc-
     tion. British Med. J. 1: 435-440.

49. Boston Collaborative Drug Surveillance Group. 1974. Regular
     aspirin intake and acute myocardial infarction. British
     Med. J. 1: 440-443.

50. Rowsell, H.C., E.A.Murphy and J.F.Mustard. 1965. Heparin
     dosage and atherogenesis in the rabbits. Arch. Path.80:
     63-69.

51. Harman, D. 1962. Atherosclerosis: Inhibiting effect of an
     antihistamine drug, chlorpheniramine. Circ. Res. 11: 277-282.

52. Harman, D. 1969. Pig atherosclerosis. Effect of the anti-
     histamine, chlorpheniramine, on atherogenesis and serum lipids.
     J. Atheroscler . Res. 10:77-84.

53. Kwak, Y.S. and K.T.Lee. 1975. Suppression of cholesterol-
     induced atherosclerosis in rabbits by antimetabolites. Fed.
     Proc. 34: 247.

54. Kwak, Y.S. unpublished data.

55. Nam, S.C., R.A.Florentin, K.Janakidevi, K.T.Lee, J.M.Reiner
     and W.A.Thomas. 1974. Population dynamics of arterial smooth
     muscle cells. III. Inhibition by aortic tissue extracts of
     proliferative response to intimal injury in hypercholestero-
     lemic swine. Exptl. Mol. Pathol. 21: 259-267.

56. Kellner, A., J.W.Correll and A.T.Ladd. 1949. Sustained
     elevation of blood cholesterol and phospholipid levels in
     rabbits given detergent intravenously. Fed. Proc. 8: 359.

57. Ladd, A.T., A. Kellner and J.W.Correll, 1949. Intravenous
     detergents in experimental atherosclerosis with special
     reference to the possible role of phopholipids. Fed. Proc.
     8: 360.

58. Kellner, A., J.W.Correll and A.T.Ladd. 1949. Modification of
     experimental atherosclerosis by means of intravenous deter-
     gents. Am. Heart J. 38: 460-461.

59. Payne, T.P.B. and G.L.Duff. 1950. The effect of Tween 80 on
     the serum lipids and the tissues of cholesterol-fed rabbits.
     Circulation 2: 471.

60. Payne, T.P.B. and G.L.Duff. 1951. Effect of Tween 80 on the
     serum lipids and the tissues of cholesterol-fed rabbits.
     Arch. Path. 51: 379-386.

61. Weigensberg, B.I., R.H.More, A. Sumiyoshi and B. Mullen.
     1974. Effects of sufactant on thromboatherosclerosis and
     cholesterol atherosclerosis. Exptl. Mol. Pathol. 20:154-167.

62. Stafford, W.W. and C.E.Day. 1975. Regression of atheroscler-
     osis effected by intravenous phospholipid. Artery 1: 106-114.

63. Adams, C.W.M., Y.H.Abdulla, O.B.Bayliss and R.S.Morgan. 1967
     Modification of aortic atheroma and fatty liver in cholesterol-
     fed rabbits by intravenous injection of saturated and poly-
     unsaturated lecithins. J. Path. Bact. 94: 77-87

64. Kwak, Y.S. and D.N.Kim. 1974. Acceleration of cholesterol-
     induced atherosclerosis in rabbits by lysosome stabilizers.
     Fed. Proc. 33: 623.

65. Hollander, W., H.L.McCombs, C. Franzblau, B. Kirkpatrick and
    K.Schmid. 1974. Influence of the anti-calcifying agent,
    ethane-1-hydroxy-1, 1-diphosphonate (EHDP) on pre-established
    atheromata in rabbits. Circulation. 50:III-93.

66. Carrier, O., Jr., B.R.Clower and P.J.Whittington. 1968.
    Inhibition of cholesterol-induced vascular lesion by dietary
    reserpine. J. Atheroscler. Res. 8: 229-236.

67. Chung, T.H. 1969. The effects of Lysium Chinense, Pachyma
    Hoelen and Acorus Calamus on serum lipoprotein cholesterol and
    cholesterol induced atherosclerosis in rabbits. J. Korean
    Med. Assoc. 12: 138-144.

68. Morrison, L.M., G.S.Bajwa, R.B. Alfin-Slater and B.H. Ershoff.
    1972. Prevention of vascular lesions by chondroitin sulfate
    A in the coronary artery and aorta of rats induced by a
    hypervitaminosis D, cholesterol-containing diet. Atheroscler-
    osis 16: 105-118.

69. Morin, R.J., G.G.Edralin and J.W.Woo. 1974. Esterification of
    cholesterol by subcellular fractions from swine arteries and
    inhibition by amphipathic and polyanionic compounds.
    Atherosclerosis 20: 27-39.

TURNOVER AND AORTIC UPTAKE OF VERY LOW DENSITY LIPOPROTEINS (VLDL) FROM HYPERCHOLESTEREMIC RABBITS AS A MODEL FOR TESTING ANTIATHEROSCLEROTIC COMPOUNDS

J. Rodriguez*, A. Catapano, G.C. Ghiselli and C.R. Sirtori

Center E. Grossi Paoletti for the Study of Metabolic Disease and Hyperlipidemias, University of Milano - 20129 Milano, Italy

*Visiting Scientist from the University of LaHabana, Cuba

ABSTRACT - VLDL from hypercholesteremic (HC) rabbits display features which are suggestive of inherent atherogenicity. The lipid composition, compared to that of control VLDL, shows an enrichment of cholesterol esters, which have a very high 18:1/18:2 ratio in their fatty acids, and an increased sphingomyelin content, with decreased PC/Sph ratio. This lipid composition is very similar to that of the atherosclerotic plaque. Apoprotein peptides of HC VLDL show a predominance of arg-rich proteins, similar to human conditions (Type III hyperlipoproteinemia and hypothyroidism) character- ized by early and severe atherosclerosis. Turnover of ^{125}I-labelled HC VLDL is significantly slower than that of control VLDL, both when the lipoprotein is injected into the donor animals and into controls. Conversion of HC VLDL into lipoproteins of higher density is also very small, as compared to control VLDL. Uptake of radioac- tivity into the aortic wall after injection is about doubled, as compared to control VLDL, when HC rabbits receive their own lipo- protein, and almost tripled when control rabbits receive HC VLDL. This experimental model suggests that structural modifications of HC VLDL make them poorly metabolizable, and possibly more akin to the recently described arterial lipoprotein complexing factor (ALCF). Metformin was selected as the test compound, because it has been shown to decrease aortic and liver lipid accumulation in cholesterol fed rabbits, while only slightly affecting plasma cholesterol levels. VLDL from rabbits fed cholesterol and metformin (HC+Met), while still enriched in cholesterol esters, have a higher protein content, less sphingomyelin and more phosphatidylethanola- mine and phosphatidylinositol than HC VLDL, while fatty acid compo- sition of cholesterol esters does not differ. Turnover of HC+Met VLDL is extremely rapid, with a t½ even shorter than that of control VLDL.

Apoprotein composition shows a decrease of both arg-rich and C
peptides. Affinity for the ALCF of this lipoprotein is very low,
as shown by the very small percentage of aortic uptake of radioactivity after injection, and by <u>in vitro</u> studies with isolated
ALCF.

INTRODUCTION

The formation of abnormal Very Low Density Lipoproteins (VLDL)
in rabbits after cholesterol feeding has been reported by several
authors (1,2) as well as by us (3). VLDL from hypercholesteremic
(HC) rabbits, as compared to control VLDL, have a 12-fold increase
of cholesterol esters, a markedly higher concentration of sphingomyelin, with a correspondent decrease of phosphatidylcholine/sphin-
gomyelin (PC/Sph) ratio, and almost a doubling of the 18:1 percentage in cholesterol esters.

These findings are reminiscent of the lipid composition of
the atherosclerotic plaque. In particular, the increase of sphingomyelin, with decreased PC/Sph ratio, is very similar to that
observed in the arterial wall phospholipids in aged subjects (4)
as well as in aged rabbits (5). Physicochemical data also indicate
that molecular configuration and cohesional forces tend to favour
a complex between sphingomyelin and cholesterol (6). The increased
18:1/18:2 ratio in cholesterol esters is considered a very sensitive prognostic index of clinical atherosclerosis (7), and it is
also found in the atherosclerotic plaques (8).

The apoprotein composition of HC VLDL shows a marked increase
of the R2 and R3 peptides, and a decrease of C peptides (1). By
separating HC VLDL into two subfractions, VLDL-1 and VLDL-2, we
noted that the former is practically only composed of R2 and R3
(3). These two peptides are rich in arginine and may correspond
to the arg-rich peptides found in conditions, such as human type
III hyperlipoproteinemia and hypothyroidism, where an increase of
cholesterol esters is accompanied by early and severe atherosclerosis (9,10).

The hypothesis of the intrinsic atherogenic   properties of

HC VLDL was further confirmed by turnover studies of ^{125}I labelled lipoproteins and by the determination of the aortic uptake of labelled lipoproteins in vivo (11). HC VLDL had a significantly longer t½ in the log normal phase that control lipoprotein, both when injected into the donor animals and into controls. Conversion of VLDL into low density lipoproteins (LDL), and into high density lipoproteins (HDL), while very rapid and almost complete for control VLDL, was very slow for HC VLDL. Up to 48 hours after the injection, in fact, about 60% of the remaining radioactivity was recovered in the VLDL fraction. Aortic radioactivity, determined one and two hours after injection, was more than doubled with HC VLDL, as compared with control VLDL.

Studies on the turnover and uptake of labelled lipoproteins, and particulary of HC VLDL, in rabbits provide therefore a model for the testing of drugs which affect the development of atherosclerosis.

We report here data on metformin, a biguanide drug in clinical use for the management of maturity onset diabetes (12), which has been shown to markedly reduce the development of atherosclerosis in cholesterol fed rabbits, while only moderately reducing cholesterol levels (13). This seemed to be a favourable situation to verify whether structural modifications of lipoproteins may be related to the development of atherosclerosis. Biochemical composition and turnover of lipoproteins are reported as well as results from studies on the interaction of lipoproteins with the recently described arterial lipoprotein complexing factor (ALCF) (14).

MATERIALS AND METHODS

Male New Zealand rabbits (2.8-3 kg) were used in all experiments. They received either a control pellet diet (Control group); or the same with the addition of 2 g cholesterol (adsorbed on 25 g of pellets

after being dissolved in diethyl ether), fed every morning after
an overnight fast (HC group); or metformin (135 mg/kg per day)
mixed with the normal diet and divided into two daily administrations
(Met group); or cholesterol and metformin (HC+Met group). After
4 weeks of treatment, rabbits were bled from an ear vein, and
cholesterol (14), triglycerides (15), phospholipids (16), and glucose[+] were determined.   A preparative ultracentrifugation was
carried out to separate lipoproteins with density: <1.019 (VLDL);
1.019-1.063 (LDL); and 1.063-1.21 (HDL) (18). Each lipoprotein,
after separation, was recentrifuged at the same density used
for isolation.

Lipoproteins were extensively dialysed against NaCl 0.15 M+
EDTA-Na$_2$ 0.01 M (pH 7.4) prior to lipid and protein analysis.
Chemical composition was assessed for each lipoprotein class of the
control, HC, Met, HC+Met groups. Fatty acids of cholesterol esters,
triglycerides and phospholipids, were determined by gas liquid
chromatography after direct transesterification (19). The apoprotein peptide composition was analysed by polyacrylamide gel
electrophoresis (20). Electron microscopy was carried out according
to Stange et al. (21).

VLDL from each group of rabbits were labelled with Na^{125}I
according to McFarlane (22), as modified by Bilheimer and Eisenberg
(23), and reinjected i.v. into the donor animals, or, in the case
of lipoproteins from the HC and HC+Met groups, also into control
rabbits. Each animal received 1.2-1.5 mg of protein in a volume of
0.4-0.5 ml, containing 10^7 cpm. Blood samples were collected from
the ear veins at intervals up to 48 hours. Labelled VLDL had the
same electrophoretic mobility in agarose as unlabelled material·
Labelled lipids never exceeded 14.6% of the total radioactivity,
and more than 96% of the total radioactivity was TCA precipitable.

The radioactivity of collected plasma samples was determined,
and the t$\frac{1}{2}$ of the distribution and log-normal phase was calculated,

---

[+]Enzymatic Glucose Kit, Carlo Erba Milano

as well as the fractional catabolic rates (24). Plasmas at different
intervals were pooled and adjusted to the proper densities to
determine radioactivity distribution in plasma lipoproteins. Aortic
radioactivity was measured two hours after injection (25): this
interval had provided the most reproducible findings in our previous
experiments (11). Aortic and liver lipids were also determined.

ALCF was prepared according to Camejo _et al_. (14), with some
modifications. We noted that complexing properties and protein
composition (26) did not differ in the various treatment groups.
Data reported here refer to ALCF isolated from rabbits with only
initial atheromatosis. ALCF-lipoprotein complexes were examined by
electron microscopy (21) before and after incubation and ultracentrifugation. Fig. 1 shows typical complexes of human LDL with an ALCF

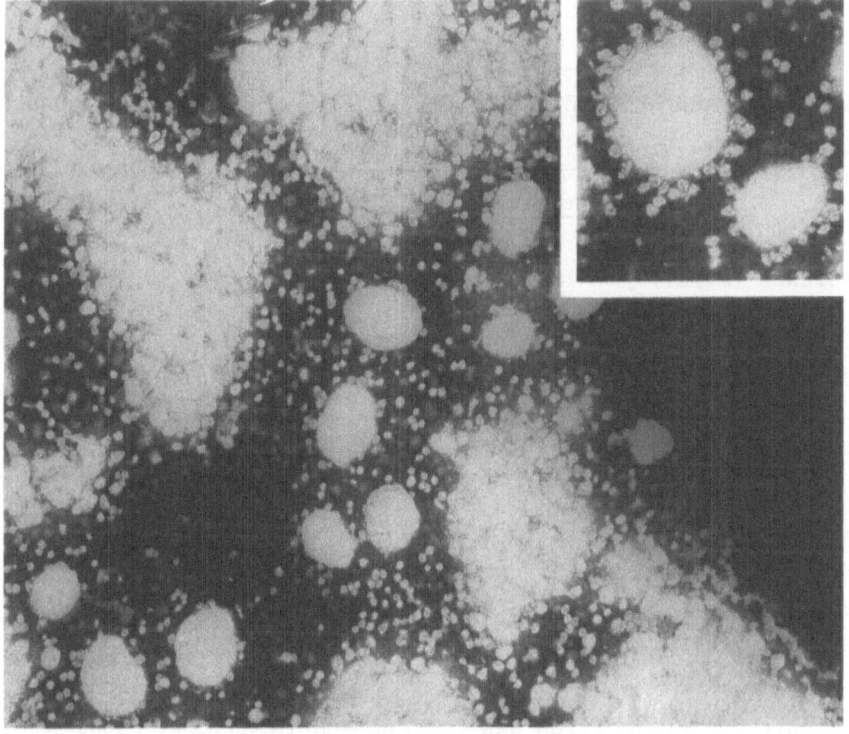

FIGURE 1

Complexes between human arterial lipoprotein complexing factor
and human LDL. x 20,000 (Insert x 40,000). (Reduced 15% for
reproduction.)

isolated from a human aorta. Cholesterol concentration was measured
in each insoluble complex after a brief ultracentrifugation.

RESULTS

Metformin administration significantly lowered plasma cholesterol and phospholipids, but not triglycerides,in rabbits on a normal
diet (Met group) (Table 1). On the other hand, in the HC+Met
group, cholesterol was lowered about 30% on the average, as
compared to the HC group, but levels remained generally high with
several rabbits in the two groups having practically overlapping
levels. Triglycerides in the HC+Met group were higher than in
the HC group, while phospholipids were significantly decreased by
the pharmacological treatment. Glucose levels did not differ
significantly in any of the four groups.

TABLE I

PLASMA LIPID AND GLUCOSE LEVELS IN THE FOUR EXPERIMENTAL GROUPS
    (data after 4 weeks; 6 rabbits per group; $\overline{X} \pm$ S.D.)

	Control	Met	HC	HC+Met
CHOLESTEROL (mg/dl)	74$\pm$11	26$\pm$4 [+]	1403$\pm$297 [++]	978$\pm$89°
TRIGLYCERIDES (mg/dl)	74$\pm$8	83$\pm$21	55$\pm$37	134$\pm$61
PHOSPHOLIPIDS (mg/dl)	150$\pm$10	96$\pm$9 [+]	506$\pm$34 [++]	300$\pm$55°°
GLUCOSE (mg/dl)	94$\pm$8	98$\pm$10	86$\pm$13	98$\pm$4

[+] $P < 0.05$; [++] $P < 0.01$ compared to controls.
° $P < 0.05$; °° $P < 0.01$ compared to HC

Lipoprotein composition was not changed in control rabbits
treated with Met (Met Group). On the other hand, composition of
VLDL of the HC and HC+Met groups differed markedly (Table II).

TABLE   II

% COMPOSITION OF DIFFERENT VLDL ($\bar{X}$+SD)

(data from 4 different samples)

	Control	HC	HC+Met
PROTEIN	18.50+1.2	8.10+0.8[+]	20.5+1.8
PHOSPHOLIPIDS	17.30+0.9	19.41+1.1	20.5+0.5
TRIGLYCERIDES	52.98+1.7	13.13+1.2[++]	7.5+0.6°°
FREE CHOL.	9.12+0.9	10.87+1.1	14.5+0.9°
CHOL. ESTERS	5.14+0.6	63.10+1.8[++]	36.7+1.8°°

[+]P <0.05; [++]P <0.01 compared to controls.

°P <0.05; °°P <0.01 compared to HC

In VLDL from the HC+Met group, protein concentration is
practically normal, the percentage of cholesterol esters is lower
than in the HC group, and the free cholesterol is significantly
higher. Concentrations of VLDL triglycerides and phospholipids in
these two groups of rabbits do not differ. Electrophoretic mobilities in agarose gel of HC and HC+Met VLDL are similar, i.e. both
lipoproteins show β mobility. By electron microscopy HC+Met VLDL,
in contrast to HC VLDL, appears to be very homogeneous, with few
particles of large size.

Phospholipid distribution, as already pointed out, shows, in
HC VLDL, a marked increase of sphingomyelin, with a decreased
PC/Sph ratio. In VLDL from the HC+Met group (Table III), sphingomyelin concentration is significantly lower than in HC VLDL. While
the PC/Sph ratio is still reduced, there is a remarkable increase

TABLE III

PHOSPHOLIPID DISTRIBUTION OF VLDL IN CONTROL (C), HYPERCHOLESTEREMIC (HC), AND
HYPERCHOLESTEREMIC TREATED WITH METFORMIN (HC+Met) GROUPS ($\overline{X}$+SEM)

	C(n=5)	HC(n=5)	HC+Met(n=5)
Origin of chromatograms	2.32+0.26	1.95+0.1	1.29+0.42
Phosphatidylcholine	72.16+1.13	62.49+0.5$^+$	62.15+1.07
Lysophosphatidylcholine	4.16+0.6	5.57+0.6	6.20+0.81
Phosphatidylinositol	3.03+0.05	2.68+0.06	6.98+0.82$^{\circ\circ}$
Sphingomyelin	6.68+0.42	21.58+0.4^{++}	16.74+0.42$^{\circ\circ}$
Phosphatidylethanolamine	12.14+0.44	3.66+0.2^{++}	6.12+0.61$^{\circ\circ}$

$^+$p <0.05 as compared to controls

$^{++}$p <0.01 as compared to controls

$^{\circ\circ}$p <0.01 as compared to the HC group

in these lipoproteins of phosphatidylinositol, which is twice as
high as in control VLDL. Phosphatidylethanolamine concentration is
intermediate between that of control and HC VLDL.

Fatty acid composition of cholesterol esters, tryglicerides,
and phospholipids does not differ in HC and HC+Met VLDL. Also in
drug treated animals there is an increase of 18:1 percentage in
cholesterol esters, similar to that in HC VLDL.

Apoprotein composition of VLDL from the HC+Met group is
different from that of control and HC VLDL (Fig.2).

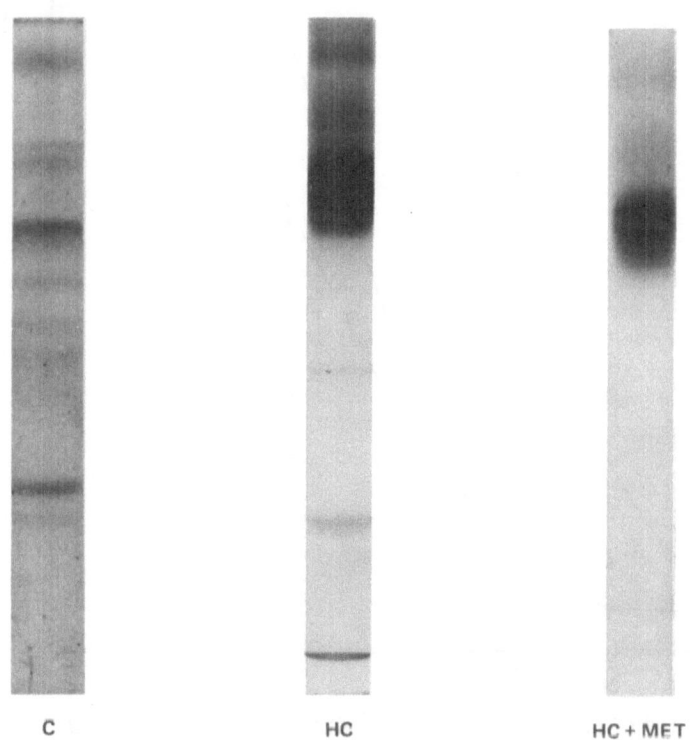

C   HC   HC + MET

FIGURE 2

Gel electrophoresis of VLDL from control (C), hypercholesteremic
(HC), and hypercholesteremic+metformin (HC+Met) groups.200 γ of
protein were applied to the first two gels, 100 γ to the third.

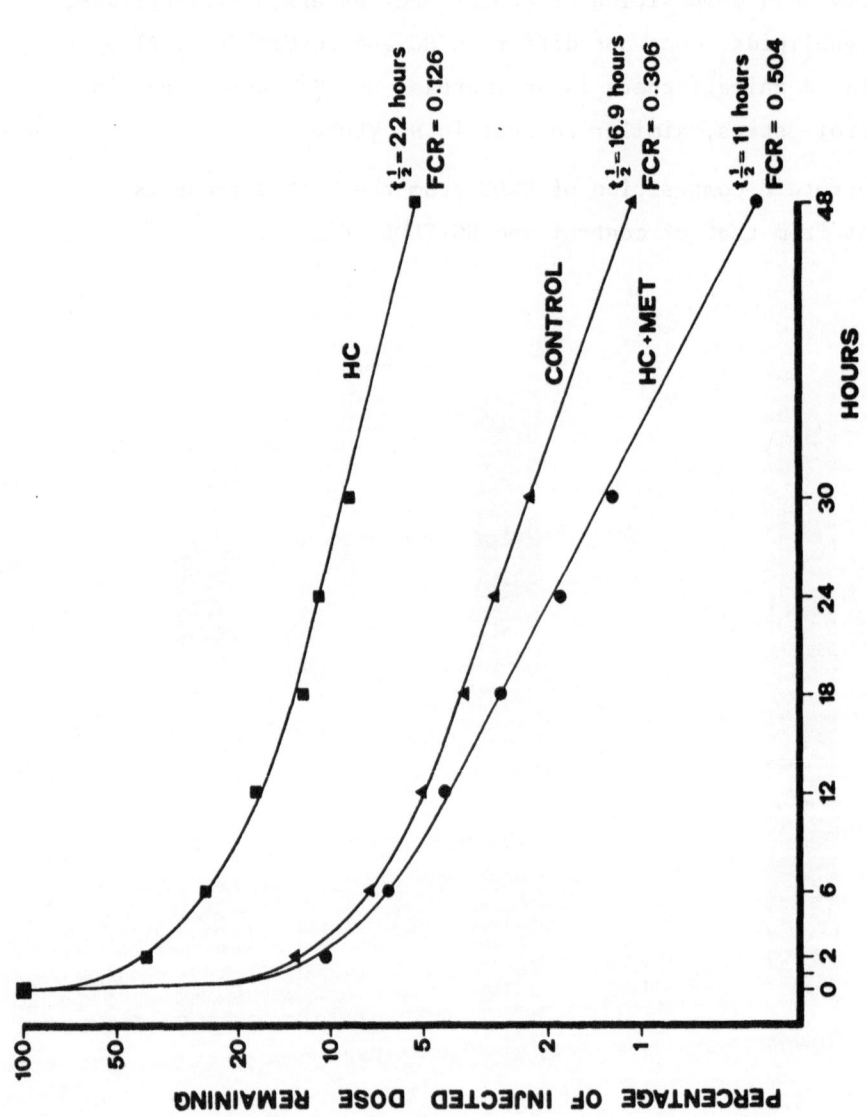

FIGURE 3

Plasma decay curves of ^{125}I labeled very low density lipoproteins when injected into control rabbits.

HC VLDL is characterized by an increase of arg-rich proteins
(R2-R3), and a decrease of C peptides. VLDL from the HC+Met group
has a lower concentration of peptides with the same mobility of
arg-rich proteins, and a practically complete absence of fast C
peptides. It may be noted, that in our electrophoretic system
arg-rich proteins appear to be constituted by more than two
peptides; separation of HC VLDL peptides by anion exchange
chromatography had indicated that R2-R3 were composed of at least
four different peptides (1).

Studies on the turnover of ^{125}I labelled VLDL provided evidence for an extremely rapid turnover of the lipoproteins from the
HC+Met rabbits. While, in fact, VLDL of the Met group behave
identically to control lipoproteins, HC+Met VLDL has a significantly shorter $t\frac{1}{2}$ in the log-normal phase than both control and
HC lipoproteins. This is true both when HC and HC+Met lipoproteins
are injected into the same donor animals or into controls. Fig. 3
reports plasma radioactivity decay curves of control, HC and
HC+Met VLDL when injected into control rabbits.

Analysis of the distribution of radioactivity in plasma
lipoproteins at different intervals indicates that control and
Met VLDL behave similarly, i.e. radioactivity is immediately
transferred to HDL. On the other hand, the largest portion of
radioactivity of HC VLDL, both when injected into the donor animals
or into controls, remains in VLDL. The behaviour of VLDL from the
HC+Met group is similar to that of control VLDL, i.e.there is a
rapid transfer of radioactivity to LDL, and later to HDL. Table IV
reports the distribution of radioactivity at different intervals
when VLDL from the various groups are injected into control rabbits.

Aortic uptake of radioactivity, measured one and two hours
after the injection of labelled lipoproteins, is highest in the
case of HC VLDL, and lowest with HC+Met VLDL, even lower than the
uptake observed after the injection of control VLDL (Fig. 4).

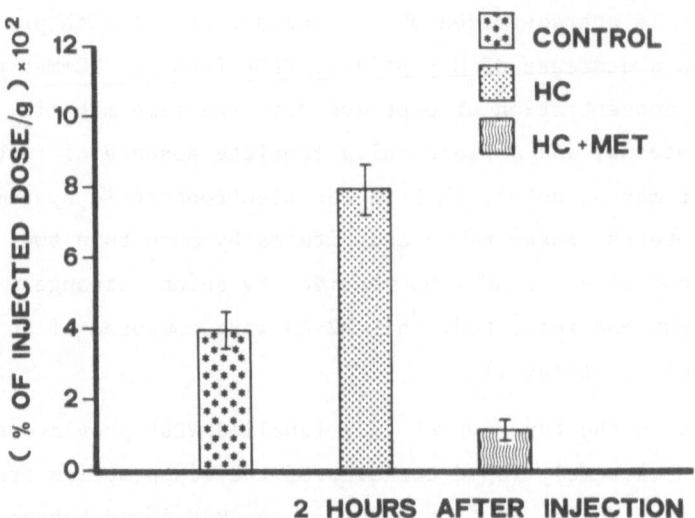

FIGURE 4

Aortic uptake of radioactivity following injection of different VLDL
into control rabbits. ($\overline{X}$+S.D. of six experimental data)

Interaction of the ALCF with different lipoproteins (Table V)
was also investigated, by measuring cholesterol bound in the
insoluble complex, after incubation and a brief ultracentrifugation.
While both VLDL and LDL from control rabbits have a negligible
interaction, lipoproteins from the HC rabbits form very thick
precipitates, with a very large cholesterol concentration. Both LDL
and VLDL from HC+Met rabbits, when added to the ALCF, cause the
formation of insoluble precipitates. These are, however, far less
conspicuous than with HC VLDL and LDL, and complexed cholesterol
is about half that seen with HC VLDL and LDL.

TABLE IV

DISTRIBUTION OF RADIOACTIVITY AMONG PLASMA LIPOPROTEINS FOLLOWING
INJECTION OF DIFFERENT ^{125}I-VLDL INTO CONTROL RABBITS

(each figure is the mean of three experiments; at each interval,
from top to bottom, control VLDL, HC VLDL, HC+Met VLDL).

TIME	VLDL	LDL	HDL	
1/20 hr	27.66	37.38	36.95	C
	52.50	38.22	9.26	HC
	12.86	55.18	31.96	HC+Met
1/2 hr	27.30	28.15	44.54	
	56.90	37.32	5.88	
	17.07	50.26	32.67	
1 hr	27.94	20.95	51.09	
	57.80	36.10	6.10	
	23.57	40.56	35.87	
2 hr	32.12	19.60	48.28	
	52.52	42.30	5.18	
	30.50	31.40	38.10	
6 hr	34.01	17.31	48.68	
	51.00	44.40	5.60	
	30.18	24.72	45.09	
12 hr	35.42	17.19	47.45	
	50.60	43.20	6.20	
	27.44	30.05	47.49	
24 hr	38.29	17.60	44.10	
	50.81	43.00	6.19	
	26.98	22.20	50.82	
30 hr	34.11	16.06	49.83	
	51.82	43.52	5.66	
	27.36	22.09	50.55	
48 hr	34.11	16.10	48.79	
	52.20	41.20	6.60	
	26.01	22.55	51.49	

TABLE V

INSOLUBLE COMPLEXES BETWEEN AORTIC COMPLEXING FACTOR AND DIFFERENT
PLASMA LIPOPROTEINS

Lipoproteins	Chol. in complex[+] ($\overline{X}$+SEM)	No. of Expt
A) CONTROL		
VLDL	0	(5)
LDL	11.2+4.7	(5)
B) HC GROUP		
VLDL	461+102	(7)
LDL	583+ 98	(7)
C) HC+Met GROUP		
VLDL	201+ 25 °°	(7)
LDL	376+ 31 °°	(7)

[+] μg of cholesterol/mg of aortic protein
°° P <0.01 as compared to HC group

DISCUSSION

Investigations on the mode of action of drugs affecting the
development of the atherosclerotic process, both in man and in
experimental animals, have generally considered quantitative
changes in biochemical parameters, such as plasma lipid and lipoprotein levels, or quantitative and qualitative changes of
coagulative mechanisms. Little attention has been paid to changes
of lipid and lipoprotein metabolism, when these are not accompanied
by marked quantitative changes. Our data report an experimental
situation where a reduction in severity of cholesterol induced
atherosclerosis is likely to be related to changes in structure
and turnover of specific lipoprotein classes.

Turnover studies with labelled lipoproteins in man have pointed out that delayed clearances are generally due to removal defects. Langer et al. (27), in type II patients, noted a remarkable prolongation of the apparent $t\frac{1}{2}$ of LDL. Although conflicting data had been previously reported (28), very recent studies have pointed out a delayed clearance of LDL in homozygous and heterozygous type II patients (29). Moreover, LDL from type II patients is cleared at a normal rate by normal individuals, while the opposite takes place in type II patients receiving normal LDL (30).

Similar studies on VLDL have shown that triglyceride-rich lipoproteins have a rapid turnover rate, as compared to other lipoproteins, and are efficiently converted to higher density classes both in vivo and in vitro (31). Our data on the metabolic fate of normal (triglyceride-rich) ^{125}I-VLDL in rabbits confirm a rapid transfer of radioactivity to both LDL and HDL (see Table IV), similar to human (23) and rat (32) VLDL. These results are attributed to an exchange of low molecular weight peptides (C proteins) between VLDL and HDL, while the LDL apoprotein moiety of VLDL moves to LDL (33).

Our observation of a delayed clearance of HC VLDL in rabbits may not be explained by a removal defect, since both normal and HC rabbits clear these lipoproteins at a similar rate (11). Structural modifications of these lipoproteins are the most likely cause for their delayed clearance. This has also been suggested for VLDL of human type III hyperlipoproteinemia, in a preliminary study by Bilheimer et al. (34), where a delayed clearance as well as a delayed conversion to lipoproteins of higher density were demonstrated.

Structural changes of HC VLDL include: enrichment of cholesterol esters, increased sphingomyelin content, with decreased PC/Sph ratio, increased percentage of 18:1 in cholesterol esters, presence of arginine rich apoproteins, similar to those occurring in type III disease and hypothyroidism. HC VLDL also shows a β mobility in

agarose electrophoresis, and lipoprotein particles are larger and
more heterogeneous than those of control VLDL.

Metformin was tested on this experimental model to investigate
the relationship between structural modifications of lipoproteins,
independent of plasma total lipid levels, and the development of
atherosclerotic lesions. It had, in fact, been reported that
administration of this drug together with cholesterol (13) only
slightly affects plasma lipids, while markedly reducing the extent
of atherosclerotic lesions. We could confirm both an inconstant
(approximately 40%) reduction of plasma total cholesterol, as well
as a clear-cut decrease of atherosclerotic lesions and aortic
cholesterol content.

VLDL from rabbits fed cholesterol and metformin (HC+Met) have
an increased protein content, some decrease of cholesterol esters
(which are, however, about 6 times higher than in controls), and
maintain a β mobility in electrophoresis. The major differences
between HC VLDL and HC+Met VLDL are found in the phospholipid
distribution and in the apoprotein composition.

The decreased sphingomyelin concentration, as already pointed
out (4,5,6) makes the lipoprotein composition less similar to that
of the atherosclerotic plaque, and may also be related to the decreased cholesterol content of the lipoproteins. The significance
of the phosphatidylinositol increase, even above the percentage
found in control lipoproteins, is very difficult to explain. Although
several data are available on the possible role of phosphatidylinositol in brain function (35), information on the relationship between
this phospholipid and atherosclerosis in general, are scanty. We
can only report here that phosphatidylinositol concentration is
higher in the arteries of women (36), and that an inhibitory effect
on cholesterol biosynthesis has been demonstrated (37).

Apoprotein composition of HC+Met VLDL shows a reduction of
proteins with mobility corresponding to R2-R3 (arg-rich), as well as

of C peptides. Similar changes had been reported for VLDL from
sucrose fed rats treated with clofibrate (38). These apoprotein
changes, although not clarifying the mechanism by which HC+Met VLDL
is so rapidly metabolized, may be consistent with a more efficient
interaction of these lipoproteins with peripheral removal mechanisms.
It has been recently demonstrated that the liver is the major site
of removal for VLDL cholesterol esters (39). And, possibly, only in
the case of control and HC+Met VLDL is this mechanism fully operant,
while, with HC VLDL, liver removal is inadequate, and both liver
infiltration and atheromatosis may take place.

The other interesting finding is the very low uptake of HC+Met
VLDL into the arterial wall. This was demonstrated both in vivo,
by measuring the fraction of radioactivity remaining in the aorta
at different intervals after injection, and in vitro, on the isolated
ALCF. The data in vivo indicate that aortic radioactivity is even
lower after labelled HC+Met VLDL than after control VLDL. On the
other hand, data in vitro with the ALCF, show significantly less
formation of insoluble complexes with HC+Met lipoproteins (both
VLDL and LDL) than with HC. A discrepancy between these findings
is that, while radioactivity uptake of HC+Met is significantly
below that of control lipoproteins, the interaction of HC+Met
lipoproteins with the ALCF is far from negligible. This apparent
discrepancy is due to the different parameter which is measured in
each case (protein radioactivity in the experiment in vivo, bound
lipids in the case of the ALCF), as well as to the still enigmatic
role of the ALCF. It is not known whether this arterial structure
only binds lipoproteins or also catabolizes them, similar to the
LDL receptor described by Brown et al. (40).

In conclusion, our study points out a situation of decreased
atherogenicity in the presence of elevated plasma lipid levels.
Structural modifications of VLDL, leading to a rapid turnover and
a decreased interaction with arterial wall binding components, are
the tentative explanations for these experimental findings. This

study also shows that HC rabbits may provide a valuable test
for antiatherosclerotic compounds by allowing, within the same
experiment, determination of lipid and lipoprotein level, structure,
turnover, and interaction, both in vivo and in vitro with arterial
wall complexing factors.

ACKNOWLEDGMENTS

Mr. and Mrs. Gino and Gina Caliari are gratefully acknowledged for
taking care, patiently and competently, of our animals. Dr. Lisa
Innocenti, Miss Claudia Fragiacomo, and Miss Donatella Moltoni
carefully collaborated in the laboratory work. Metformin was
a gift of Spemsa Aron (Florence), through the kind interest of
Drs. Nesi and Cocuzza.

REFERENCES

1. Camejo, G. and A. Lopez. 1974. The very low density lipoproteins
   of cholesterol-fed rabbits: a study of their structure and in vivo
   changes in plasma. Atherosclerosis 19: 139-152.

2. Shore, V.G., B. Shore, and R.G. Hart. 1974. Changes in apolipoproteins andproperties of rabbit very low density lipoproteins on
   induction of cholesteremia. Biochemistry 13: 1579-1586.

3. Rodriguez, J., G.C. Ghiselli, D. Torreggiani, and C.R. Sirtori.
   1975. Very low density lipoproteins in normal and cholesterol
   fed rabbits: lipid and protein composition and metabolism. I.
   Chemical composition of very low density lipoproteins in rabbits.
   Atherosclerosis, in press.

4. Smith, E.B. 1965. The influence of age and atherosclerosis on
   the chemistry of the aortic intima. J. Atheroscler. Res. 5: 224-
   240.

5. Eisenberg, S., Y. Stein, and O. Stein. 1969. Phospholipases in
   arterial tissue: III Phosphatide acyl-hydrolase, lysophosphatide-
   acyl hydrolase and sphingomyelin cholinephosphohydrolase in rat
   and rabbit aorta in different age groups. Biochim. Biophys. Acta
   176: 557-572.

6. Patton, S. 1970. Correlative relationship of cholesterol and
   sphingomyelin in cell membranes. J. Theoret. Biol. 29: 489-496.

7. Kingsbury, K.J., D.M. Morgan, R. Stovold, C.G. Brett, and J.
   Anderson. 1969. Polyunsaturated fatty acids in myocardial
   infarction. Lancet ii: 1325-1328.

8. Chalvardjan, A.M., and J.S. Still. 1964. Fatty acid composition of tissues in cholesterol fed rabbits. J. Atheroscler. Res. 4: 507-514.

9. Havel, R.J. and J.P. Kane. 1973. Primary dysbetalipoproteinemia: Predominance of a specific apoprotein species in triglyceride-rich very low density lipoproteins. Proc. Nat. Acad. Sci. 70: 2015-2019.

10. Shore, B., V. Shore, A. Salel, D. Mason, and R. Zelis. 1974. An apolipoprotein preferentially enriched in cholesteryl ester-rich very low density lipoproteins. Biochem. Biophys. Res. Comm. 58: 1-7.

11. Rodriguez, J., A. Catapano, G.C. Ghiselli, and C.R. Sirtori. 1975. Very low density lipoproteins in normal and cholesterol fed rabbits. II. Metabolism of very low density lipoproteins in rabbits. Atherosclerosis, in press.

12. Sterne, J. 1964. The present state of knowledge on the mode of action on the antidiabetic diguanides. Metabolism 13: 791-798.

13. Agid, R., and G. Marquiè. 1969. Effects préventifs du NN'diméthyl-biguanide sur le developpement de l'athérosclérose induite par le cholesterol chez le lapin. C.R. Acad. Sci. Paris 269: 1000-1003.

14. Camejo, G., A. Lopez, H. Vegas, and H. Paoli. 1975. The participation of aortic proteins in the formation of complexes between low density lipoproteins and intima-media extracts. Atherosclerosis 21: 77-91.

15. Block, V.D., J. Jarrett, and J.B. Levine. 1965. Use of a single color reagent to improve the automated determination of serum cholesterol. Technicon Symposia on Automation in Analytical Chemistry. New York, Mediad Inc., pp. 345-349.

16. Noble, R.P., and F.M. Campbell. 1970. Improved accuracy in automated fluorimetric determination of plasma triglycerides. Clin. Chem. 16: 166-170.

17. Rouser, G., S. Fleischer, and A. Yamamoto. 1970. Two dimensional thin layer chromatographic separation of polar lipids and determination of phospholipids by phosphorus analysis of spots. Lipids 5: 494-496.

18. Havel, R.J., H. A. Eder, and J.H. Bragdon. 1955. The distribution and chemical composition of ultracentrifugally separated lipoproteins in human serum. J. Clin. Invest. 34: 1345-1353.

19. Christie, W.W. 1973. Lipid Analysis. Pergamon Press, New York.

20. Kane, B.J. 1973. A rapid electrophoretic technique for identification of subunit species of apoproteins in serum lipoproteins. Anal. Biochem. 53: 497-506.

21. Stange, E., B. Agostini, and J. Papenberg. 1975. Changes in rabbit lipoprotein properties by dietary cholesterol, and saturated and

polyunsaturated fats. Atherosclerosis 22: 125-148.

22. Mc Farlane, A.S. 1958. Efficient trace-labelling of proteins
    with iodine. Nature 182: 53-54.

23. Bilheimer, D.W., S. Eisenberg, and R.I. Levy. 1972. Metabolism
    of very low density lipoproteins. I. Preliminary in vitro and
    in vivo investigations. Biochem. Biophys. Acta. 260: 212-224.

24. Sniderman, A.D., T.E. Carew, J.G. Chandler, and D. Steinberg.
    1974. Paradoxical increase in rate of catabolism of low density
    lipoproteins after hepatectomy. Science 183: 526-528.

25. Klimov, A.M., A.D. Denisenko, and E. Ya. Magracheva. 1974. Prepa-
    ration of tissue fluids of the vessel wall and determination of
    its lipoproteins. Atherosclerosis 19: 243-251.

26. Sirtori, C.R., L. Innocenti, A. Catapano, G.C. Ghiselli, and
    J. Rodriguez, to be published.

27. Langer, T., W. Strober, and R.I. Levy. 1972. The metabolism
    of low density lipoproteins in familial type II hyperlipoproteinemi
    J. Clin. Invest. 51: 1528-1535.

28. Walton, V.W., P.J. Scott, J. Verrier Jones, R.F. Fletcher, and
    T. Whitehead. 1963. Studies on low density lipoprotein turnover
    in relation to Atromid therapy. J. Atheroscler. Res. 3:396-414.

29. Feldman, H.A., H. Torsvik, A.M. Gifford, and R.S. Lees. 1974. Low
    density lipoprotein turnover in homozygous hyperbetalipoproteinemia.
    Circulation 50:III-71.

30. Reichl, D.S., L.A. Simons, and M.B. Myant. 1974. The metabolism
    of low density lipoproteins in a patient with familial hyperbeta-
    lipoproteinemia. Clin. Sci. 47: 635-639.

31. Eisenberg, S., D.W. Bilheimer, and R.I. Levy. 1972. The metabolism
    of very low density lipoprotein proteins. II. Studies on the
    transfer of apoproteins between plasma lipoproteins. Biochem.
    Biophys. Acta. 280: 94-112.

32. Eisenberg, S., and D. Rachmilewitz. 1973. Metabolism of rat plasma
    very low density lipoproteins. I. Fate in circulation of the whole
    lipoprotein. Biochem. Biophys. Acta. 326: 378-396.

33. Gydyl, N.E. 1974. A review of methods and metabolic studies asso-
    ciated with the radioiodination of lipoproteins. Clin. Chim. Acta
    52: 5-23.

34. Bilheimer, D.W., S. Eisenberg, and R.I. Levy. 1971. Abnormal metabo
    lism of very low density lipoproteins (VLDL) in type III hyperlipo-
    proteinemia. Circulation 44:II-196.

35. Ansell, G.B., R.M.C. Dawson, and J.N. Hawthorne. 1973. Form and
    Function of Phospholipids. Elsevier, Amsterdam, pp. 377-415.

36. Rouser, G., and R.D. Solomon. 1969. Changes in phospholipid compo-
    sition of human aorta with age. Lipids 4: 232-234.

37. Haven, G.T., and H.P. Jacobi. 1971. Effects of renal factors on in vitro hepatic cholesterol synthesis. Lipids 6: 751-757.

38. Roheim, P.S., D. Edelstein, and P. Segal. 1974. The effect of clofibrate on serum apolipoproteins in sucrose induced hyperlipo-proteinemia . Circulation 50: III-1044.

39. Faergeman, O., and R.J. Havel. 1975. Metabolism of cholesteryl esters of rat very low density lipoproteins. J. Clin. Invest. 55: 1210-1218.

40. Brown, M.S., S.E. Dana, and J.L. Goldstein. 1973. Regulation of 3-hydroxy-3-methylglutaryl coenzyme A reductase activity in human fibroblasts by lipoproteins. Proc. Nat. Acad. Sci. 70: 2162-2166.

EVALUATION OF THE PERMEABILITY PARAMETERS (INFLUX, EFFLUX AND VOLUME

OF DISTRIBUTION) OF ARTERIAL WALL FOR LDL AND OTHER PROTEINS

S. Ghosh, J.N. Finkelstein, D.B. Moss and J.S. Schweppe

Departments of Biochemistry and Medicine

Northwestern University Medical School, Chicago, IL

Atherosclerosis is generally considered to be a multifactorial disease; as such, the prevention or cure of the disease may be
approached at different levels, control of serum cholesterol or β-
lipoprotein being an important one. However, the ultimate manifes-
tation of the disease is in the arterial wall, and any prospective
drug will have to be effective in producing the beneficial action
at the arterial level. From this point of view it is of great importance to be able to monitor the effect of a drug on the relevant
processes at the arterial wall. For the present discussion the arterial permeability to serum proteins, low density lipoprotein (LDL)
in particular, will be taken as the relevant process.
    Permeability of arterial tissue to plasma macromolecules and
its alteration under different conditions have been invoked as important in atherosclerosis (1,2). Unfortunately, very often the
published data on permeability represent uptake of a label after one
given time (3-5). The uptake is a net effect and represents the
difference between at least two independent parameters, influx and
efflux. We shall describe the approach we took for measuring the
rates of influx and efflux of different serum proteins at the arterial wall with a view to formulating a kinetic model of the process
as well as establishing the minimum number of independent parameters
that can describe the process. It should be understood at the outset
that these parameters will be those coming out of kinetic analyses
and will only be macroscopic quantities for the whole tissue; none-
theless, our understanding of the physical process will have to await
such quantitative information.
    Several workers have attempted to characterize the process by
the use of cholesterol (6-8) as tracer and measured the uptake of
cholesterol radioactivity by arterial tissue. It has, however,
been shown that free cholesterol exchanges reversibly between lipo-

proteins and membranes (9,10) and the observed uptake of radioactivity in these studies cannot be readily interpreted as a net
transfer of LDL into the tissue. In a review Dayton and Hashimoto
remarked: "There exists no direct and totally convincing evidence
for net influx of cholesterol or its esters from plasma into intima"
(11). An approach to this problem may be to calculate the net influx
of LDL cholesterol esters into arterial wall as attempted by
Zilversmit and Hughes (12). We have, on the other hand, used radioactive iodine (I) label on the protein moiety to trace the movement
of LDL, as has been attempted by several previous investigators (13-
15).

There is still another important aspect of atherosclerosis research that we would like to mention at this point. Looking for the
cause of atherosclerosis very often one compares the tissue or metabolism say of normal rabbits with that of rabbits fed high cholesterol and with experimentally induced atherosclerosis. It is sometimes not appreciated that difference between the two may not necessarily be the cause but the effect of the trauma or disease. It is
possible that atherogenesis is a normal but slow process accompanying
aging (16); it may be accelerated by different insults to the organism, like dietary cholesterol, or by immunological or mechanical injury to the arterial wall. But the "normal" individual may be slowly
accumulating lipid in the arterial wall and giving way to a chain
of events leading to a well developed atheroma.

It is with this rationale that we focussed our attention on
studying arterial permeability in normal rabbits, not just as control
animals.

The basic questions we ask are: assuming that retention of
plasma LDL in the arterial wall is the primary event in atherogenesis,
is the influx of LDL or any other serum protein into the arterial wall
a normal process? If so, do they come in and go out fast, with the
difference between them for LDL being equal to the slow accumulation;
or does LDL enter only at the rate it accumulates, the removal being
almost ineffective?

We use for this purpose a simple model that can be solved on
the basis of the experiments. The model is similar to one used by
several workers earlier, in particular by Duncan et al.(17),and the
mathematical analysis follows in part their approach. The model does
not assume any particular molecular mechanism for the influx or efflux,
and aims only at quantitating the parameters that determine them under
a given condition.

KINETIC MODEL

The simplest model for the flux of a substance that is not ir-
reversibly retained in the wall, may be represented as follows:

$$\boxed{\text{Blood}} \underset{K_2}{\overset{K_1}{\rightleftharpoons}} \boxed{\text{Tissue}}$$

where K_1 and K_2 are fractional rate constants for unidirectional flux. This scheme is suitable not only for the flux of a substance like albumin or inulin but possibly also for LDL flux in normocholesteremic rabbit artery, assuming negligible irreversible deposition (vide supra).

The second aspect of this model is that the arterial wall is regarded here as a single compartment. This is not to regard it as a well-mixed homogeneous pool. Even if the tissue may have different regions with nonidentical permeability properties, it is always possible to describe the overall property of the tissue by an equivalent parameter.

Thirdly, both K_1 and K_2 may include more than one process. However, as long as the influx or efflux is proportional to the concentration at the originating side, and there is no phase difference between the component processes that can be important within the time limits of the experiment, this assumption is also a necessary one. A test of the validity of the second and third assumptions will be the accuracy with which the equations derived on this basis describe the experimental data.

The following equations may be derived from this model to be used for calculating the values of K_{in} and K_{out} from experimental data: We define

$$K_{app} \; (\mu l/cm^2/hr) = W_t/C_{pt} dt \qquad\qquad \text{equation 1}$$

Where W_t is the arterial uptake at time t in dpm/cm^2 and C_{pt} is the concentration in plasma in dpm/ml at time t. It can be shown that:

$$K_{app} = K_{in} - K_{out} \frac{\int (W_t/C_{po}) \; dt}{\int (C_p/C_{po}) \; dt} \qquad\qquad \text{equation 2}$$

Where $K_{in} = K_1 \cdot T$, C_{po} the plasma radioactivity at zero time, and $1/T$ the surface area of the artery per μl of interstitial fluid; K_{out} is the same as K_2 of the model. From normalized data on arterial uptake at different times and the serum decay of radioactivity, the two integrals can be evaluated. A plot of K_{app} vs. "Q", the coefficient of K_{out} in equation 2, is expected to be linear if scheme 1 is correct, and K_{in} and K_{out} can be obtained from the plot.

It can be shown that for a two compartment open system like in our model, the steady state levels of W (moles/cm²) and C_p (moles/ml) are given by:

$$W/C_p = K_{in}/K_{out} \qquad\qquad \text{equation 3}$$

From a knowledge of K_{in} and K_{out} one may thus estimate the tissue level of the substance (moles/cm² of tissue) as obtained by partitioning with plasma at steady state. A comparison between the ratio W/C_p for LDL and albumin, would indicate whether, compared to albumin,the lipoprotein is relatively enriched in concentration in the arterial tissue.

Since the model does not have net retention explicitly, the analysis cannot directly calculate it. Atherogenic potential in this model can only be correlated with the tissue level of LDL (i.e., K_{in}/K_{out}).

MATERIALS AND METHODS

The animals used in this study were New Zealand White male rabbits maintained on standard rabbit chow diet with an average serum cholesterol of 60 mg %.

Crystallized rabbit serum albumin (RSA) and γ-globulin were purchased from Miles Laboratory, Elkhart, Indiana, and used without further purification.

LDL (d 1.006-1.063) was isolated by ultracentrifugation (18) from mildly hyper-cholesterolemic (300 mg. % Cholesterol) rabbits maintained on lab chow with 1% cholesterol and 4% corn oil. The details of the experimental procedure will be published elsewhere. LDL used gave a single band by gel electrophoresis, immunoelectrophoresis and immunodiffusion.

The proteins were iodinated by a modification (19) of the ICl method of McFarlane (20) with high molar ratios of ICl to protein and at a relatively high pH (∿10) to maximize the protein/lipid iodination ratio. TCA soluble radioactivity of the preparations was in general less than 0.4% and a lipid bound radioactivity extractable by chloroform methanol was about 1-2%. The iodinated samples were rechecked for purity and denaturation by agarose gel electrophoresis, SDS-polyacrylamide gel electorophoresis and biological screening, as described below.

Autoradiography of the agarose gel electrophoretogram showed the protein band to be as sharp and having the same mobility as the original sample of protein. Counting of sections of SDS-PAGE column showed most (>95%) of the radioactivity to be confined to the apo-B peptide region (Fig. 1). For the biological screening, the iodinated LDL was injected into one rabbit and after allowing sufficient time for the disappearance of any denatured protein contaminant, LDL was re-isolated later from the rabbit and re-injected into a second one. The decay of the radioactivity in the plasma in the two rabbits was comparable showing that the iodinated LDL preparation behaved by and large like native LDL. A typical decay curve is shown in Fig. 2.

For experiments _in vivo_, a rabbit was injected with about 20 µCi of ^{125}I-LDL, the total quantity of LDL amounting to about 1 -2% of the plasma content. Plasma decay of radioactivity was monitored from 2 min. (∿5 X circulation time) until sacrifice of the animal. The 2 minute value of dpm/ml was regarded as the zero time value. At specified time the rabbit was anaesthesised by sodium pentobarbital (60 mg/kg i.v.) and the chest cavity opened to reach the thoracic aorta. After complete bleeding the thoracic aorta was washed with 100 ml of normal saline _in situ_ and carefully excised. The aorta was

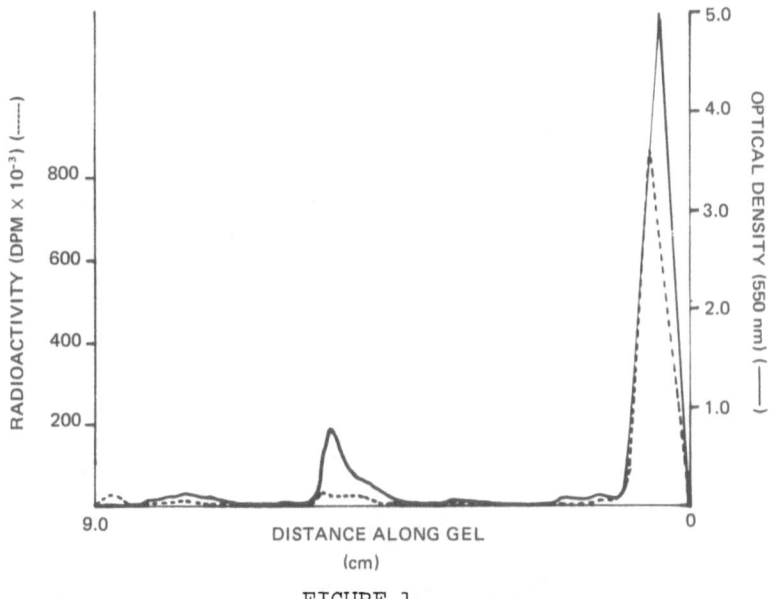

FIGURE 1

Protein and radioactivity distribution in a SDS-polyacrylamide gel
electrophoretogram of ^{125}I-LDL (———) cooamassie blue stain; (----)
radioactivity. Distance is from the top.

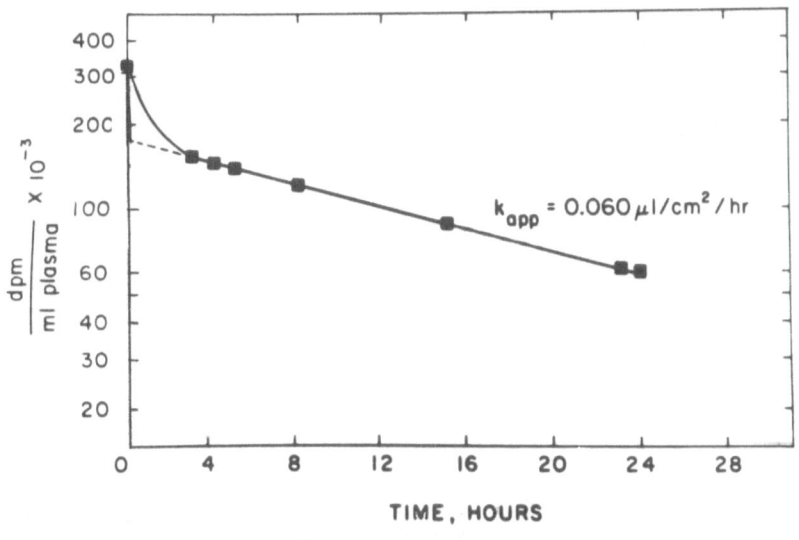

FIGURE 2

Decay of plasma radioactivity after injection of ^{125}I-LDL.

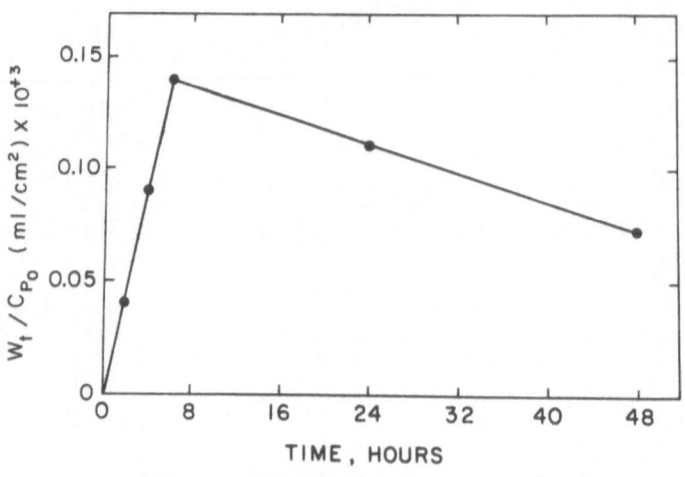

FIGURE 3

Arterial uptake of [125]I- albumin as fraction of initial dose.

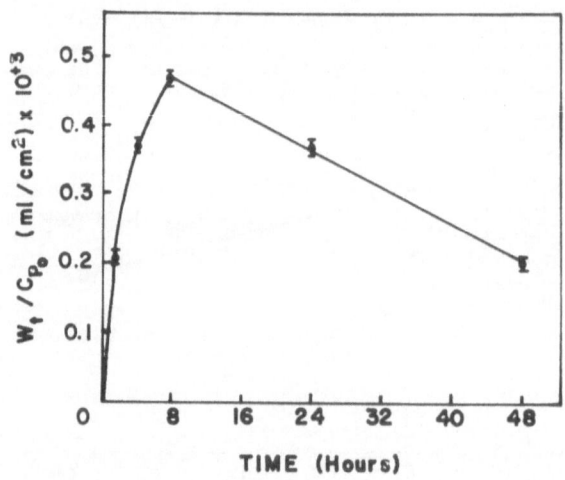

FIGURE 4

Arterial uptake of ^{125}I-LDL as fraction of initial dose.

cut longitudinally along the intercostal ostia and small punches were
cut with a small cork-borer. The intima-media was carefully separated
and counted. As defined above, K_{app} is calculated as the observed
dpm/cm^2 of the intima-media per average serum radioactivity. The
latter quantity is obtained from the area under the serum radioactivity vs. time curve (Fig. 2).

Fig. 3 shows a plot of average W/C_{p_0} vs. time for albumin showing an initial rise, a plateau at about 6 hours after injection and
then a slow decay. Fig. 4 shows a similar plot for LDL. Results of
uptake, when expressed as percent of the initial dose showed very
little variation between animals.

From these two types of curves, the integrals of equation (1)
could be evaluated. Fig. 5 shows the plot of K_{app} vs. Q for albumin
and LDL.

RESULTS OF EXPERIMENTS IN VIVO

Results of the experiments in vivo show that first, within the
time limits of the experiments, the plot of K_{app} vs. Q is linear as
expected from equation 2; and, therefore, the influx and efflux may
be described by the simple kinetic model. The values of K_{in} and
K_{out} for RSA, γ-globulin and LDL are shown in Table I. It may be
observed that while the values of K_{in} of albumin and γ-globulin are
inversely related to their sizes, LDL which is the largest of
the proteins has an anomalously high value.

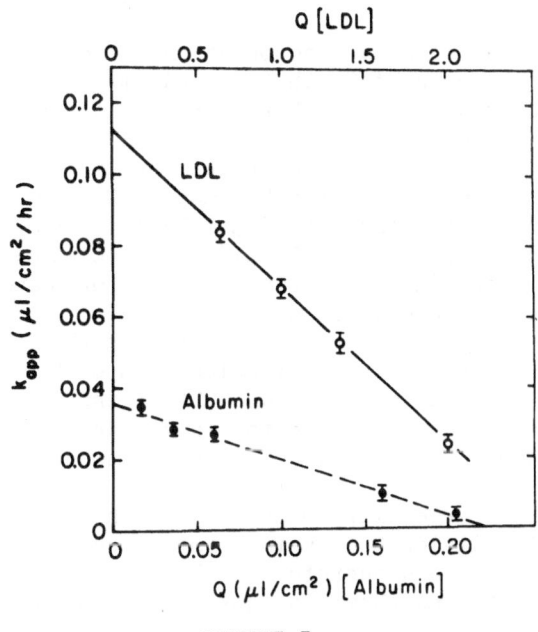

FIGURE 5

Plot of equation 2 for albumin and LDL.

TABLE I

Kinetic Parameters of in vivo Transport of Proteins into Rabbit
Thoracic Aorta.

	K_{in} ($\mu l/cm^2/hr$)	K_{out} (hr^{-1})	K_{in}/K_{out} ($\mu l/cm^2$)
LDL	0.113	0.44	2.57
RSA	0.036	0.163	0.221
γ-globulin	0.027	0.015	0.18

The inverse size dependence of the former two is in keeping with
the observations of Bell et al. (21) about the arterial uptake of
albumin and fibrinogen and suggest the possibility of a sieving
action by the gel-like extracellular matrix of the arterial wall.
The very high value of LDL may represent a distinctly different
(maybe an additional and/or parallel) pathway for LDL to get into
the tissue. Hypothetically these may be the binding sites say on
the arterial mucopolysaccharides, elastin, or even membrane receptor sites.

From the rate of accumulation of cholesterol in an artery one
may calculate the rate of accumulation of LDL, assuming cholesterol
coming only from LDL.

Based on a value of 2 µg. accumulation in 38 years, a value
obtained from the results of Smith (22) and Smith et al. (23), Stein
and Stein (24) calculated the number of LDL molecules entering arterial intima. The number turns out to be 1.35×10^8 molecules/cm^2/hr.
A K_{in} value of 0.113 $\mu l/cm^2$/hr. determined by us may also be used to
calculate the number of moles of LDL crossing 1 sq.cm per hour – and
it turns out to be of the order of 2.3×10^{11} molecules/cm^2/hr based
on a serum LDL concentration of 750 mg% and a molecular weight of 2.2
million (assuming for simplicity the same K_{in} for human as in rabbit,
and a serum cholesterol level of about 250mg%).

The rate of entry therefore is higher than the rate of retention by a factor of about 10^3. The number approaches the lower limit
of the number of vesicles calculated by Stein and Stein. We may
point out, however, that there are too many approximations involved
in these calculations and the actual numbers should be interpreted
with caution.

Because of the large difference between the influx and retention, in a normal individual or animal the situation is more like
that of a steady state and therefore influx ≃ efflux. This condition
leads to the equality, as shown in Equation (3) before:

$$\frac{\text{Concentration of LDL in arterial tissue}/cm^2}{\text{Concentration of LDL in plasma} \quad /\mu l} = \frac{K_{in}}{K_{out}} = 2.57$$

The values of this ratio for the three proteins are shown in the last column in Table I. The ratio represents the LDL concentration in the arterial tissue compared to that of plasma. The similar ratio for albumin is 0.22 so that compared to albumin, LDL is about 10 fold enriched in the wall compared to plasma. It is probable that the enrichment will be related to the ultimate retention. Although this should not be regarded as established at the moment, Dayton (25) while comparing cholesterol influx into abdominal vs. thoracic aorta in chicken came to a similar conclusion.

EXPERIMENTS IN VITRO

While the parameters K_{in} and K_{out} could be obtained from in vivo measurements alone, as shown in Equation 2, K_{in} has the unknown parameter T, $\mu l/cm^2$ - the volume of distribution or the apparent volume available to the molecule in the tissue. This can be more suitably measured by equilibrium experiments in vitro.

Measurements in vitro were performed with freshly isolated thoracic aorta of normo-cholesteremic rabbits. The aorta was washed in normal saline. Small pieces were cut out avoiding arch, bifurcation and intercostal ostia. The tissue samples were then incubated at 37° C. in lactated Ringer solution containing a marker substance with radioactive label. The markers included ^{125}I-LDL and ^{125}I-albumin as above, ^{14}C - dextran of molecular weight 16,000 and ^{14}C inulin. The uptake of radioactivity in the intima media was determined as before. From the values of the equilibrium uptake of labeled material and the external concentration, the apparent tissue space (T) available to the marker could be calculated. Table II shows the values for the different markers used. It is seen that, except for LDL, the volume is inversely proportional to the molecular size. This is to be expected if the distribution volume refers to the extracellular matrix of the arterial tissue with the excluded volume effect of the connective tissue macromolecules restricting the volume available to the marker. As in experiments in vivo, the uptake of LDL was abnormally high, suggesting the existence of a specific

TABLE II

Apparent Tissue Space in vitro for Different Markers in Rabbit Thoracic Aorta.

Marker	Apparent Tissue Space ($\mu l/cm^2$)
Inulin	8.3
RSA	4.15
I⁻	15.0
LDL	50.0
Dextran (16,000)	5.9

uptake process for the lipoprotein. This specific effect could be
binding to specific sites and may be in addition to the general mode
of entry that obtains for the other molecules tested. A specific
binding implies saturation effects as well as the possibility of competitive inhibition by similar molecules. These possibilities were
tested as follows.

Binding was determined at different concentrations of I - LDL
and the results are shown in Fig. 6. The initial rise in uptake
is like that of a saturation binding,although a constant value was
not obtained even at the highest concentration studied. Fig.7 shows
the double reciprocal plot of the data and it appears that there may
be two processes involved: one that is predominant at low concentration and is saturable and another which is not saturable and therefore is readily observed at higher concentration

Uptake of ^{125}I-LDL was also determined as a function of added
unlabeled LDL, VLDL, or RSA. At a given concentration, the uptake
of ^{125}I-LDL is inhibited by LDL and VLDL but not by HDL or albumin,
suggesting that the binding may be specific for apoB. On the other
hand the uptake of ^{125}I-albumin is not affected by unlabeled albumin
nor by any other protein like LDL, VLDL, or HDL. The non-saturable
uptake of LDL (Fig. 6) gives an apparent tissue space of 14 μl/cm^2
which is still too high to be the extracellular volume available to
LDL and is higher than that of any other protein tested. The significance of this is not clear.

The extracellular volume available to a macromolecule is an independent parameter, characteristic of the structure of the tissue, and
being in equation 2, is important in determining the total uptake of
a plasma macromolecule from the plasma. The fractional uptake of
LDL from plasma remaining the same, a tissue with a low value of T
will have higher uptake. Higher uptake thus may not necessarily
mean a higher permeability (in terms of K_1 or K_2). Atherosclerotic
tissue is often said to have higher permeability, which may be due
to this structural factor,while K_1 and K_2 may be normal.

ANTI-ATHEROSCLEROSIS DRUG AND THE KINETIC MODEL

Just as the conditions predisposing one to atherosclerosis
should increase influx and decrease efflux, anti-atherosclerosis
drugs of necessity will be such as to slow down or prevent the accumulation of lipid in the arterial wall by decreasing the influx
or increasing the efflux of LDL.

Drugs that influence serum LDL concentration may affect C_p in
equation 1; however, there may be drugs that directly affect K_{in} and
K_{out} - which are dependent on the property of the tissue.

Shimamoto and co-workers (26,27),for example, have shown that
epinephrine and other vasoactive agents that produce contraction of
endothelial cells may thereby cause an increased influx of plasma
macromolecules into the wall. On the other hand C-AMP and compounds
which act as phosphodiesterase inhibitors may act as agents inhibiting
contraction and may render the endothelial barrier more effective.

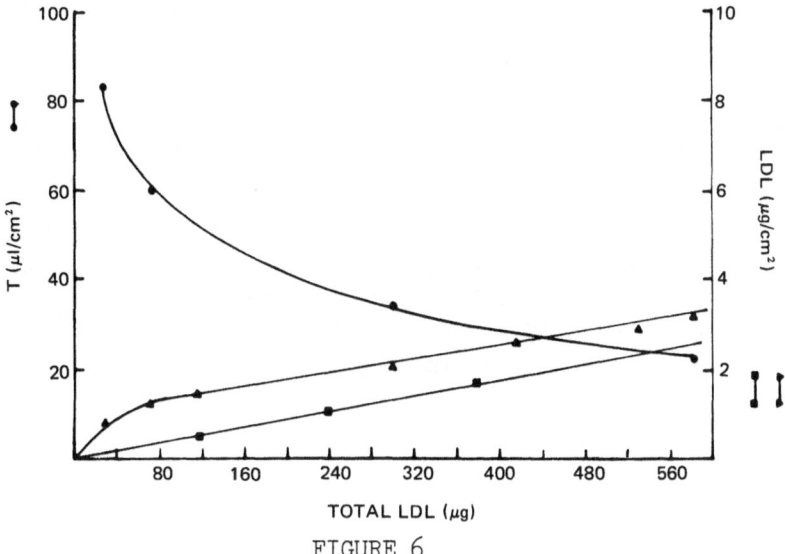

FIGURE 6

Uptake in vitro of LDL by rabbit thoracic aorta as a function of
LDL concentration (μg in a total volume of 3.2 ml). -O- Apparent
tissue space T -Δ- total LDL uptake. -□- the nonsaturable part of
LDL-uptake.

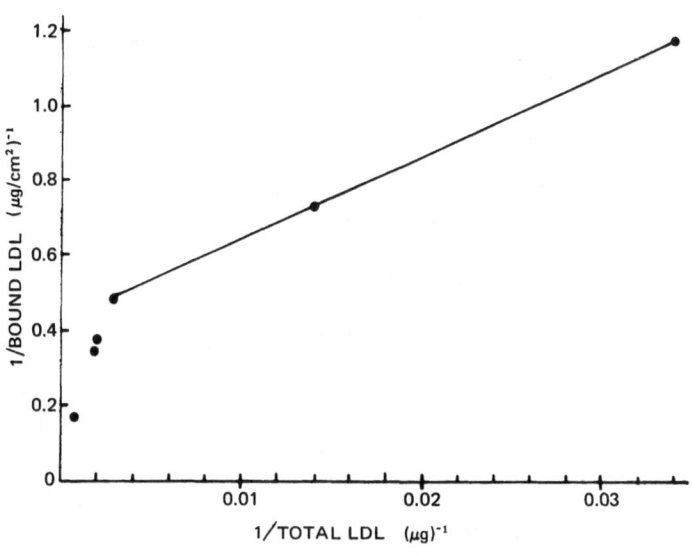

FIGURE 7

Double reciprocal plot of data in figure 6.

Robertson and Khairallah (28) have also been able to show the effect
of several vasoactive agents, especially of angiotensin II, on vascular contraction and opening up of gap junctions – events which lead
to a trapping of plasma macromolecules in the subendothelial space.

In conclusion,therefore, studies using local injection, single
point uptake and EM- technique in our opinion should be extended to
dynamic experiments to show if the "steady state" concentration and
tissue enrichment is increasing or decreasing. Preliminary in vivo
experiments done using rabbits show for example that epinephrine
(1µg/Kg i.v.) treatment may even decrease the K_{app} as well as W/C_{po}
at a particular time. One will have to determine K_{in} and K_{out} separately before concluding about the efficacy of a drug. Studies on the
effect of vasoactive agents on K_{in}, K_{out} and T, the tissue space, are
in progress.

REFERENCES

1. Packham, M.A., H.C. Rowsell, L. Jorgensen and J.F. Mustard.
    1967. Localized protein accumulation in the wall of the aorta.
    Exp. Mol. Path. 7: 214-232.

2. Hollander, W. 1967. Recent advances in experimental and mole-
    cular pathology. Influx, synthesis, and transport of arterial
    lipoproteins in atherosclerosis. Exp. Mol. Path. 7: 248-258.

3. Veress, B., A. Balint. A. Koczé, Z. Nagy, and H. Jellinek. 1970.
    Increasing aortic permeability by atherogenic diet.
    Atherosclerosis 11: 369-371.

4. Stefanovich, V. and I. Gore. 1971. Cholesterol diet and per-
    meability of rabbit aorta. Exp. Mol. Path.14: 20-29.

5. Adams, C.W.M., R.S. Morgan and O.B. Bayliss. 1970. The differ-
    ential entry of [125I] albumin into mildly and severely athero-
    matous rabbit aortas. Atherosclerosis 11: 119-124.

6. Campbell, D.J., A.J. Day, S.L. Skinner and R. Tume. 1973.
    The effect of hypertension on the accumulation of lipids and the
    uptake of [3H] cholesterol by the aorta of normal-fed and cho-
    lesterol-fed rabbits. Atherosclerosis 18: 301-319.

7. Hollander, W. and D. M. Kramsch. 1967. The distribution of
    intravenously administered [3H] cholesterol in the arteries and
    other tissues. Part 1. Tissue fractionation findings.
    J. Atheroscler. Research 7: 491-500.

8. Christensen, S. and J. Jensen. 1965. Uptake of labelled choles-
    terol from plasma by aortic intima-media in control and insulin-
    injected rabbits. J. Atheroscler. Res. 5: 258-259.

9. Newman, H.A.I. and D.B. Zilversmit. 1962. Quantitative aspects
    of cholesterol flux in rabbit atheromatous lesions. J. Biol.
    Chem. 237: 2078-2084.

10. Dayton S. and S. Hashimoto. 1966. Movement of labelled choles-
    terol between plasma lipoprotein and normal arterial wall across
    the intimal surface. Circ. Res. 19: 1041-1049.

11. Dayton S. and S. Hashimoto. 1970. Recent advances in molecular
    pathology: A review of cholesterol flux and metabolism in arterial
    tissue and atheromata. Exp. Mol. Path· 13: 253-268.

12. Zilversmit D.B. and L.B. Hughes. 1973. Incorporation in vivo
    of labeled plasma cholesterol into aortas of young and old rab-
    bits. Atherosclerosis 18: 141-152.

13. Virag, S., T. Pozsonyi, R. Denes and S. Gerö. 1968. Uptake of
    ^{125}I-labeled β-lipoprotein by the aortas of animals differently
    susceptible to cholesterol induced atherosclerosis.
    J. Atheroscler. Res. 8: 859-860.

14. Scott, P.J. and J.P. Hurley. 1970. The distribution of radio-
    iodinated serum albumin and low density lipoproteins in tissues
    and the arterial wall. Atherosclerosis 11: 77-103.

15. Okishio. T. 1961. Studies on the transfer of I^{131}-labeled serum
    lipoproteins into the aorta of rabbits with experimental atheros-
    clerosis. Med. J. Osaka Univ. 11: 367-381.

16. Wissler, R.W. 1973. Development of the atherosclerotic plaque.
    Hospital Practice __: 61-72.

17. Duncan, L.E., J. Cornfield and K. Buck. 1958. Circulation of
    iodinated albumin through aortic and other connective tissues of
    the rabbit. Circ.Res. 6: 244-255.

18. Ghosh, S., M.K. Basu, and J.S. Schweppe. 1972. Agarose gel
    electrophoresis of serum lipoproteins: Determination of true mo-
    bility, isoelectric point and molecular size.
    Anal. Biochem. 50: 592-601.

19. Langer, T., W. Strober and R.I. Levy. 1972. The metabolism of
    low density lipoprotein in familial type II hyperlipoproteinemia.
    J. Clin. Invest. 51: 1528-1536.

20. McFarlane, A.S. 1958. Efficient trace labelling of proteins with iodine. Nature 182:53.

21. Bell, F.P., A.S. Gallus and C.J. Schwartz. 1974. Focal and regional patterns of uptake and the transmural distribution of ^{131}I-fibrinogen in the pig aorta in vivo. Exp. Mol. Path. 20: 281-292.

22. Smith, E.B. 1965. The influence of age and atherosclerosis on the chemistry of aortic intima. Part 1. The lipids. J. Atheroscler. Res. 5: 224-240.

23. Smith, E.B., and P.H. Evans and M.D. Downham. 1967. Lipids in the aortic intima, the correlation of morphological and chemical characteristics. J. Atherocler. Res. 7: 171-186.

24. Stein, Y. and O. Stein. 1973. Lipid synthesis and degradation and lipoprotein transport in mammalian aorta. In: Atherogenesis: Initiating Factors. Ciba Foundation Symposium 12 (new series) Elsevier, New York, pp. 165-183.

25. Dayton, S. 1959. Turnover of cholesterol in the artery walls of normal chickens. Circ.Res. 7: 468-475.

26. Shimamoto, T., M. Kobayashi, and F. Numavo. 1972. Infiltration of γ-globulin, fibrinogen and β-lipoprotein into blood vessel walls by atherogenic stress visualized by immunofluorescence. Proc. Japan Acad. 48: 336-341.

27. Shimamoto, T., and F. Numano. 1970. Cyclic AMP phosphodiester-ase inhibitors in the prevention and treatment of atherosclerotic disorders. 2nd International Conference on C-AMP. Abstract No. ThP-33.

28. Robertson, A.L. Jr., and P.A. Khairallah. 1973. Arterial permeability and vascular disease. The "trap door" effect. Exp. Mol. Path. 18: 241-260.

OXYGEN DIFFUSION AND ATHEROSCLEROSIS

Joseph D. Pool[1], John L. Gainer[1] and Guy M. Chisolm III[2]

[1]University of Virginia, Charlottesville, Virginia and

[2]Case Western University, Cleveland, Ohio

BACKGROUND

That deprivation of oxygen may be a factor in atherogenesis is not a new theory. A review of the hypoxia phenomenon was presented by Heuper (1) in the mid 1940's. He suggested that the common action of agents which cause vascular injury leading to edema or atherosclerosis is an interference with the oxidative metabolism of the vascular wall.

Studies of the effects of prolonged hypoxia on cholesterol-fed rabbits by Kjeldsen et al.(2), Kipshidze (3), and Astrup et al.(4) indicate a pronounced worsening of edema, medial thickening and degenerative vascular lesions in lowered oxygen atmospheres. These studies indicate the occurrence of an increased permeability of the endothelium and intima to cholesterol, triglycerides and proteins (2,4), as well as impairment of the capacity for oxidation and therefore excretion of cholesterol (3).

Repeated severe exposures to anoxia also appear to cause formation of grossly visible necrotic lesions and vascular injury even in rabbits not being fed a high cholesterol diet (5,6,7). Increases in the weight of the heart and aorta as well as the inner surface area of the aorta have been reported. Disintegration, fragmentation and straightening of the elastic membranes usually associated with increased permeability were very noticeable. Constantinides (8) reports that even though extreme mechanical distension of arterial walls failed to open endothelial junctions to increase permeability, clamping of the vessel causing anoxia opened these junctions in a short period.

Oxygen supply to the luminal tissue of larger arteries is critical for many reasons. For example, the vascularization of the aorta in humans is such that the intima and the inner one-third of the media are dependent on the blood flowing through the vessel for their supply of nutrients. Only the outer two-thirds of the media and adventitia are supplied by the vasa vasorum (1,9,10,11,12). Using an average respiration rate for aortic tissue, Kirk. et al. (13) calculated that this avascular portion of the inner arterial wall is very close to the limiting penetration distance for oxygen. This suggests that the inner media is constantly on the verge of hypoxia and therefore might be expected to be very sensitive to alterations in oxygen tension and intimal thickness (7, 10, 14).

If one accepts the hypothesis that hypoxia is the main cause of atherogenesis, then how does such hypoxia come about? It must be a very common mechanism since atherosclerosis is so prevalent in the population. Some investigators have suggested that such a hypoxic state may be induced by increased levels of carbon monoxide in the blood caused by smoking, among other things (15). We have previously suggested that such hypoxia may instead be due to a decreased rate of diffusion of oxygen from the red blood cells to the vascular wall (16).

This decreased rate of oxygen diffusion through the blood may be due to several factors. For example, we have found, in vitro, that increases in plasma protein levels (16) or of serum glucose levels (17) can result in large decreases in the diffusion rate of oxygen through blood plasma. Although there is a significant correlation between the diseases of diabetes and atherosclerosis, the effect of increases of plasma protein levels has not been studied extensively. However, we have shown that increased plasma protein levels do result in more severe atherosclerosis in rabbits (16,18). In addition, we have reported a general increase in certain plasma protein levels with age (19), thus possibly accounting for the general correlation of atherosclerosis with ageing.

If diffusion-caused hypoxia does initiate atherosclerosis, one possible way to prevent it would be to use a drug which increases oxygen diffusion in plasma. Very few compounds appear to do this; however, the carotenoid crocetin has been found to bring about a large increase in the oxygen diffusivity in plasma (2). This result led us to perform a study in which we found that crocetin reduced atherosclerotic damage and reduced serum cholesterol levels in rabbits, even in the presence of increased plasma protein levels (20). Although there may be disagreement concerning the hypothesis which prompted the use of crocetin for atherosclerosis, the results of using it were so striking that we decided to further test its effects.

A more recent test (21), using rabbits, showed that both serum

cholesterol and triglyceride levels were lowered by the use of crocetin over a period of five and one-half months. At the beginning
of the test using a diet of 1% cholesterol added to regular rabbit
chow, the crocetin-treated group maintained higher levels of serum
cholesterol. However, after about three months the levels of the
controls began to exceed those of the crocetin-treated group, and
at the end of the test period the levels of the crocetin-treated
rabbits were 50% lower than those in the control group. The serum
triglyceride levels differed even more markedly between the two groups.
The triglyceride levels of the crocetin-treated group remained in the
normal range throughout the test period, while the controls increased
by 2000%. We have done further testing with the use of crocetin
which has not been published before, and those results are reported
in this paper.

EXPERIMENTS AND RESULTS

Sixteen Dutch-belted rabbits, which weighed approximately two
kilograms each, were divided into two equal groups. All rabbits were
fed a normal rabbit lab chow diet mixed with 1% cholesterol and pelleted (Teklad Mills). The diet was fed 5 days per week and the rabbits were placed on a normal rabbit chow diet for 2 days per week.
The rabbits were allowed to eat and drink water ad libitum. One
group was designated as the control group and the other group was
injected i.m. 5 days per week with 3 ml of an isotonic saline solution containing approximately 30 µg/ml of crocetin. The injections
were started 4 weeks prior to starting the cholesterol feeding.
Blood samples were taken every other week from the ear vein, and
standard clinical analyses were used to determine the serum cholesterol and triglyceride contents.

After about five months, the animals were sacrificed. The
method of sacrificing included intravenous injections of sodium pento-
barbitol and perfusion of the left heart with saline followed by a
10% formalin solution. The aorta was then excised and transferred
immediately to formalin solutions for storage. Following fixation,
a one-centimeter length of the lower thoracic aorta (above the upper
abdominal bifurcation) was removed from each sample and prepared in
the usual manner for light microscopy. The remainder of the aorta
was opened longitudinally and prepared for gross evaluation of lipid
deposits by staining with Sudan IV dye. After staining, the aortae
were divided into two sections for viewing, the thoracic section and
the abdominal section. The aortae were coded so that different groups
were not distinguishable by labels in order to eliminate as much sub-
jective bias as possible. Each section was then visually appraised
by several different people for the percentage of intima affected
by lipid deposits.

The results of the lesion coverage and lipid levels at the end of the test are given in Tables 1 and 2. Again, the use of crocetin appeared to lessen the effects of the cholesterol diet.

Table 1

Group	Cholesterol (mg/dl)	Triglycerides (mg/dl)
Control	1224	249
Crocetin	989	47

Table 2

Group	Aorta Thickness (mm)	Lesion Coverage (%) Abdominal	Thoracic
Control	0.561	45	62
Crocetin	0.436	28	37

Shorter term tests have been done using rats. Twenty-four rats, weighing about 125 grams each, of the Wistar strain, were fed the diet listed in Table 3 for 10 days. At that time, they were grouped according to weight and cholesterol levels into four groups. One group was continued on the diet as a control group, and the other groups were continued on the diet and injected daily, i.p., with various concentrations of crocetin. One group received 1 ml of an isotonic saline solution containing 30 µg of crocetin. The third group received 0.2 ml of a solution containing the sodium salt of crocetin at a concentration of 1 mg/ml, and the fourth group received 1 ml of this same crocetin salt solution. The test was continued for 12 days and then cholesterol levels were measured. There were still no differences in the cholesterol levels of the rats, so the test was continued another 12 days, at which time cholesterol levels were again obtained. Those are shown in Table 4.

Table 3

Composition	Grams per kilo
Butterfat (salt free)	400
Cholesterol	53
Sodium cholate	20
Casein	200
Sodium chloride	40
Sucrose	Remaining

Table 4

Group	Cholesterol (mg/dl)
Control	579
30 µg Crocetin	473
.2 mg Crocetin	350
1 mg Crocetin	440

The difference between the control group and the group receiving 0.2 mg of crocetin per day was statistically significant (p<.05). So another test was done using slightly larger rats.

Rats, weighing about 200 grams each, again of the Wistar strain, were fed the same diet as listed in Table 3 for 18 days. At that time, they were grouped according to weight and cholesterol levels into two groups. One group was continued on the diet as a control group, and the other group was continued on the diet and injected daily with 0.5 ml solution containing 0.5 mg of crocetin salt (sodium). The injections were i.p. This test was continued for 21 days and then cholesterol and triglyceride levels were measured. These are shown in Table 5.

Table 5

Group	Chol. (mg/dl)	p	Trigly. (mg/dl)	p
Control	407 ± 30		354 ± 36	
Crocetin	310 ± 55	0.02	128 ± 13	0.001

Thus, it would appear that the sodium salt of crocetin is effective in lowering lipid levels in rats. Although crocetin was chosen for use originally because of its enhancement of oxygen diffusion, the mechanism of its action is not completely understood at this time. Its effects may indeed be due to increasing oxygen transport, but many other possible mechanisms cannot be eliminated at the present time.

REFERENCES

1. Hueper, W. C. 1944. Arteriosclerosis, the anoximia theory. Arch. Pathol. 39: 162, 245, 350.

2. Kjeldsen, K., J. Wanstrup and P. Astrup. 1968. Enhancing influ-
    ence of arterial hypoxia on the development of atheromatosis in
    cholesterol-fed rabbits. J. Atheroscler. Res. 8: 835-845.

3. Kipshidze, N. N. 1959. The effect of oxygen deficiency on the
    development of experimental atherosclerosis of the coronary
    arteries. Bull. Exp. Biol. Med. 47: 447-453.

4. Astrup, P., K. Kjeldsen and J. Wanstrup. The effects of exposure
    to carbon monoxide, hypoxia and hyperoxia on the development of
    experimental atheromatosis in rabbits. In: Atherosclerosis,
    Proceedings of the Second International Symposium. Ed. by R.
    J. Jones, Springer-Verlag, New York, pp. 108-111.

5. Helin, P., I. Lorenzen, C. Garbarsch and M. E. Matthiessen. 1969.
    Arteriosclerosis and hypoxia, Part 2 (Biochemical changes in muco-
    polysaccharides and collagen of rabbit aorta induced by systemic
    hypoxia). J. Atheroscler. Res. 9:295-304.

6. Helin, P. and I. Lorenzen. 1969. Arteriosclerosis in rabbit
    aorta induced by systemic hypoxia. Angiology 20:1-12.

7. Garbarsch, C., M. E. Matthiessen, P. Helin and I. Lorenzen.1969.
    Arteriosclerosis and hypoxia, Part 1 Gross and microscopic
    changes in rabbit aorta, induced by systemic hypoxia. Histo-
    chemical studies. J. Atheroscler. Res. 9:283-294.

8. Constantinides, P., 1970. The role of endothelial injury in
    arterial thrombosis and atherogenesis. Adv. Cardiol. 4:67-71.

9. Wanstrup, J., K. Kjeldsen and P. Astrup. 1969. Acceleration of
    spontaneous intimal-subintimal changes in rabbit aorta by a
    prolonged moderate carbon monoxide exposure. Acta Pathol.
    Micro. Scand. 75:353-362.

10. Kjeldsen, K., P. Astrup and J. Wanstrup. 1969. Reversal of rabbit
    atheromatosis by hyperoxia. J. Atheroscler. Res. 10:173-178.

11. Dixon, K. C. 1961. Deposition of globular lipid in arterial
    cells in relation to anoxia. Amer. J. Path. 39:65-74.

12. Woener. C. A. 1959. Vasa vasorum of arteries, their demonstra-
    tion and distribution. In: The Arterial Wall. Ed. by A. I.
    Lansing, Williams and Wilkins, Baltimore, pp. 1-14.

13. Kirk, J. E. and T. J. S. Laursen. 1955. Diffusion coefficients
    of various solutes for human aortic tissue with special reference
    to variation in tissue permeability with age. J. Gerontol. 10:
    288-302.

14. Robertson, A. L., Jr. 1968. Oxygen requirements of the human
     arterial intima in atherogenesis. Progr. Biochem. Pharmacol.
     4:305-316.

15. Kjeldsen, K. 1969. Smoking and Atherosclerosis. Thesis at
     University of Copenhagen, Munksgaard, Copenhagen.

16. Chisolm, G. M., III, J. L. Gainer, G. E. Stoner and J. V. Gainer,
     Jr. 1972. Plasma proteins, oxygen transport and atherosclerosis.
     Atherosclerosis 15:327-343.

17. Chisolm, G. M. III and J. L. Gainer. 1973. Altering diffusion
     rates. In: Oxygen Transport to Tissue--Pharmacology, Mathe-
     matical Studies and Neonatology. Ed. by D. F. Bruley and H.
     I. Bicher, Plenum Press, New York, pp. 729-731.

18. Chisolm, G. M., III, J. L. Gainer and A. J. Raineri, Jr. 1973.
     Proteins and atherosclerosis. Experientia 29: 167.

19. Chisolm, G. M. III., E. N. Terrado and J. L. Gainer. 1971.
     Physiological transport in relation to ageing. Nature 230:
     390-391.

20. Gainer, J. L. and G. M. Chisolm III. 1974. Oxygen diffusion
     and atherosclerosis. Atherosclerosis 19:135-138.

21. Gainer, J. L. and J. R. Jones. 1975. The use of crocetin in
     experimental atherosclerosis. Experientia 31:548-549.

SECTION 3

RODENT MODELS

HIGH VOLUME SCREENING PROCEDURES FOR

HYPOBETALIPOPROTEINEMIC ACTIVITY IN RATS

Paul E. Schurr, John R. Schultz, and Charles E. Day

The Upjohn Company

Kalamazoo, Michigan 49001

ABSTRACT. We describe high volume screening tests for hypobetalipoproteinemic agents in which compounds are administered orally
to cholesterol-cholic acid fed (hypercholesterolemic) or normally
fed weanling rats for 4 days. In these tests total serum cholesterol levels and heparin precipitating lipoproteins (HPL) are determined by automated analyses interfaced with a computer which
eliminates all manual data reduction and provides necessary reports.
The hypercholesterolemic rat test detects compounds which specifically reduce HPL (beta and pre beta lipoproteins) causing a decrease
in the HPL:cholesterol ratio. Such activity is called hypobetalipo-
proteinemia. This activity is exhibited by bicyclo(2.2.2)-
octyloxyaniline (U-26328) but not by any of the familiar hypocholesterolemic agents including clofibrate, lifibrate, nicotinic
acid, probucol, triparanol, lentysine, D-thyroxine or the estrogens
estrone and diethylstilbestrol.

INTRODUCTION

Although hyperlipemia has not been proved to be the causative
factor in human atherosclerosis, the circumstantial case against
excessive serum lipids is quite strong as determined by both epidemiological and experimental animal studies. Excessive serum lower
density lipoproteins (the beta or LDL and the pre-beta or VLDL
lipoproteins) are generally implicated as at least one of the
causative factors in this major disease problem.

The feasibility of lowering serum cholesterol levels in man by
chemotherapeutic means has been well established. However, none of

these has achieved the desired effectiveness of levels below normal. Thus, we reasoned that it may be more advantageous to search for a different type of agent. Levy and Day (1) demonstrated that the interaction of LDL with polyanions is an electrostatic phenomenon. They suggested that deposition in the arterial wall may be due to nonspecific electrostatic enmeshment of these molecules in the briar patch of charged macromolecular colloids in the arterial intima. Furthermore, it has been demonstrated that lipoproteins can be modified to inhibit precipitation by mucopolysaccharides (2). Therefore, we decided to search for an agent that would alter LDL in some manner which might inhibit their well known property of being precipitated from diluted serum by heparin in the presence of calcium ions. Toward this end we searched for a suitable animal model by examining lipoprotein electrophoretic patterns of numerous animal species (3). However, only pigs, opossums, and snakes possessed moderately high concentrations of LDL, but these are unsuitable for screening purposes, so we settled for the dietary induced hyperbetalipoproteinemic rat.

Cholesterol-cholic acid fed weanling rats develop a fairly severe hypercholesterolemia within 3 days. Most of the serum cholesterol is in the VLDL density range of $d<1.006$ g/ml. This lipoprotein has many of the properties of both VLDL and LDL and has been designated β-VLDL or cholesterol ester rich VLDL (4). Although not ideal as a model of either type II or IV hyperlipoproteinemia in humans, such lipoproteins are atherogenic in rabbits, pigeons, and other animal species.

In this communication we describe our screening test for agents that modify LDL. To accomplish this we measure serum heparin precipitating lipoproteins (HPL) turbidimetrically and compare the values to total serum cholesterol levels. Although we have not detected the ideal hypobetalipoproteinemic agent, we have detected drugs which depress HPL values to a much greater extent than their hypocholesterolemic activity indicates. Subsequently, it has been shown that this activity consists of reductions in HPL and increases in high density lipoproteins which do not precipitate with heparin (5).

METHODS

Weanling albino rats (Upj:TUC(50)spf) derived from the Sprague-Dawley strain and obtained from the Upjohn rodent colony were fed a semipurified diet containing 1.5% cholesterol and 0.5% cholic acid (Table I) to induce hypercholesterolemia. After 3 days, they were evenly distributed by weight into treatment groups, with each group housed together in a metal cage. Compounds were dispersed in vehicle by either shaking with glass beads in sealed vials or by maceration in a glass tissue grinder. Drug concentrations were adjusted to provide the daily dosage with oral administration of 1 ml per 50 ± 2.5 gm rat. Average body weight per each group of rats was used to determine dosage. The animals were dosed for 4 days, fasted overnight, anesthetized with Cyclopal® sodium (80 mg/kg I.P.), and bled into 12 x 75 mm test tubes from severed throats.

TABLE I

Composition of Hypercholesterolemic Diet

	g/100 g
Dextrin	48.0
Casein	18.0
Sucrose	15.0
Coconut oil	10.0
Salts (Jones & Foster)†	4.0
Cellu flour	2.0
Cholesterol	1.5
Cholic acid	0.5
Liver Concentrate Powder (N.F.)	0.4
Choline Chloride	0.2
Methionine	0.2
Inositol	0.1
Vitamins*	0.1

*Composition per 100 mg is as follows: thiamine HCl 0.5 mg, riboflavin 1.0 mg, pyridoxine HCl 0.5 mg, Ca-pantothenate 2.5 mg, niacin 0.5 mg, p-aminobenzoic acid 30.0 mg, α-tocopherol 2.5 mg, menadione 0.2 mg, folic acid 0.01 mg, biotin 0.01 mg, vitamin A (34,000 USP units) and vitamin D_3 (650 USP units) to 56 mg in corn oil, vitamin B_{12} 1.5 µgm to 6.3 mg with Ca-phosphate.

†Formulated per Jones and Foster, J. Nut. 24:245, 1942 by ICN Nutritional Biochemicals, Cleveland, Ohio.

Three studies were conducted to determine the sensitivity and repeatability of the test system. The specific objective of Study I was to obtain data which could be used to determine the number of animals required to evaluate each test compound. Each of the 12 screening runs in this study consisted of 30 groups of 6 male rats each. On the basis of random selection, four of these groups received vehicle (0.25% aqueous methylcellulose), one group was treated with positive standard, one with negative standard, and the remaining 24 groups received test compounds.

In addition to confirming results obtained in Study I, the purpose of Study II was to evaluate the effect of sex on test results. Each screening run was made up of 30 groups each containing 4 rats. Four of these groups served as vehicle controls, one group received negative standard, one received positive standard, one received 270 mg/kg clofibrate, and the remaining groups received test compounds. Five of these runs were conducted with male rats, and female rats were used in eleven runs.

The purpose of Study III was to compare the effects of cholesterol-cholic acid feeding with normal feeding on the detection of known hypolipidemic drugs. The normal fed animals also received the diet given in Table I, except that cholesterol and cholic acid were replaced by dextrin. With each type of feeding, groups of 4 male rats were used. Four groups were selected as vehicle controls, one group received negative standard, and the remaining groups were treated with various dosages of the hypolipidemic agents. In all studies the negative standard was 50 mg sodium carbonate/kg, and in hypercholesterolemic studies the positive standard was 50 mg U-41792/kg (5).

SERUM ANALYSES

Individual serum samples were analyzed for total cholesterol by the method of Block et al. (6) and for heparin precipitating lipoproteins (HPL) by a method quite similar to that of Lopez et al. (7), even though our method was developed independently. Our procedure is depicted by the flow diagram in Figure 1. All components except the spectrophotometer and reference DC voltage were from Technicon Instruments Corp., Tarrytown, N.Y. The Technicon recorder requires a standard reference voltage usually supplied by a Technicon N-cell colorimeter. A special electronic component supplying this reference voltage was necessary to make the Turner spectrophotometer compatible with the Technicon recorder.

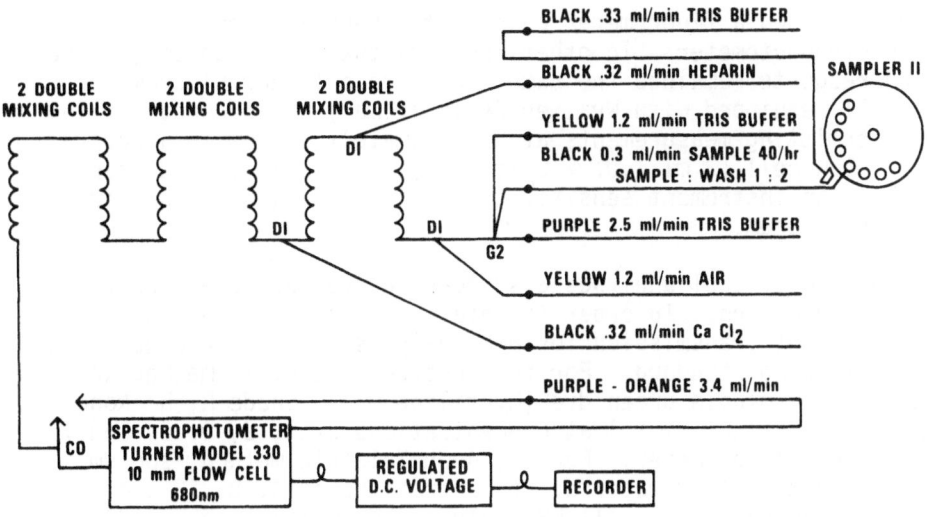

Figure 1.   Flow diagram for automated turbidimetric
analysis of lower density lipoproteins.

Reagents were:

Tris buffer: 0.02$\underline{M}$ Tris (hydroxymethyl) aminomethane
adjusted to pH 7.4 with concentrated
hydrochloric acid.

Heparin solution: 0.2% solution of the sodium salt
of bovine lung heparin (The Upjohn
Company) in Tris buffer at pH 7.4.

Calcium chloride solution: 0.4$\underline{M}$ $CaCl_2$ in Tris buffer
at pH 7.4.

Whenever possible only fresh serum samples (0.3 ml) were used.
Frozen serum was not used. It is important to use serum because
fibrinogen in plasma is precipitated by polyanions and interferes
with the lipoprotein analysis.

Serum samples that generate high absorbance values (O.D. 0.5-
1.0 at 680 nm) tend to coat the flow cell with time, thereby causing
a progressive elevation of the baseline. To alleviate this a 20%
sodium chloride wash preceded and followed by a buffer wash was used
between every 28 samples, or the baseline was manually reset. At
the end of each run the flow cell was thoroughly cleaned by flushing
with 6N HCl.

For serum samples, such as normal rat serum that generate very
slight heparin precipitates (O.D. < 0.1 at 680 nm) by the above

method, we used a fluorometer adapted for nephelometry in place of
the spectrophotometer. In other respects the flow diagram (Figure
1) and reagents remained the same. We used a Turner Fluorometer
Model III equipped with Wratten 2A-12 primary and secondary filters, permitting measurements at approximately 510 nm in a square
quartz flow cell (3 ml I.D. x 5 mm O.D.) with 12 mm masked adapter
insert[1]. An instrument sensitivity setting of 1 X was required for
normal rat serum.

For cholesterol analyses a standard curve was generated for
each screening run. In order to obtain values expressed in absorbance or light transmission for HPL analyses, curves were generated
using a working standard. For the spectrophotometric method we
used a water soluble green dye (Myrtiline Green Shade R, H. Kohn-
stamm and Co., Inc., N.Y.) at concentrations of 1, 2, 4, 8, and 16
mg/ml in distilled water. For the nephelometric method, sodium
fluoride in distilled water at concentrations of 4, 8, 12 and 16
mg/ml were appropriate. All HPL values were multiplied by 10^3 to
eliminate fractional values.

DATA COLLECTION AND ANALYSIS

Analog signals from the automated instruments were converted
to digital form by a Digital Equipment Corp. PDP-8 computer. Data
were then transmitted to an IBM 370/155 computer for processing and
reporting. A coding form prepared for each screening run identified
sample sequence and treatment group. This form also included both
initial and final body and food weights. Data from the samples and
the coding form were then integrated to produce the reports.

The first of seven reports generated was a listing of all raw
data in the sequence run, with values identified by cup number and
sample type (standard, unknown or wash). This report was compared
to recorder charts to assure data integrity. Following this, a
report presented standard curves which were used to calculate serum
values. Another listed each group, identified by sequence number,
treatment (control, compound name or code number, standards), and
dosage. This printout also showed individual values (cholesterol,
HPL, and HPL/cholesterol ratios) for each serum sample within that
group. In addition, weight gains and food intakes, calculated from
initial and final animal and food weights recorded on the coding
sheet, were presented. The 4th, 5th, and 6th reports were summaries
of the results of statistical analyses on the cholesterol, HPL, and

[1]Catalog numbers B16-63019 and A363-62140, American Instrument Co.,
Barrington, Ill.

HPL/cholesterol data. The 7th report, presented in duplicate, was
an overall summary of the test data, derived from the other reports.
This report summary was suitable to paste on one page of a research
notebook. In this manner indexing and reference to test results
was facilitated. The other reports were stored in a looseleaf
binder.

Data from each run were statistically analyzed as a one-way
classification (8). All values were transformed to logarithms to
achieve more homogeneous within-group variances. The mean response
for each test compound was compared with the mean observed in the
control animals with the LSD test (9). An unknown compound was
declared "active" if the mean response was significantly ($P \leq 0.05$)
less than the control mean.

Data from Study I were analyzed separately for vehicle control, negative standard, and positive standard. The one way
classification was also used for these analyses to obtain estimates
of within-run and between-run variances. This procedure was also
followed in Study II for both male and female animals. The within-
run variance estimated from Study I was used to construct operating
characteristic curves according to the method described by Pearson
and Hartley (9).

RESULTS AND DISCUSSION

Study I

Results of analyses are shown in Table II. The observed
difference between mean logarithms of cholesterol values for vehicle and positive standard was 0.266 and that for HPL values was
0.430. Values obtained for the negative standard were very similar
to control values for both cholesterol and HPL. Within-run standard deviations were also comparable in these two groups. Operating
characteristic curves given in Figure 2 were constructed with standard deviations obtained from vehicle treated rats. These curves
give the probability of declaring a significant difference, at the
0.05 level, between control and drug as a function of the true (but
unknown) difference between the two groups. In effect, this is the
probability of declaring a test compound active. Curves are shown
for tests consisting of 4, 5, and 6 animals per group having 16,
20, and 24 control animals, respectively. Since analyses are performed on logarithms, the activity scale is expressed as the difference (Δ) between logarithms of control and drug means. These
curves apply to both cholesterol and HPL because within-run standard
deviations were almost identical for both endpoints. Figure 2
shows that the probability of detecting hypocholesterolemic activity equaling or greater than the positive standard ($\Delta = 0.266$) is

0.985 with 4 rats per group. The corresponding probability for detecting HPL reductions is greater than 0.999.

TABLE II

Mean Responses and Within- and Between-Run Standard Deviations for Cholesterol and HPL from 12 Tests Using 6 Male Rats per Group

		Vehicle	Negative Standard	Positive Standard
Cholesterol	mean log	2.724	2.720	2.458
	antilog	520	525	287
	SD (within)	0.118	0.113	0.070
	SD (between)	0.055	0.069	0.033
HPL	mean log	2.898	2.871	2.468
	antilog	791	743	294
	SD (within)	0.119	0.106	0.115
	SD (between)	0.044	0.055	0.090

Since the objective of the screen was to detect compounds with activities comparable to that of the positive standard, it was apparent that only 4 rats per group were sufficient. Under conditions of routine testing it would be predicted that the false negative rate for cholesterol would be 0.015; and less than 0.001 for HPL. The false positive rate would be 0.05 for both endpoints.

Study II

Results with male and female test animals are given in Table III. In terms of mean reductions by the standards and within and between-run standard deviations, there was no consistent advantage for either sex. Furthermore, these values are in very close agreement with those found in Study I (Table II).

TABLE III

Mean Responses and Within- and Between-Run Standard
Deviations for Serum Cholesterol and HPL in Tests
Using 4 Male or Female Rats per Group

		Vehicle	Negative Standard	Positive Standard	Clofibrate 270 mg/kg
		4 male rats per group, 5 runs			
Choles-terol	mean log	2.773	2.816	2.493	2.644
	antilog	593	655	311	441
	SD (within)	0.118	0.106	0.061	.117
	SD (between)	0.021	0.038	0.066	0.022
HPL	mean log	2.938	2.967	2.479	2.793
	antilog	867	927	301	621
	SD (within)	0.107	0.100	0.104	0.127
	SD (between)	0.042	0.036	0.052	0.029
		4 female rats per group, 11 runs			
Choles-terol	mean log	2.748	2.777	2.454	2.599
	antilog	560	598	284	397
	SD (within)	0.110	0.125	0.058	0.105
	SD (between)	0.026	0.120	0.037	0.026
HPL	mean log	2.927	2.941	2.352	2.753
	antilog	845	873	225	566
	SD (within)	0.120	0.125	0.080	0.140
	SD (between)	0.028	0.035	0.076	0.022

The data (Table III) indicate that this test system would
detect 270 mg clofibrate/kg with a probability of 0.5-0.6. Obviously the test was not ideal for drugs with this degree of
activity.

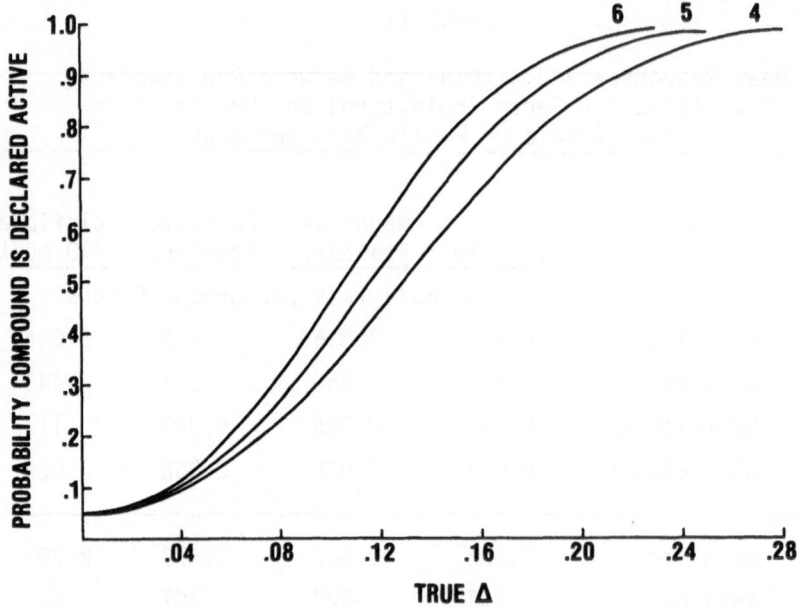

Figure 2.   Operating characteristic curves for group
            sizes of 4, 5, and 6.

Study III

Results obtained in hypercholesterolemic rats given various
compounds with previously demonstrated serum lipid lowering activity
in experimental animals and/or man are given in Table IV. Probucol
(10) and triparanol (11) were not active in this test system. Other
drugs, clofibrate (12), and the clofibrate-like Sandoz drug lifibrate (13), nicotinic acid (14), lentysine (15), D-thyroxine (16)
and the estrogens, estrone (17) and diethylstilbestrol (18) were
hypocholesterolemic. However, none of these drugs depressed HPL
values to a greater extent than cholesterol values as can be noted
by failures to depress HPL/cholesterol ratios. Only U-26328
(bicyclo(2,2,2)-octyloxyaniline) (19) demonstrated hypobetalipoproteinemic activity. The positive standard is even more active
than U-26328.

The effects of the drugs in normal fed male rats are shown in
Table V. It may be noted that only 25 mg triparanol per kg depressed HPL levels significantly, but to no greater extent than
cholesterol levels. Hypocholesterolemic activities for clofibrate,
lifibrate, probucol, triparanol, D-thyroxine, estrone, and diethylstilbestrol were obtained. We did not obtain cholesterol reductions

TABLE IV

Effects of Hypolipidemic Agents in the
Hypercholesterolemic Male Weanling Rat

TREATMENT	DRUG DOSE mg/kg	WIEGHT GAIN gms (1)	FOOD INTAKE gms (1)	CHOLES- TEROL T/C	HPL T/C	CHOLES- TEROL T/C
Control		49	95	1.00 $(703)^2$	1.00 $(1110)^2$	1.00 $(1.58)^2$
Clofibrate	400	54	102	0.51**	0.50**	0.99
	200	54	97	0.61**	0.71	1.16
	100	51	99	0.77	0.76	0.98
Lifibrate	50	42	93	0.50**	0.53**	1.05
	25	54	94	0.63**	0.78	1.23*
	12.5	48	96	0.79	0.94	1.19
Niacin	400	44	86	0.64**	0.74	1.15
U-26328	100	45	96	0.52**	0.42**	0.81*
	50	50	114	0.68*	0.66*	0.97
U-41792(+St.)	50	53	103	0.50**	0.34**	0.69**
Probucol	200	51	111	0.84	0.86	1.03
Triparanol	25	39	89	0.79	1.06	1.34**
	12.5	37	86	0.80	0.89	1.11
Lentysine	25	51	95	0.53**	0.54**	1.01
	3	50	94	0.63**	0.59**	0.94
D-thyroxine	3	45	94	0.28**	0.29**	1.04
Estrone	6	39	87	0.38**	0.47**	1.25*
	3	41	98	0.57**	0.60**	1.04
Diethylstil- bestrol	1.0	24†	82	0.42**	0.47**	1.12
	0.1	49	94	0.52**	0.52**	0.99
	0.01	54	105	0.68*	0.69*	1.02
Na_2CO_3(-St.)	50	50	110	0.84	1.05	1.26*
% Standard Deviation				26.6	32.1	18.2

[1]Weight gains and food intakes are 3 day amounts for 4 rats.
[2]Values in parenthesis are cholesterol mg/dl, HPL (heparin precipi-
tating lipoproteins) 680 nm x 10^3 and HPL/cholesterol ratio.
*Significantly different from control P≦.05.
**Significantly different from control P≦.01.
†Weight gain and food intake T/C≦0.63 and 0.73 respectively.

TABLE V

Effects of Hypolipidemic Agents in the Normal Male Weanling Rat

TREATMENT	DRUG DOSE mg/kg	WEIGHT GAIN gms (1)	FOOD INTAKE gms (1)	CHOLES- TEROL T/C	HPL T/C	CHOLES- TEROL T/C
Control		58	107	1.00 $(123)^2$	1.00 $(417)^2$	1.00 $(3.39)^2$
Clofibrate	400	65	112	0.71**	0.84	1.18
	200	71	126	0.79**	0.77	0.97
	100	60	110	0.71**	0.88	1.25
Lifibrate	50	64	112	0.68**	0.96	1.40*
	25	60	106	0.70**	0.93	1.33
	12.5	68	113	0.74**	1.01	1.36*
Niacin	400	65	113	0.93	1.70**	1.83**
U-26328	100	55	111	1.03	0.96	0.92
	50	60	115	0.95	1.09	1.16
Probucol	200	70	116	0.78**	0.81	1.03
Triparanol	25	50	95	0.65**	0.67**	1.03
	12.5	46	97	0.65**	0.80	1.24
Lentysine	25	61	114	1.00	0.88	0.88
	3	59	107	0.88	1.03	1.16
D-thyroxine	3	51	107	0.85*	1.18	1.40*
Estrone	6	39	85	0.61**	1.47**	2.43**
	3	44	94	0.56**	1.23	2.19**
Diethylstil- bestrol	1.0	22†	114	0.36**	1.21	3.33**
	0.1	52	103	0.61**	1.23	2.00**
	0.01	59	99	1.05	1.76**	1.67**
Na_2CO_3(-St.)	50	65	110	0.91	1.12	1.24
% Standard Deviation				13.1	25.0	25.8

[1]Weight gains and food intakes are 3 day amounts for 4 rats.
[2]Values in parenthesis are cholesterol mg/dl, HPL (heparin precipitating lipoproteins) % light transmission x 10 and HPL/cholesterol
  ratio.
 *Significantly different from control $P \leqq .05$.
**Significantly different from control $P \leqq .01$.
 †Weight gain and food intake $T/C \leqq 0.63$ and 0.73 respectively.

with nicotinic acid, U-26328, or lentysine. We have no explanations for the hyper HPL responses obtained with nicotinic acid and the estrogens.

On the basis of these studies, the test system in its final form consists of 16 control rats, 4 rats treated with a positive standard (U-41792, 50 mg/kg), 4 rats given negative standard (50 mg sodium carbonate/kg), and 24 groups of 4 rats given test compounds. The activity of each compound is evaluated by comparing its mean response with that of controls.

Control charts are maintained for the positive and negative standards to monitor performance of the test system. Comparison of expected responses (Figure 2) with actual responses from 214 consecutive tests showed that the positive standard was declared hypocholesterolemic in 98% of the tests and hypobetalipoproteinemic in 100%. The negative standard was declared active in 8% of the tests.

Compounds that selectively decrease lower density lipoproteins, which are precipitated by heparin (HPL), are designated as hypo-betalipoproteinemic agents. This activity is exemplified by results for the positive standard which show that HPL values were reduced from controls to a much greater extent than cholesterol levels. For example, in male rats the treatment/control ratio (T/C) for HPL values is 301/876=0.35 whereas the T/C for cholesterol values is 311/593=0.52 (Table III). These results indicate a selective decrease in the atherogenic HPL and/or an increase in cholesterol content of HDL. In the screening results these agents are indi-cated by significant decreases in the ratio of HPL/cholesterol. No familiar hypocholesterolemic agent (Table IV) has been shown to exhibit this phenomenon in our test system.

ACKNOWLEDGEMENTS

Computer programming was provided by A. Probutsky and tech-nical assistance by J. Stuut Jr. and T. Watkins.

REFERENCES

1. Levy, R.S. and C.E. Day. 1970. Low density lipoprotein structure and its relation to atherogenesis. In: Athero-sclerosis: Proceedings of the Second International Symposium. Ed. by R.V. Jones, Springer-Verlag, New York, pp. 186-189.

2. Day, C.E. and R.S. Levy. 1975. Control of the precipitation reaction between low density lipoproteins and polyions. Artery 1:150-164.

3. Alexander, C. and C.E. Day. 1973. Distribution of serum
    lipoproteins of selected vertebrates. Comp. Biochem. Physiol.
    46B:295-312.

4. Day, C.E., B. Barker, and W.W. Stafford. 1974. Composition
    of very low density lipoproteins from cholesterol fed animals.
    Comp. Biochem. Physiol. 49B:501-505.

5. Day, C.E., P.E. Schurr, W.E. Heyd, and D. Lednicer. 1976.
    Biological activity of a hypobetalipoproteinemic agent. In:
    Atherosclerosis Drug Discovery Ed. by C.E. Day, Plenum Press,
    New York, pp. 231-249.

6. Block, W.D., K.J. Jarrett Jr., and J.B. Levine. 1965. Use of
    a single color reagent to improve the automated determination
    of serum total cholesterol. In: Automation in Analytical
    Chemistry, Ed. by L.T. Skeggs Jr., Mediad Inc., New York, pp.
    345-347.

7. Lopez. A., R. Vial, L. Gremillion, and L. Bell. 1971. Auto-
    mated simultaneous turbidimetric determination of cholesterol
    in β- and pre-β-lipoproteins. Clin. Chem. 17:994-997.

8. Snedecor, G.W., and W.G. Cochran. 1969. Statistical Methods.
    Iowa State University Press, Ames, Iowa, pp. 258-296.

9. Pearson, E.S. and H.O. Hartley. 1951. Charts of the power
    function for analysis of variance tests, derived from the non-
    central F-distribution. Biometrika 38:112-130.

10. Barnhart, J.W., V.A. Sefranka, and D.D. McIntosh. 1970. Hypo-
    cholesterolemic effect of 4,4'-(isopropylidenedithio)-bis
    (2,6-di-t-butylphenol) (Probucol). Am. J. Clin. Med. 23:1229-
    1233.

11. Blohm, T.R. and R.D. MacKenzie. 1959. Specific inhibition of
    cholesterol biosynthesis by a synthetic compound (MER-29).
    Arch. Biochem. Biophys. 85:245-249.

12. Thorp, J.M. 1963. An experimental approach to the problem of
    disordered lipid metabolism. J. Atheroscler. Res. 3:351-360.

13. Timms, A.R., L.A. Kelly, R.S. Ho, and J.H. Tropold. 1969.
    Laboratory studies of 1-methyl-4-piperidyl bis (p-chloro-
    phenoxy) acetate (SaH 42-348) - a new hypolipidemic agent.
    Biochem. Pharmacol. 18:1861-1871.

14. Levy, R.I., J. Morganroth, and B.M. Rifkind. 1974. Treatment
    of hyperlipidemia. N. Engl. J. Med. 290:1295-1301.

15. Takashima, K., K. Izumi, and H. Iwai. 1973. The hypocholesterolemic action of eritadenine in the rat. Atherosclerosis 17:491-502.

16. Cohen, B.M. 1970. Sodium dextrothyroxine. Clin. Med. 77:25-32.

17. Merola, A.J. and A. Arnold. 1964. Estrone inhibition of cholesterol biosynthesis at the mevalonic acid stage. Science 144:301-302.

18. Robinson, R.W., N. Higano, and W.D. Cohen. 1963. Long-term effects of high dosage estrogen therapy in men with coronary heart disease. J. Chron. Dis. 16:155-161.

19. Day, C.E., P.E. Schurr, D.E. Emmert, R.E. Ten Brink, and D. Lednicer. 1975. Hypobetalipoproteinemic agents. I. Bicyclo (2.2.2.)octyloxyaniline and its derivatives. J. Med. Chem. 18:1065-1070.

BIOLOGICAL ACTIVITY OF A HYPOBETALIPOPROTEINEMIC AGENT

Charles E. Day, Paul E. Schurr, William E. Heyd, and
Daniel Lednicer
The Upjohn Company
Kalamazoo, Michigan 49001

ABSTRACT. A new kind of pharmacologic activity called hypobeta-
lipoproteinemia is described. Operationally the activity consists
of a marked reduction of heparin precipitating lipoproteins (beta
and/or pre-beta electrophoretic mobility) in hypercholesterolemic
animals with a simultaneous decrease in the heparin precipitating
lipoprotein:cholesterol ratio. As determined by ultracentrifugal
fractionation of the lipoproteins from hypercholesterolemic rat
serum, this activity consists of both a reduction in heparin precipitating lipoproteins and an increase in high density lipoproteins
that are not precipitated by heparin. Changes in composition were
also induced in both lipoprotein fractions. The greatest changes
were observed for free and esterified cholesterol, which were
markedly reduced in the heparin precipitating lipoproteins and
concomitantly increased in the high density lipoproteins. The
hypobetalipoproteinemic agent exhibiting this activity is 1-[p-
(1'-adamantyloxy)phenyl]-piperidine (U-41792). This agent is
active in hypercholesterolemic rats, mice, quail, and pigeons.

INTRODUCTION

Excessive concentration of serum low density, or beta, lipoprotein (LDL) is generally regarded as a primary pathogenetic
factor in the development of atherosclerosis. Pre-beta, or very
low density, lipoproteins (VLDL) also enhance the development of
atherosclerosis. Of the three classes of lipoproteins found in
normal, fasting, human serum, only LDL and VLDL are atherogenic.
It seems desirable to develop therapeutic agents which specifically
lower these atherogenic lipoproteins. Since total serum cholesterol

concentration represents a composite of that of all serum lipoproteins, measuring serum cholesterol alone does not allow a
distinction between reduction in atherogenic or nonatherogenic
lipoproteins,or both, to be made.

Heparin in the presence of divalent calcium specifically precipitates the atherogenic LDL plus VLDL from human serum (1). The
resulting precipitate can be quantitated conveniently by turbidi-
metry or nephelometry. Utilizing these techniques, we have developed automated and computer interfaced methodologies to rapidly
and inexpensively assay for agents that specifically reduce atherogenic serum lipoproteins (2). As a result of the application of
these procedures, we discovered a new class of agents that reduce
serum LDL and VLDL concentrations and increase high density lipoprotein (HDL) levels. We have designated these compounds as hypobetalipoproteinemic agents since they decrease the beta family
(beta plus pre-beta) of lipoproteins in serum.

The first hypobetalipoproteinemic agent that we discovered
was p-(bicyclo[2.2.2]oct-1-yloxy)-aniline (3). The present report
deals exclusively with the biological activity of the more potent
hypobetalipoproteinemic agent, U-41792, or 1-[p-(1'-adamantyloxy)-
phenyl]-piperidine, which has been studied in four animal systems:
rats, mice, quail, and pigeons. The effect of U-41792 on the serum
lipoprotein composition of cholesterol-cholic acid fed rats was also
examined.

EXPERIMENTAL METHODS

Rats

Male, UPJ:TUC(SD)spf, 80-100 g rats were fed a semi-purified
diet with 1.5% cholesterol and 0.5% cholic acid (2). After 6 days,
they were evenly distributed by weight into groups of 10, housed
singly in metal cages,and started on treatment. Compounds were
administered orally, suspended in 0.25% aqueous methyl cellulose
at concentrations adjusted to provide the daily dosage with the
administration of 1 ml per 100 g body weight. Controls received
comparable volumes of vehicle. The rats were weighed twice a week
and dosages were adjusted accordingly. Following the final dose,
the animals were weighed and then fasted overnight (approximately
17 hr). Rats were anesthetized with Cyclopal® sodium (80 mg/kg
I.P.) and bled from the abdominal aorta. Livers were removed,
blotted, and weighed. Individual serum samples were analyzed for
total cholesterol by the method of Block et al. (4) and for heparin
precipitating lipoproteins (HPL) by the turbidimetric method of
Schurr et al. (2).

Duplicate pooled serum samples were used for lipoprotein
analyses. Two 5 ml pools of each rat group were prepared by com-
bining 0.5 ml of serum from each animal. One ml of each pool was
saved for unfractionated serum analyses. To 4.0 ml serum in a 6 ml
preparative ultracentrifuge tube, 2.0 ml of NaCl solution was added
to give a final, non-protein solution density of 1.040 g/ml. The
tubes were spun for 23 hr at 36,000 rpm at 18°C in a type 40 rotor
in a Beckman-Spinco Model L preparative ultracentrifuge. From tubes
containing sera from drug treated rats, 1.0 ml was quantitatively
aspirated for analyses, and the next 2.0 ml were discarded. From
control sera, the top 3.0 ml were saved for analyses. To the remaining 3.0 ml of solution in each tube, 3.0 ml of NaBr solution
were added to give a non-protein density of 1.21 g/ml. After centrifugation for 50 hr under the same conditions as before, the top
1.0 ml was removed for analyses, the next 2.0 ml discarded, and the
remaining 3.0 ml saved for analyses. Protein was analyzed by the
colorimetric methods of Lowry et al. (5). Cholesterol was determined by gas liquid chromatography employing a Hewlett-Packard
series 5700A chromatograph containing an 18 x 1/8" O.D. U-shaped
glass column packed with 3.8% silicone rubber UC-W98 on 60-80 mesh
diaport S at a column temperature of 220°C. Gas flow rates were
helium 30, hydrogen 30, and air 240 ml per minute. Aliquots of
isopropyl alcohol extracts of samples were analyzed. For free
cholesterol, an aliquot was dried and the residue dissolved in
chloroform containing the internal standard cholestane. For total
cholesterol an aliquot was dried, saponified, and extracted
according to the method of Abell et al. (6). Aliquots of the
petroleum ether extract were dried and redissolved in chloroform
containing the internal standard. Esterified cholesterol was calculated as the difference between free and total cholesterol.
Esterified cholesterol was multiplied by 1.67 (7) to give total
weight of cholesterol ester. Triglycerides were determined by the
automated method of Royer and Ko (8). Phospholipids (lipid phos-
phorous X 25) were determined colorimetrically by the methods of
Steward and Hendry (9).

For data on individual animals (Table I), statistical differences from control means (P≤0.05) were determined by Student's
test using pooled error variance (10). In these statistical analyses all values except weight gains are transformed to logarithms
to achieve more homogeneous within group variance and are reported
as antilogs of the logarithm means.

Mice

Male, albino, Carworth (CF1) mice (20 ± 2g) were housed in
groups of 10 and fed a semipurified diet (2) containing 1.5%
cholesterol and 0.5% cholic acid for 10 days. During the last 5

days, U-41792 suspended in 0.25% aqueous methyl cellulose was administered by stomach tube at concentrations to provide the daily
dosage in 1 ml per 20 g body weight. Control groups received
similar volumes of vehicle only. After the final dosage the mice
were weighed, fasted overnight, anesthetized with Cyclopal® sodium
(0.1 cc of 2% solution I.P.), and sacrificed. Livers were removed,
blotted, and weighed. Blood was collected in 12 x 75 mm test tubes
from severed throats. Individual serum samples were analyzed for
total cholesterol (4) and heparin precipitating lipoproteins (2).
Statistical analyses were the same as those performed on individual
rat data.

Quail

     Male Japanese quail (*Coturnix coturnix japonica*), 3 months old
with an average weight of 112 g, were individually caged and fed a
diet of chicken mash (11) supplemented with 2% crystalline cholesterol. Each bird was on cholesterol diet for 9 days and on each
of those days received a single dose of U-41792, suspended in 0.25%
methyl cellulose, by gastric intubation. Control birds received
only the aqueous vehicle. Blood was drawn from the right jugular
vein after animals had been fasted overnight. Blood was placed in
a test tube containing 10 µl of topical bovine thrombin solution
(500 IU/ml) to insure adequate clotting. Individual serum samples
were assayed for total cholesterol (4) and heparin precipitating
lipoproteins (2). Statistical analyses were performed as before.

Pigeons

     Male, White Carneau pigeons were placed on a diet of mixed
pigeon grains supplemented with 5% lard and 1% cholesterol. After
1 year birds were randomly distributed into several groups. The
positive control was continued on the cholesterol diet. The regression group was placed on a grain only diet. The treated group
was continued on the cholesterol plus lard diet to which was added
0.2% U-41792. Animals were on these regimens for an additional 6
months. The negative control had never been on cholesterol or lard
throughout the experiment. Non-fasting birds were bled just prior
to drug treatment (time 0) and after 6 months. Total cholesterol
(4) and turbidimetric heparin precipitating lipoprotein analyses
(2) were determined on individual serum samples. Samples for
heparin precipitating lipoprotein assay were diluted with 2 volumes
of 0.9% NaCl prior to analysis. Statistical analyses were the same
as those described above.

TABLE I

Effects of Six Daily Doses of U-41792 in Hypercholesterolemic Rats

Dose U-41792 (mg/kg/day)	Surviving Rats/Group (initial=10)	Serum Cholesterol (mg/dl)	Serum HPL ($A_{680}\times10^3$)	HPL/Cholesterol Ratio	Weight Gain (g)	Food Intake (g)	Liver Weight (g)
0	10	784	1034	1.32	30.6	66.6	6.90
50	10	180*	172*	0.96	31.5	73.3	7.40
100	10	167*	57*	0.34*	26.2	66.5	8.14*
200	10	258*	46*	0.18*	16.9*	52.5	9.14*
400	10	330*	68*	0.20*	-3.5*	31.2*	8.87*
800	6	395*	62*	0.16*	-13.8*	18.8*	8.50*
% Pooled Standard Deviation		17.8	40.9	36.8	54.4	10.0	11.2

*Significantly different (p≤0.05) from control means.

RESULTS

Rats

In a dose response study, U-41792 was orally administered to hypercholesterolemic rats in the dose range of 50 to 800 mg/kg/day for six days. The drug effectively reduced serum cholesterol and heparin precipitating lipoproteins (HPL) at all doses tested (Table I). HPL concentrations were reduced as much as twenty-fold. At 100 mg/kg/day and above, the HPL/cholesterol ratio was dramatically reduced also. Significant decreases in weight gains were noted at levels above 200 mg/kg/day. Hepatomegaly was noted from 100 to 800 mg/kg/day. Food intakes were not affected significantly until the 400 mg/kg/day level was reached. Four animals on 800 mg/kg/day died.

Determination of the esterified and non-esterified fractions of serum cholesterol showed that the decrease of greatest magnitude had occurred in the cholesterol esters (Table II). After an initial drop in free cholesterol (FC) at 50 mg/kg/day, FC rose in a dose dependent fashion until at 800 mg/kg/day of drug it actually exceeded the control level. Serum triglycerides were increased at all drug levels. Phospholipids were reduced at all doses. Total serum protein concentrations were not affected.

The reduction in HPL/cholesterol ratio could be interpreted several ways. One possibility is that the HPL are selectively reduced while the HDL remain unchanged. Another explanation is that HDL may be increased when HPL are reduced. Or a qualitative change may occur in the HPL so that they are no longer precipitated by heparin. To distinguish among these and other possibilities, the lipoproteins from duplicate pools of rat serum were fractionated by preparative ultracentrifugation. Two fractions of lipoproteins were isolated. The first fraction isolated by ultracentrifugation at a solvent density of 1.040 g/ml contained all the lipoproteins that could be precipitated with heparin. The material sedimenting at 1.040 g/ml was adjusted to 1.21 g/ml and recentrifuged. The resulting lipoprotein (1.040<D<1.21 g/ml) was designated HDL. After each centrifugation, with one exception, the top 1.0 ml of solution containing the floating lipoprotein could be quantitatively aspirated into a 1 ml volumetric flask. The exception was the 1.040 spin of the control sera. The concentration of lipoprotein was so great that it was necessary to aspirate 3.0 ml to quantitatively remove it.

Compositional analyses of the two lipoprotein fractions revealed that U-41792 exerted effects on both fractions. The question of interpretation of reduction in HPL/cholesterol ratio effected by

TABLE II

Effect of U-41792 on Lipid Composition and Concentration
of Unfractionated Serum in Hypercholesterolemic Rats

Dose U-41792 (mg/kg/day)	Protein (g/dl)	Free Cholesterol (mg/dl)	Cholesterol Esters (mg/dl)	Triglycerides (mg/dl)	Phospholipids (mg/dl)
0	6.0	136	1049	16	519
50	6.2	49	256	28	224
100	6.5	64	225	25	223
200	7.5	108	284	27	207
400	6.0	152	317	48	292
800	5.1	204	326	47	342

TABLE III

Effect of U-41792 on the Composition and Concentration of Lipoproteins with Density Less Than 1.040 g/ml in Hypercholesterolemic Rat Serum

Dose U-41792 (mg/kg/day)	Protein (mg/dl)	Free Cholesterol (mg/dl)	Cholesterol Esters (mg/dl)	Triglycerides (mg/dl)	Phospholipids (mg/dl)	Total Lipoprotein (mg/dl)
0	148	144	1064	6	442	1804
50	28	34	158	28	104	352
100	19	21	52	20	81	193
200	16	22	33	24	58	153
400	27	30	53	38	84	232
800	25	28	47	33	79	212

drug treatment was clearly answered. Not only did U-41792 cause a dramatic reduction in D<1.040 g/ml lipoproteins, from 1804 to as low as 153 mg/dl (Table III), it also caused an increase in HDL from 87 to as high as 811 mg/dl (Table IV). Absolute concentrations of protein, free cholesterol, cholesterol esters, and phospholipids in the D<1.040 g/ml lipoproteins were all reduced, with the greatest absolute and relative reduction occurring in cholesterol esters (Table III). Triglycerides were elevated. In the HDL fraction the absolute concentrations of protein, free cholesterol, cholesterol esters, and phospholipids were all elevated (Table IV). The greatest relative increase (with respect to control levels) was in free cholesterol. No effect on the negligible amount of triglyceride could be detected.

Lipid analyses were performed on the D>1.21 g/ml ultracentrifugal fraction (presumably lipoprotein free serum) to determine whether U-41792 might produce abnormal very high density lipoproteins. No cholesterol, free or esterified, or triglycerides could be detected in this fraction (Table V). U-41792 appeared to cause a small increase in the lipid phosphorus associated with the D>1.21 g/ml proteins.

Pronounced but not so dramatic compositional changes were also produced in the lipoproteins. The greatest change was in the triglyceride content of D<1.040 g/ml lipoproteins which rose from 0.3% in controls to 16% in treated animals (Table VI). In addition the per cent protein, free cholesterol, and phospholipid all increased. Only cholesterol esters were reduced. The most striking qualitative change in HDL was the increase in free cholesterol from 2% to 18% (Table VII). An increase in cholesterol esters was also observed. Protein and phospholipid levels were reduced.

Mice, Quail, Pigeons

Definite toxic effects of U-41792 in mice were seen only at 1600 mg/kg/day. Two animals died at this dose. U-41792 reduced serum cholesterol, HPL, and HPL/cholesterol ratios in hypercholesterolemic mice (Table VIII). The effects on HPL and HPL/cholesterol ratio were dose dependent.

In Japanese quail U-41792 significantly reduced the serum HPL and HPL/cholesterol ratio (Table IX). No significant reduction in serum cholesterol occurred.

In White Carneau pigeons the drug caused a significant reduction in serum cholesterol and HPL (Table X). The HPL/cholesterol ratio was not affected.

TABLE IV

Effect of U-41792 on the Composition and Concentration of High
Density Lipoproteins* in Hypercholesterolemic Rat Serum

Dose U-41792 (mg/kg/day)	Protein (mg/dl)	Free Cholesterol (mg/dl)	Cholesterol Esters (mg/dl)	Triglycerides (mg/dl)	Phospholipids (mg/dl)	Total Lipoprotein (mg/dl)
0	33	2	23	<1	28	87
50	120	10	116	<1	89	336
100	140	29	149	1	110	429
200	172	68	205	1	111	557
400	174	96	187	1	178	636
800	200	146	225	1	239	811

*1.040<D<1.21 g/ml

TABLE V

Effect of U-41792 on the Composition of Lipoprotein
Free Serum* in Hypercholesterolemic Rats

Dose U-41792 (mg/kg/day)	Protein (g/dl)	Free Cholesterol (mg/dl)	Cholesterol Esters (mg/dl)	Triglycerides (mg/dl)	Phospholipids (mg/dl)
0	5.4	0	0	0	16
50	5.5	0	0	0	32
100	5.5	0	0	0	32
200	5.6	.0	0	0	38
400	5.5	0	0	0	30
800	5.1	0	0	0	24

*D>1.21 g/ml

TABLE VI

Effect of U-41792 on the Percent Composition of Lipoproteins with
Density Less Than 1.040 g/ml in Hypercholesterolemic Rat Serum

Dose U-41792 (mg/kg/day)	Protein	Free Cholesterol	Cholesterol Esters	Triglycerides	Phospholipids
0	8	8	59	0.3	24
50	8	10	45	8	30
100	10	11	27	10	42
200	10	14	22	16	38
400	12	13	23	16	36
800	12	13	22	16	37

TABLE VII

Effect of U-41792 on the Percent Composition of High
Density Lipoproteins* in Hypercholesterolemic Rat Serum

Dose U-41792 (mg/kg/day)	Protein	Free Cholesterol	Cholesterol Esters	Triglycerides	Phospholipids
0	38	2	26	<1	32
50	36	3	35	<1	26
100	33	7	35	<1	26
200	31	12	37	<1	20
400	27	15	29	<1	28
800	25	18	28	<1	29

*1.040<D<1.21 g/ml

TABLE VIII

Effects of Five Daily Doses of U-41792 in Hypercholesterolemic Mice

Dose U-41792 (mg/kg/day)	Surviving Mice/Group (initial=10)	Serum Cholesterol (mg/dl)	Serum HPL (A_{680}x10^3)	HPL/Cholesterol Ratio	Weight Change (g)	Food Intake (g)	Liver Weight (g)
0	9	410	541	1.32	-0.5	11.2	1.30
25	10	396	410	1.03	-0.2	9.7	1.36
50	10	415	377	0.91*	0.5	12.8	1.37
100	10	340	282*	0.83*	-0.4	10.1	1.36
200	10	268*	206*	0.77*	-0.1	9.2	1.42
400	10	301*	206*	0.68*	-0.4	11.9	1.54
800	10	221*	139*	0.63*	-2.7	6.1	1.51
1600	8	314*	83*	0.26*	-3.4	5.6	1.59*

*Significantly different ($p \leq 0.05$) from control means.

TABLE IX

Effects of Nine Daily Doses of U-41792 in Hypercholesterolemic Japanese Quail

Dose U-41792 (mg/kg/day)	Birds/Group	Serum Cholesterol (mg/dl)	Serum HPL ($A_{680} \times 10^3$)	HPL/Cholesterol Ratio	Weight Loss (g)
0	9	460	459	1.00	9.4
25	9	405	372	0.92	14.4*
50	9	378	265*	0.70*	12.0
100	9	441	215*	0.49*	11.9

*Significantly different ($p \leq 0.05$) from control means.

TABLE X

Effect of U-41792 in Hypercholesterolemic White Carneau Pigeons

Group	Starting			Final (6 months)		
	Serum Cholesterol (mg/dl)	Serum HPL ($A_{680} \times 10^3$)	HPL/Cholesterol Ratio	Serum Cholesterol (mg/dl)	Serum HPL ($A_{680} \times 10^3$)	HPL/Cholesterol Ratio
Positive Control	3486	3780	1.08	4248	4415	1.04
Regressing	3303	3933	1.19	398*	285*	0.72*
U-41792 Treated	3873	4037	1.04	1260*	1277*	1.01
Negative Control	310*	173*	0.57*	312*	194*	0.62*

*Significantly different ($p \leq 0.05$) from positive control means.

DISCUSSION

We have identified a new kind of hypolipidemic activity that we have designated hypobetalipoproteinemic. 1-[p-(1'-adamantyloxy) phenyl]-piperidine, or U-41792, possessed good hypobetalipoprotein-emic activity. Operationally this activity is defined as a re-duction in lipoproteins that are precipitated by heparin (HPL) with a concomitant reduction in the HPL/cholesterol ratio.

U-41792 exhibited a broad spectrum of species activity. It was hypobetalipoproteinemic in cholesterol-cholic acid fed rats and mice and in cholesterol fed quail. Although it significantly reduced both serum cholesterol and HPL in White Carneau pigeons, the HPL/cholesterol ratio was not reduced at the dose studied. Thus some interspecies differences in activity were noted.

The significance of the U-41792-induced reduction of the HPL/ cholesterol ratio was evaluated in cholesterol-cholic acid fed rats by lipoprotein fractionation by ultracentrifugation. The HPL was reduced markedly while the HDL was increased significantly. In terms of the composition of the HPL, the percent cholesterol ester decreased dramatically, while the triglycerides rose significantly. In the HDL the percent free cholesterol increased while the percent protein decreased. Although it was possible to descriptively define the effect of U-41792 in this manner, it was not possible from these data to gain an insight into the mechanism of this activity.

Of greater importance is the potential human relevance of hypobetalipoproteinemic activity. The composition of HPL in choles-terol-cholic acid fed rats (Table VI) is unlike that of any human lipoprotein. The distinguishing characteristic of HPL is its very high concentration of cholesterol esters. The predominant lipopro-tein in cholesterol fed quail and pigeon serum is quite similar in composition to the hypercholesterolemic rat HPL reported here (12). Since the lipoproteins in animal models in which U-41792 exhibits its activity are so vastly different from those that occur in human hyperlipoproteinemias (with the possible exception of Type III hyper-lipoproteinemia), activity in these models certainly cannot be ex-trapolated to indicate activity in humans. Regardless, hypobeta-lipoproteinemic activity is a new phenomenon that may provide a useful tool for exploring the complex area of lipoprotein metabolism.

ACKNOWLEDGEMENT

We are gratefully indebted to J. Stuut, W.W. Stafford and W.S. Cantrall for technical assistance.

REFERENCES

1. Burstein, M. and H.R. Scholnick. 1973. Lipoprotein-polyanion-metal interactions. In Advances in Lipid Research, ed. by R. Paoletti and D. Kritchevsky, Academic Press, New York, pp. 68-108.

2. Schurr, P.E., J.R. Schultz, and C.E. Day. 1976. High volume screening procedures for hypolipoproteinemic activity in rats. In Atherosclerosis Drug Discovery, ed. by C.E. Day, Plenum Press, New York, pp. 215-229.

3. Day, C.E., P.E. Schurr, D.E. Emmert, R.E. Ten Brink, and D. Lednicer. 1975. Hypobetalipoproteinemic agents. I. Bicyclo [2.2.2]octyloxyaniline and its derivatives. J. Med. Chem. 18: 1065-1070.

4. Block, W.D., K.J. Jarrett, Jr., and J.B. Levine. 1965. Use of a single color reagent to improve the automated determination of serum total cholesterol. In Automation in Analytical Chemistry, ed. by L.T. Skeggs, Jr., Mediad Inc., New York, pp. 345-347.

5. Lowry, O.H., N.J. Rosebrough, A.L. Farr, and R.J. Randall. 1951. Protein measurement with the Folin phenol reagent. J. Biol. Chem. 193:265-275.

6. Abell, L.L., B.B. Levr, B.B. Brodie, and F.E. Kendall. 1952. A simplified method for the estimation of total cholesterol in serum and demonstration of its specificity. J. Biol. Chem. 195:357-367.

7. Mills, G.L. and C.E. Taylaur. 1971. The distribution and composition of serum lipoproteins in eighteen animals. Comp. Biochem. Physiol. 40B:489-501.

8. Royer, M.E. and H. Ko. 1969. A simplified semi-automated assay for plasma triglycerides. Anal. Biochem. 29:405-416.

9. Stewart, C.P. and E.B. Hendry. 1935. The phospholipids of blood. Biochem. J. 29:1683-1689.

10. Steel, R.G.D. and J.H. Torrie. 1960. Principles and Procedures of Statistics, McGraw-Hill, New York, p. 106.

11. Tennent, D.M., H. Siegel, G.W. Kuron, W.H. Ott, and C.W. Mushett. 1957. Lipid patterns and atherogenesis in cholesterol fed chickens. Proc. Soc. Exptl. Biol. Med. 96:679-683.

12. Day, C.E., B. Barker, and W.W. Stafford. 1974. Composition of very low density lipoproteins from cholesterol fed animals. Comp. Biochem. Physiol. 49B:501-505.

NONISOTOPIC METHOD FOR ESTIMATING CHOLESTEROGENESIS IN THE RAT

W.A. Phillips, J.M. Ratchford and J.R. Schultz

Diabetes and Atherosclerosis Research

The Upjohn Company, Kalamazoo, Michigan 49001

ABSTRACT. Influence of several compounds on sterol production was determined from serum desmosterol (D) levels in rats treated with U-18666A:3β-(2-diethylaminoethoxy)androst-5-en-17-one HCl. U-18666A blocks biosynthesis of cholesterol (C) by inhibiting conversion from D to C. Diets containing C (2%), the bile acid sequestrant colestipol HCl (1%), clofibrate (0.2%), combination of colestipol HCl and clofibrate, or basal diet were fed to normal or U-18666A (3 mg/kg/d) male rats for 2 weeks. In normal rats, C feeding increased serum C levels (39%), colestipol HCl had no significant effect, while clofibrate or the combination with colestipol HCl reduced C levels to the same extent (37%). In U-18666A-treated rats, C feeding reduced D concentration (30 to 13 mg/dl) indicating inhibition of synthesis via negative feedback system. Colestipol HCl increased D level (33%) and reduced C (60%) indicating increased synthesis; results are compatible with an agent capable of binding bile acids in the rat which can compensate for loss of these acids by increasing sterol synthesis. Compared to control, clofibrate reduced serum C (33%) and D (43%); in combination with colestipol HCl it inhibited the increased synthesis caused by the latter. Clofibrate appears to be an inhibitor of C biosynthesis. Also, tests with other compounds make it apparent that the U-18666A-treated rat model system can be useful in evaluating cholesterogenesis.

INTRODUCTION

The primary purpose of the present study was to determine the feasibility of employing serum desmosterol concentrations of

U-18666A[1]-treated rats to evaluate the influence of compounds on
cholesterogenesis. It appears that the principle site of action
of U-18666A is at the very last step in cholesterol biosynthesis,
that is, in the reduction of the side chain double bond of desmosterol (1). Since desmosterol is not consumed in the diet nor
readily detectable in the serum of normal rats, then this sterol
should serve as an easily measurable, nonisotopic index of endogenous sterol production. Giver et al. (2-4) have suggested a
similar model system with the cholesterol biosynthesis inhibitor
AY-9944 which acts by blocking the conversion of 7-dehydrocholes-
terol to cholesterol. The levels of 7-dehydrocholesterol, elevated
in nephrotic rats and in mice receiving thyroxine and reduced in
rats fed cholesterol, illustrate the usefulness of this system for
estimating the rate of cholesterol biosynthesis. Bricker et al. (5)
have proposed a similar assay in which blood desmosterol levels are
measured after 7 to 14 days administration of triparanol. Cholesterol feeding causes a marked diminution of blood desmosterol indicating a virtually complete disappearance of endogenous sterols
from the blood and demonstrates the operation of the cholesterol
negative feedback system in the intact animal.

METHODS

Ten male rats[2] with an average initial fasted weight of
approximately 220 g were used in each group. Control and treated
groups were fed a basic diet (6); treated groups received supplements of 2% cholesterol[3], 1% cholestyramine[4], 1% colestipol HCl[5],
0.2% clofibrate[6] or a combination of colestipol HCl and clofibrate
for 13 days. U-21743[7] (10 mg/kg/day), nicotinic acid[8] (200 mg/kg/
day), nicotinamide[9] (200 mg/kg/day), L-thyroxine[10] (0.3 mg/kg/day)
and U-21892[11] (5 mg/kg/day) were administered by gavage for 14 days.

[1]3β-(2-diethylaminoethoxy)androst-5-en-17-one, hydrochloride
[2]Upjohn:TUC(SD)spf
[3]Cholesterol USP, lot 3141A
[4]Cuemid® corrected for 8.5% inert material, Merck, Sharpe & Dohme,
  division of Merck & Co., West Point, PA, Lot no. P2999
[5]Colestid®, Lot 387-AT
[6]Ethyl-p-chlorophenoxyisobutyrate, synthesized at The Upjohn Co.
[7]p-chlorophenyl methanesulfonate, synthesized at The Upjohn Co.
[8]Niacin NF Lot no. 647A
[9]Niacinamide USP Lot no. 426B
[10]L-thyroxine Nutritional Biochemicals, Cleveland, Ohio
[11]4-(4-hydroxy-3,5 xylyloxy)-3,5-diiodo-phenethyl alcohol
  synthesized at The Upjohn Co.

Two groups of rats received each treatment, one was stomach-tubed with U-18666A in 0.25% methylcellulose vehicle at 3 mg/kg/day, the other with vehicle alone. At the end of the 13th day rats receiving drugs in the diet were stomach-tubed with their respective dietary supplements based on prior mg/kg/day consumption of the compounds. All animals were fasted overnight and blood samples (0.7 ml) were taken without anesthesia from the external jugular vein (7). Weight changes, liver weights, and food intakes were recorded at the end of the 14-day test period.

Serum samples (0.2 ml) were saponified according to the method of Abell et al. (8). Aliquots of the petroleum ether extracts were taken to dryness and residues dissolved in chloroform containing the internal standard androstane-diol at 0.21 mg per ml. Concentrations of cholesterol and desmosterol were determined by gas chromatography by comparing peak areas[12] of the sterols to that of the internal standard with standard solutions. The F and M Model 400 Biomedical Flame Ionization Gas Chromatograph was used with an 18" x 1/4" O.D. U-shaped glass column packed with 3% OV-225 on 100-120 mesh Gas-Chrom Q[13].

Under our gas chromatographic conditions desmosterol and campesterol have the same relative retention times. These sterols can be separated with a 6 foot column packed with 3% OV-17 on 80-100 mesh Gas Chrom Q. The average contribution of campesterol to desmosterol values was determined from pooled aliquots of petroleum ether extracts from each group.

Separate analyses of variance were performed on the data from each experiment (9). The within-group variances for sterol values tended to be proportional to the square of the means and were transformed to logarithms prior to statistical analysis. Sterol values are therefore reported as the antilog of the logarithm means. Treatment comparisons were made within normal rat groups and those treated with U-18666A. Tests of statistical significance were made at the 0.05 probability level.

RESULTS

In all experiments the endogenous inhibitor U-18666A significantly reduced serum cholesterol and increased serum desmosterol levels; total serum sterols were reduced from the normal untreated control.

[12]Model 3373B Integrator, Hewlett-Packard, Avondale, PA
[13]Applied Science Laboratories Inc., State College, PA

The effects of cholesterol feeding to normal and U-18666A-treated rats are shown in Table I. In normal animals, cholesterol treatment significantly increased serum cholesterol concentration from 85 to 116 mg/dl. In U-18666A-treated animals, cholesterol feeding significantly increased serum cholesterol from 34 to 102 mg/dl and reduced desmosterol level from 29 to 13 mg/dl; total sterol concentration was increased from 63 to 115 mg/dl. Cholesterol feeding caused a significant increase in body weight change, food intake, and liver weight in normal animals; these end-points did not significantly vary from control in animals given U-18666A.

TABLE I

Effects of Dietary Cholesterol in Normal and U-18666A-Treated Rats

| RAT GROUP | TREAT-MENT[†] | SERUM STEROLS (mg/dl)[‡] | | | BODY WEIGHT CHANGE g | FOOD INTAKE g | LIVER WEIGHT g |
		CHOLES-TEROL	DESMOS-TEROL	TOTAL			
NORMAL	CONTROL	85	--	85	73	227	8.2
	CHOLES-TEROL	116[a]	--	116[a]	83[a]	256[a]	10.1[a]
U-18666A TREATED	CONTROL	34	29	63	83	245	9.9
	CHOLES-TEROL	102[a]	13[a]	115[a]	81	241	9.8
% STANDARD DEVIATION		17.2	13.2	17.1	13.0	8.0	9.5

[†]Cholesterol supplemented at 2% in the basal diet. Ten rats per treatment group.
[‡]In all tables serum sterols are expressed as antilog of logarithm means.
[a]Significantly different from respective control, $P < 0.05$.

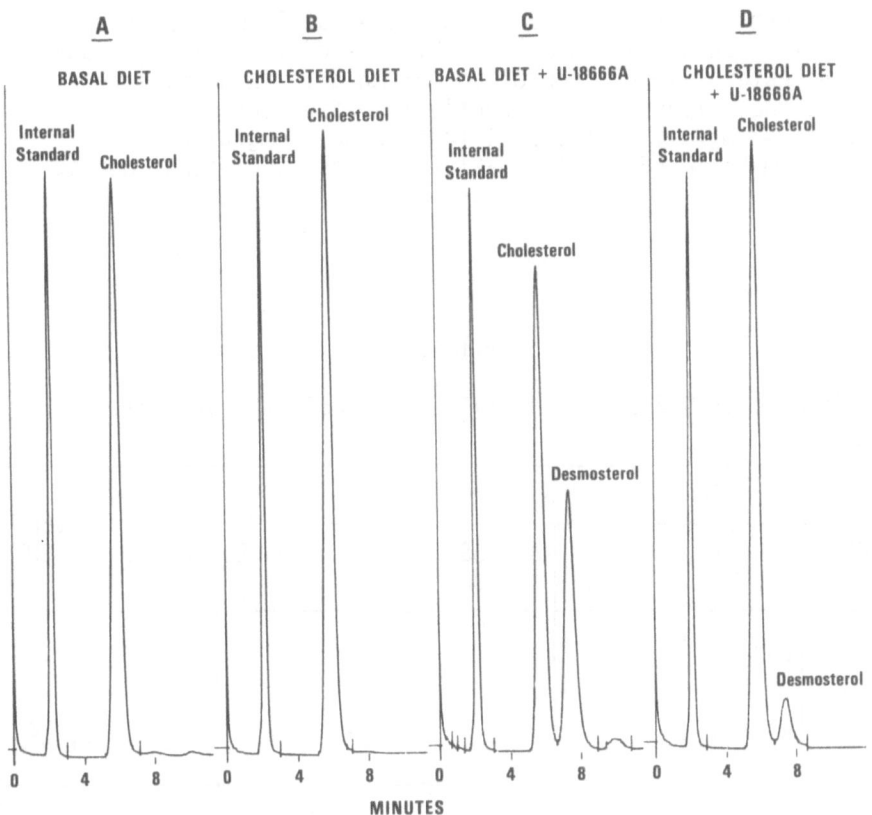

Figure 1
GLC analysis of cholesterol and desmosterol in serum of normal,
U-18666A, and cholesterol-fed rats.

As shown by gas chromatographic analyses illustrated in
Figure 1, in the normal rat (Figure 1A) or rat fed 2% cholesterol
in the basal diet (Figure 1B), cholesterol represents the major
sterol detected in the serum. The first small peak after cholesterol is campesterol, which has the same retention time as desmosterol, followed by β-sitosterol. Mass spectroscopic analysis
shows no detectable desmosterol in the serum of normal animals.
After treatment with U-18666A, the animal fed basal diet develops
a significant desmosterol peak (Figure 1C). However, as shown in
Figure 1D, feeding cholesterol to a U-18666A-treated animal causes
a suppression of serum desmosterol. The contribution of campesterol to desmosterol values in U-18666A-treated rats is less than
1 mg/dl in all experiments.

The results with U-21743 administered at 10 mg/kg/day appears in Table II. In normal animals, U-21743 significantly increased serum cholesterol level from 81 to 125 mg/dl. In animals receiving U-18666A, the compound significantly increased serum cholesterol from 29 to 43 mg/dl, desmosterol from 26 to 45 mg/dl, and total sterols from 55 to 88 mg/dl. U-21743 causes significant hepato-megaly.

TABLE II

Effects of U-21743 in Normal and U-18666A-Treated Rats

RAT GROUP	TREAT-MENT[†]	SERUM STEROLS (mg/dl)			BODY WEIGHT CHANGE g	FOOD INTAKE g	LIVER WEIGHT g
		CHOLES-TEROL	DESMOS-TEROL	TOTAL			
NORMAL	CONTROL	81	--	81	76	248	9.1
	U-21743	125^a	--	125^a	79	257	11.4^a
U-18666A TREATED	CONTROL	29	26	55	86	273	10.4
	U-21743	43^a	45^a	88^a	76	258	12.9^a
% STANDARD DEVIATION		13.6	18.3	11.8	13.5	7.5	10.5

[†]U-21743 given by gavage at 10 mg/kg/day; controls received vehicle only. Ten rats per treatment group.
[a]Significantly different from respective control, $P<0.05$.

TABLE III

Effects of Colestipol HCl or Clofibrate, Singly or in Combination
in Normal and U-18666A-Treated Rats

RAT GROUP	TREAT-MENT[†]	SERUM STEROLS (mg/dl)			BODY WEIGHT CHANGE g	FOOD INTAKE g	LIVER WEIGHT g
		CHOLES-TEROL	DESMOS-TEROL	TOTAL			
NORMAL	CONTROL	82	--	82	90	256	9.3
	COLESTI-POL HCl	89	--	89	92	281	9.9
	CLOFI-BRATE	54[a]	--	54[a]	85	266	16.5[a]
	COLESTI-POL HCl CLOFI-BRATE	50[a]	--	50[a]	90	267	15.8[a]
U-18666A TREATED	CONTROL	30	29	59	94	267	10.9
	COLESTI-POL HCl	12[ab]	40[ab]	52[b]	92	275	11.9[b]
	CLOFI-BRATE	19[ab]	16[ab]	35[a]	93	269	17.6[ab]
	COLESTI-POL HCl CLOFI-BRATE	8[a]	23[a]	31[a]	84	255	15.6[a]
% STANDARD DEVIATION		17.9	18.8	16.0	12.9	9.5	10.4

[†]Colestipol HCl and clofibrate supplemented at 1.0 and 0.2%,
respectively, in the basal diet. Ten rats per treatment group.
[a]Significantly different from respective control, P<0.05.
[b]Significantly different from combination of colestipol HCl and
clofibrate, P<0.05.

In normal animals, 1% colestipol HCl in the diet did not significantly alter serum cholesterol concentration from control (Table III). Clofibrate supplemented at 0.2% in the diet significantly reduced serum cholesterol from 82 to 54 mg/dl; in combination with colestipol HCl it caused a similar reduction in cholesterol level (50 mg/dl). In U-18666A-treated animals, colestipol HCl reduced serum cholesterol from 30 to 12 mg/dl and increased desmosterol level from 29 to 40 mg/dl; total sterol concentration did not differ significantly from control. Compared to control, clofibrate reduced serum cholesterol and desmosterol 37 and 45%, respectively. Compared with the colestipol HCl group, clofibrate in combination with colestipol HCl significantly reduced serum cholesterol from 12 to 8 mg/dl and desmosterol from 40 to 23 mg/dl. Clofibrate caused a significant reduction in total sterol concentration; in all animals it caused significant hepatomegaly.

TABLE IV

Effects of Cholestyramine in Normal and U-18666A-Treated Rats

RAT GROUP	TREAT-MENT[†]	SERUM STEROLS (mg/dl)			BODY WEIGHT CHANGE g	FOOD INTAKE g	LIVER WEIGHT g
		CHOLES-TEROL	DESMOS-TEROL	TOTAL			
NORMAL	CONTROL	92	--	92	80	229	8.8
	CHOLES-TYRAMINE	93	--	93	88	254[a]	9.0
U-18666A TREATED	CONTROL	38	26	64	81	228	9.6
	CHOLES-TYRAMINE	12[a]	43[a]	55	70	223	10.1
% STANDARD DEVIATION		16.4	16.3	14.0	16.7	10.7	7.5

[†]Cholestyramine supplemented at 1% in the basal diet. Ten rats per treatment group.
[a]Significantly different from respective control, $P < 0.05$.

NONISOTOPIC METHOD FOR ESTIMATING CHOLESTEROGENESIS IN THE RAT   259

The effects of cholestyramine supplemented at 1% in the diet are shown in Table IV. In normal animals, cholestyramine did not significantly alter serum cholesterol from control; in U-18666A-treated animals the resin reduced serum cholesterol from 38 to 12 mg/dl and increased desmosterol from 26 to 43 mg/dl; total sterol concentration did not differ significantly from control. Similar results were obtained with colestipol HCl (Table III).

TABLE V

Effects of Several Compounds in Normal Rats

TREATMENT	DOSE mg/kg/day	SERUM CHOLESTEROL mg/dl	BODY WEIGHT CHANGE g	FOOD INTAKE g	LIVER WEIGHT g
CONTROL	0	81	76	248	9.1
NICOTINIC ACID	200	80	82	266[a]	9.4
NICOTIN-AMIDE	200	85	57[a]	241	8.7
L-THYROXINE	0.3	89	61[a]	273[a]	9.8
U-21892	5	103[a]	67	284[a]	9.1
% STANDARD DEVIATION		15.3	15.7	7.4	10.3

Ten rats per treatment group.

[a]Significantly different from control, P<0.05.

The effects of nicotinic acid (200 mg/kg), nicotinamide (200 mg/kg), L-thyroxine (0.3 mg/kg) or the thyroxine analog U-21892 (5 mg/kg) are shown in normal animals (Table V) and animals treated with U-18666A (Table VI). In normal animals, U-21892 increased serum cholesterol by 27%; other cholesterol values did not differ significantly from control. Body weight change was reduced by nicotinamide and L-thyroxine; food intake was increased with nico-tinic acid, L-thyroxine, or U-21892.

TABLE VI

Effects of Several Compounds in U-18666A-Treated Rats

TREATMENT	DOSE mg/kg/day	SERUM STEROLS (mg/dl)			BODY WEIGHT CHANGE g	FOOD INTAKE g	LIVER WEIGHT g
		CHOLES-TEROL	DESMOS-TEROL	TOTAL			
CONTROL U-18666A	3	29	26	55	86	273	10.4
NICOTINIC ACID	200	28	26	54	78	268	10.4
NICOTIN-AMIDE	200	33	32^a	65^a	64^a	254	9.9
L-THYROXINE	0.3	33	35^a	68^a	53^a	275	10.2
U-21892	5	40^a	41^a	81^a	59^a	276	9.5
% STANDARD DEVIATION		18.3	16.9	14.2	18.5	8.4	9.9

Ten rats per treatment group.
[a]Significantly different from control, $P<0.05$.

In U-18666A-treated animals, nicotinamide, L-thyroxine, and U-21892 increased serum desmosterol; only serum cholesterol varied significantly from control with U-21892. Total sterols were in-creased with all three compounds. Body weight change was decreased with the same three compounds; food intake and liver weights did not differ significantly from control.

DISCUSSION

We have examined the validity and usefulness of employing desmosterol concentrations in the serum of U-18666A-treated rats as a means of determining the contributions of endogenous sterols to the serum cholesterol pool. No desmosterol was detected in the serum of the normal control rat. After 2 weeks of U-18666A treatment, serum desmosterol reached average concentrations of 26-29 mg/dl, i.e. levels of desmosterol that constitute 41-49% of the total serum sterol concentration. Dietary cholesterol caused a suppression of the level of serum desmosterol in the U-18666A-treated animals and demonstrates the operation of the cholesterol negative feedback system in the intact animal. It is well established that exogenous cholesterol depresses the rate of hepatic cholesterol synthesis by inhibiting the conversion of β-hydroxy-β-methylglutarate to mevalonate (10,11). In the rat the liver is the major source of serum cholesterol (12) although extra-hepatic tissues insensitive to inhibition by exogenous cholesterol, such as the intestine (13), might be expected to make a significant contribution to the serum sterol pool. However, in rats fed cholesterol Bricker et al. (5), using both plasma desmosterol levels caused by feeding triparanol and acetate-2-^{14}C incorporation into cholesterol as indications of endogenous sterol production, conclude that the intestine does not represent a significant source of plasma sterols in the rat. Although in our test feeding 2% cholesterol the mean desmosterol levels were only decreased from 29 to 13 mg/dl, it nevertheless is apparent that exogenous cholesterol causes a suppression in serum desmosterol in our animals.

Normal animals treated with U-21743 were hypercholesterolemic; in U-18666A-treated animals serum desmosterol and cholesterol were elevated indicating increased sterol synthesis. The results are consistent with the increase in concentration and specific activity of hepatic cholesterol in animals treated with U-21743 and acetate-1-^{14}C reported previously (14). No unusual sterols were detected in the serum or liver of these animals. In a cholesterol turnover study, U-21743 caused significant increases in the turnover of cholesterol (production rate) and size of the rapidly exchangeable pool in the rat (15). The compound may increase the activity or quantity of liver enzymes concerned with the biosynthesis of cholesterol resulting in an increase in cholesterol and desmosterol in the rat.

The decrease in serum desmosterol and cholesterol in animals treated with the hypocholesterolemic agent clofibrate suggests inhibition of cholesterol biosynthesis. There is abundant evidence that clofibrate both in vivo and in vitro markedly inhibits acetate incorporation into liver cholesterol (16-18). Colestipol HCl and cholestyramine increased serum desmosterol levels indicating increased synthesis which is consonant with the reports of increased acetate incorporation into hepatic cholesterol (19,20). The reduced cholesterol levels may reflect the limited amount of cholesterol available for conversion to bile acids. Neither resin altered serum cholesterol concentrations in normal animals. These results can be ascribed to the capacity of the rat to compensate the fecal loss of bile acids by a corresponding increase in sterol synthesis. Clofibrate in combination with colestipol HCl suppressed the increase in synthesis caused by the latter. Cayen and Dvornik (21) also showed that clofibrate can reduce the cholestyramine-induced increase in hepatic cholesterol synthesis. The rate of acetate-2-^{14}C incorporation into cholesterol after treatment with both drugs was significantly lower than that of cholestyramine alone, and significantly higher than that obtained with clofibrate alone.

Nicotinic acid did not alter serum sterols in both normal and U-18666A-treated rats. The results are in agreement with Duncan and Best (22) who reported no significant effect of nicotinic acid on the incorporation of acetate-1-^{14}C into serum and liver cholesterol. Nicotinamide, however, caused a small but significant increase in serum desmosterol levels in the U-18666A-treated animals but did not affect serum cholesterol concentrations in normal animals. The nicotinamide effect may be related to the loss of weight in both animal test systems or to an increase in activity of the NADPH dependent mixed-function oxygenases in liver microsomes leading to enhanced hydroxylation of cholesterol and more rapid conversion to bile acids. The rat can compensate for the cholesterol loss by increasing synthesis of the sterol.

The increase in cholesterol synthesis by L-thyroxine as reflected in the increase in serum desmosterol is consistent with the report of increased cholesterol synthesis using tritium in the hyperthyroid rat (23). Furthermore, hyperthyroidism is associated with increased destruction and intestinal excretion of cholesterol (24). The L-thyroxine treatment produced symptoms typical of hyperthyroidism, e.g. an increase in food consumption and a decrease in body weight in normal animals; in U-18666A-treated animals only weight gain was reduced,while food intake was unchanged from control. The thyroxine analog U-21892, at 17 times the dose used for L-thyroxine, caused an increase in both cholesterol and desmosterol levels in the U-18666A-treated animals; cholesterol levels were also significantly elevated in normal animals. Apparently, cholesterol synthesis exceeded the animals' capacity to excrete the sterol.

Our results which are consistent with the known effects of various treatments on cholesterogenesis indicate the U-18666A-treated rat model can be useful in evaluating mechanisms of action of hypocholesterolemic agents.

REFERENCES

1. Phillips, W.A. and J. Avigan. 1963. Inhibition of cholesterol biosynthesis in the rat by 3β-(2-diethylaminoethoxy)androst-5-en-17-one, hydrochloride. Proc. Soc. Exp. Biol. Med. 112:233-236.

2. Dvornik, D., M.L. Giver, and J.G. Rochefort. 1965. AY-9944, an inhibitor of cholesterol biosynthesis, as tool in the estimation of the rate of cholesterogenesis. Circulation 32: Suppl. II, 10-11.

3. Giver, M.L., J.G. Rochefort, and D.M. Dvornik. 1966. Tool for the estimation of the rate of cholesterol biosynthesis. Circulation 34:Suppl. III, 12.

4. Dvornik, D., M. Kraml, and J.F. Bagli. 1966. Agents affecting lipid metabolism. XVIII. A 7-dehydrocholesterol Δ^7-reductase inhibitor (AY-9944) as tool in studies of Δ^7-sterol metabolism. Biochemistry 5:1060-1064.

5. Bricker, L.A., H.J. Weis, and M.D. Siperstein. 1972. In vivo demonstration of the cholesterol feedback system by means of a desmosterol suppression technique. J. Clin. Invest. 51:197-205.

6. Phillips, W.A. and C.P. Berg. 1954. Effect upon growth of the D isomers in synthetic mixtures of the essential amino acids. J. Nutr. 53:481-498.

7. Phillips, W.A., W.W. Stafford, and J. Stuut Jr. 1973. Jugular vein technique for serial blood sampling and intravenous injection in the rat. Proc. Soc. Exp. Biol. Med. 143:733-735.

8. Abell, L.L., B.B. Levy, B.B. Brodie, and F.E. Kendall. 1953. A simplified method for the estimation of total cholesterol in serum and demonstration of its specificity. J. Biol. Chem. 195:357-366.

9. Snedecor, G.S., and W.G. Cochran. 1967. Statistical Methods, The Iowa State University Press, Ames, Iowa, pp. 258.

10. Siperstein, M.D. and M.J. Guest. 1960. Studies on the site of the feedback control of cholesterol synthesis. J. Clin. Invest. 39:642-652.

11. Siperstein, M.D., and V.M. Fagan. 1966. Feedback control of mevalonate synthesis by dietary cholesterol. J. Biol. Chem. 241:602-609.

12. Hotta, S., and I.L. Chaikoff. 1955. The role of the liver in the turnover of plasma cholesterol. Arch. Biochem. Biophys. 56:28-37.

13. Dietschy, J.M. and M.D. Siperstein. 1967. Effect of cholesterol feeding and fasting on sterol synthesis in seventeen tissues of the rat. J. Lipid Res. 8:97-104.

14. W.A. Phillips. 1971. Studies with known hypocholestermic agents in U-21743 (p-chlorophenyl methanesulfonate)-induced hyperlipidemic rats. Fed. Proc. 30:369.

15. Phillips, W.A. and G.L. Elfring. Effect of U-21743 (p-chlorophenyl methanesulfonate) on cholesterol turnover in the rat (in preparation).

16. Azarnoff, D.L., D.R. Tucker, and G.A. Barr. 1965. Studies with ethyl chlorophenoxyisobutyrate (Clofibrate). Metabolism 14:959-965.

17. Gould, R.G., E.A. Swyryd, D. Avoy, and D.M. Coan. 1967. The effects of α-p-chlorophenoxyisobutyrate on the synthesis and release into plasma lipoproteins in rats. Prog. Biochem. Pharmacol. 2:345-357.

18. Hill, P. and D. Dvornik. 1971. Agents affecting lipid metabolism. XL. Effect of ethyl chlorophenoxyisobutyrate on liver lipids and serum lipoproteins in rats. Can. J. Biochem. 49:903-910.

19. Honohan, T. and T.M. Parkinson. 1975. Enhancement of cholesterol turnover in rats by a catatoxic steroid (PCN) and a bile acid sequestrant (Colestipol-HCl). Biochem. Pharmacol. 24:899-903.

20. Huff, J.W., J.L. Gilfillan, and V.M. Hunt. 1963. Effect of cholestyramine, a bile acid binding polymer on plasma cholesterol and fecal bile acid excretion in the rat. Proc. Soc. Exp. Biol. Med. 114:352-355.

21. Cayen, M.N. and D. Dvornik. 1970. Agents affecting lipid metabolism. XXXIX. Effect of combined administration of ethyl chlorophenoxyisobutyrate and cholestyramine on cholesterol biosynthesis in the rat. Can. J. Biochem. 48:1022-1023.

22. Duncan, C.H. and M.M. Best. 1960. Lack of nicotinic acid effect on cholesterol metabolism of the rat. J. Lipid Res. 1:159-163.

23. Byers, S.O., R.H. Rosenman, M. Friedman, and M.W. Biggs. 1952. Rate of cholesterol synthesis in hypo- and hyperthyroid rats. J. Exptl. Med. 96:513-516.

24. Rosenman, R.H., S.O. Byers, and M. Friedman. 1952. The mechanism responsible for the altered blood cholesterol content in deranged thyroid states. J. Clin. Endocrinol. Metabolism 12:1287-1299.

CHOLESTEROL METABOLISM IN RATS SENSITIVE TO HIGH CHOLESTEROL DIET

Nozomu Takeuchi, Masami Ito and Yuichi Yamamura

The Third Department of Internal Medicine, Osaka University Hospital, Fukushima, Osaka, JAPAN 553

ABSTRACT

There was great individual variation in the elevations of serum cholesterol concentrations in a Wistar strain of rats by the ingestion of a large amount of cholesterol, although their cholesterol concentrations were almost identical while under the feeding of a regular stock diet. Their serum total phospholipid and dextran precipitable beta-lipoproteins showed the same tendencies, but serum triglyceride concentration was not affected by the dietary supplement in both groups.

So, the rats with the different elevation rates of serum cholesterol concentrations were divided into good, normo and poor responding groups to cholesterol ingestion by the degrees of the elevations and bred for several generations. Serum lipid levels in the descendants from hyperresponding rats were not different from those from hyporesponding rats during the observed period, when they were given a stock diet. However, the response of serum cholesterol level to oral cholesterol ingestion in the former was larger than that in the latter. Therefore, it is suggested that the susceptibility of serum cholesterol to cholesterol ingestion may be heritable from parents to their offsprings.

By the results of the tracer experiments, it was demonstrated that neither hepatic cholesterol synthesis nor absorption was affected in hyperresponding rats. On the other hand, a half life of labeled cholesterol was prolonged in this selected group. The relative fractional turnover rate was 17.8 per cent in hyporesponding rats and 15.8 per cent in hyperresponding rats. Excretion of the radioactivity from labeled cholesterol into the bile in good

responding rats with bile fistula was slower than that in poor responding rats.

When 1 g per 100 g body weight of glucose was given to the rats
after 40 hours fasting, hepatic cholesterol synthesis increased at
the same rate in both groups of rats, but the induction of hepatic
cholesterol 7α-hydroxylation in hyperresponding groups was slower
than that in hyporesponding groups.   The distribution rates of the
radioactivities into livers seemed to be delayed in good responders
after the labeled cholesterol was ingested orally.   It means that
some disturbances in cholesterol transport may exist which induce the
metabolic abnormality in such animals.

It was shown that cholesterol metabolism was impaired in aged
animals as compared with young ones.   Serum cholesterol concentrations were elevated in good responders more than in poor responders by aging. The inborn errors of cholesterol metabolism in such
animals might be emphasized from the fact of the impairment of cholesterol metabolism by the aging process.

INTRODUCTION

In order to elucidate the regulatory mechanism of cholesterol
metabolism or evaluate the effects of hypocholesterolemic agents,
many have used rats most frequently as an experimental animal.
However, many differences have been suggested to exist between the
cholesterol metabolism in rats and human beings.   Actually, the dietary composition of rats is different from that of humans.   From
the view point of the cholesterol metabolism, absorption rate of
cholesterol from the intestine of rats is larger than that of humans
(1,2).   The synthetic rates of cholesterol and bile acids in
the livers are also quite different (2,3).   A negative feedback control of cholesterol synthesis by the ingestion of cholesterol
in the rats is considered to be more sensitive than that of humans
(2,4).   The serum cholesterol concentration in rats is about one
third of that of humans.

Therefore, an unusually large amount of cholesterol, with agents
affecting the cholesterol metabolism, or a detergent must be
administered to the animals to elevate the serum cholesterol concentration and to make a hypercholesterolemic state.   Under these experimental conditions, cholesterol metabolism is known to be altered
markedly by the metabolic regulations.   When a large amount of
cholesterol is ingested by rats or dogs, hepatic cholesterogenesis
is inhibited completely (5-7), and cholesterol degradation to bile
acids is accelerated (8,9).   An injection of detergent stimulates the hepatic cholesterol synthesis markedly and impairs
cholesterol degradation (10-13).

Etiology of human hypercholesterolemia is still obscure at present, and might be different from these experimental models.   There have been some reports concerning hypercholesterolemic animals in pigeons, mice, rabbits or monkeys (15-22).   In some of these animals, the atherosclerotic changes were found in their aortas (18-20, 22-25).   However, a more suitable model of spontaneous hyper-cholesterolemia has not been reported in rats.

We have often examined the availabilities of drugs or the meta-bolic changes of cholesterol under some experimental conditions us-ing such artificial hypercholesterolemic animals, and have found that the elevations of serum cholesterol concentrations by feeding of an atherogenic diet containing a very high cholesterol concentra-tion were different in individual animals.   Therefore, we bred hyperresponding rats whose serum cholesterol concentrations were ele-vated markedly by the feeding of such an atherogenic diet and examin-ed the cholesterol metabolism in such rats with tracers.   From these experiments some heritable metabolic abnormalities were found in these animals.   The effect of aging on serum lipid levels in these rats was also observed.

MATERIALS AND METHODS

Animals and Methods

Wistar-King strain rats were supplied from a commercial supp-lier, Osaka Junkei (Osaka, JAPAN).   Rats of both sexes, aged 1.5-2 months, were given a stock diet (Oriental Kobo Ltd. Osaka, JAPAN) containing   1.5 per cent cholesterol and 0.5 per cent sodium cholate for a week.   Before and after the feeding of the high cholesterol diet, blood was obtained by cardiac puncture after an overnight fast, and the serum lipid concentrations were deter-mined.   Thereafter, the rats were fed with the regular stock diet containing   0.1 per cent cholesterol for the preceding 4 weeks and with the high cholesterol diet for a week again.   Serum lipid levels before and after the cholesterol ingestion were repeatedly determined.   When differences of serum cholesterol concentrations before and after the cholesterol administration were more than 100 per cent of the basal levels by the dietary change, the rats were desig-nated hyperresponders (good responder), and those less than 30 per cent elevation were selected as the hyporesponders (poor respond-er).   The rats who showed the average elevations of serum chole-sterol of all animals examined were regarded as normo responding control. All of these groups were bred for several generations, and the responses of serum cholesterol of their offspring to the high cholesterol diet were also examined by the same manner at the age of 1.5-2 months.   There were no significant differences between good, normo and poor responder rats as regards the physical activi-ties, food consumptions (13-14 g/day/rat during the age of 1-3 months) and the increases of body weights.

Determinations of serum cholesterol, phospholipid and triglyceride were followed by the methods described by Leffler et al. (26)
Haeflmayr et al.(27) and Fletcher (28).   Separation of beta-
and prebeta-lipoproteins from other serum proteins was followed by
the dextran precipitation method (29).   Protein concentration
in the lipoprotein was determined by Lowry's method (30).

Metabolic Studies of Cholesterol

For the metabolic experiments,   rats of both sexes weighing
about 200g from poor and good responder groups (aged   2-3.5 months) were used.

In order to investigate the absorption of cholesterol from intestine, 0.5 µCi 4-^{14}C cholesterol (55.8 mCi/mM, The Radiochemical
Centre, Amersham ENGLAND) in 0.5 ml of 5 per cent Tween 80 solution
was administered orally by stomach tube to good and poor responder
rats who had been fed with a stock diet and fasted   overnight.
One and a half, 2.5 and 5 hours after the ingestion of the label,
blood and liver were obtained, and the radioactivities of free and
total cholesterol in serum and liver were determined by liquid scintillation spectrometer with toluene scintillation fluid as previously
reported (31).

Incorporation of 1-^{14}C sodium acetate (40 mCi/mM, The Radiochemical Centre, Amersham ENGLAND) into the hepatic total lipid and
cholesterol in both groups of   rats were determined with liver
slices in vitro.   From these results of the incorporation rates,
the hepatic cholesterol synthesis was estimated.   The detailed
descriptions for the methods of the incubation, analysis of lipid
and determination of radioactivity were reported previously (31).

For the determination of clearance of labeled cholesterol from
the peripheral circulation, 1.5 µCi of 4-^{14}C cholesterol dissolved
in 4 per cent bovine serum albumin in saline was injected into the
tail vein of the rat fed with either a regular or a high cholesterol diet for 4-5 days.   Blood was obtained by cardiac puncture at
the appropriate intervals during 5-6 weeks to determine the decline
of the radioactivity in the blood.

Biliary bile of both groups were fractionally collected from the
bile fistulae during 48 hours.   A small poly-ethylene tube was put
into the bile duct of the rat, and 0.5 µCi of labeled cholesterol was
injected via the tail vein. Excreted radioactivity into the bile
was determined after deproteinization.

After the fasting for 40 hours, the rats were given 1 g/100 g

body weight of glucose orally by a stomach tube to investigate the
induction of cholesterol synthesis and degradation in the liver.
The rats were sacrificed at 0, 3 and 5 hours after the glucose administration.   Cholesterol syntheses in the liver slices were determined in vitro as described above.   Cholesterol 7α-hydroxyla-
tion in the liver microsome was estimated by the method described by
Mitropoulos and Balasubramaniam (32) at the same time.

Effect of Aging on Cholesterol Metabolism

Some of the rats belonging to both good and poor reponder groups
were brought up by a stock diet as long as 15 months, and their serum
lipid levels were determined by the methods described above at the
age of 6, 8 and 15 months.

Subcellular fractions of normal liver cells from young (1 month
old) and old (7-8 months old) were obtained by the usual method.
Namely, the liver tissues were homogenized with 4 volume of 250 mM
cold sucrose solution containing   75 mM nicotinamide and 1.0 mM
EDTA.   The homogenate was cetrifuged at 800 G for 10 min and the
supernatant fraction was centrifuged at 9,500 G for 10 min.   The
precipitate at 9,500 G was washed with 1.15 per cent cold KCl solution and recentrifuged at 6,700 G for 10 min to obtain the mitochondrial fraction.   Washing was repeated once more and the mitochondria were suspended to 0.1 M potassium phosphate buffer containing 10 mM $MgCl_2$ (pH 7.4) to make the mitochondrial suspension up to
the same concentration as the original liver tissue.   The supernatant at 9,500 G was centrifuged at 105,000 G for 60 min by Hitachi
50-P ultracentrifuge apparatus with 50-123 rotor.   The precipitate was washed with 1.15 per cent cold KCL solution and again centrifuged at 105,000 G to obtain the microsomal fraction. The microsomes
were   suspended to 3 ml of the potassium phosphate buffer.

Cholesterol synthesis from acetate was examined in the combined
incubation mixture of each 1 ml of microsomes, mitochondrial suspension and cytosol fractions with 2 μ moles NADP, 10 μ moles G6P,
10 μ moles ATP, 0.4 μ moles Co A, 2.5 U G6PDH and 5 μCi 1-^{14}C sodium acetate and 5.0 μ moles non-labeled sodium acetate.   For the
cholesterol synthesis from mevalonate, 1 ml of the microsomal suspension and 1 ml of cytosol fraction were incubated with 0.1 μCi 2-
^{14}C mevalonic acid and 0.5 μ moles non-labeled mevalonic acid.
Co A in the cofactors described above was omitted from the incubation medium.   Incubations were carried out at 37.5°C for 1 hour
at atmospheric pressure.   The reactions were terminated with
additions of 10 ml of chloroform-methanol (2:1 v/v).   Extraction, analysis and determination of the labeled cholesterol were
followed by above mentioned procedures .   Determination of 7α-hydro-
xylase activity was carried out by the method of Mitropoulos using
the microsome fractions from young or old rats.

RESULTS

Table I demonstrates the typical changes of the serum lipid
concentrations of the female rats of three groups at the age of 2
months, before and after the feeding of a high cholesterol diet for
one week. When they were fed with a regular stock diet, lipid concentrations of hyporesponding rats were not significantly different
from those of poor and normoresponder rats as shown in the table.
After the feeding of a high cholesterol diet for one week, the serum
cholesterol concentration in good responders was about twice that in
the case of the poor responder. The serum phospholipid and dextran-
precipitable beta-lipoprotein of good responders became higher in concentration than those of poor responders to the cholesterol ingestion.
The serum triglyceride concentration was not changed by the short
term feeding of a high cholesterol diet in both groups. So, there
was no significant difference between two groups in serum triglyceride concentration even at the high serum cholesterol levels.

TABLE I

Serum Lipid and Beta-Lipoprotein of Poor and Good Responder
Rats Fed with Either a Stock or High Cholesterol Diet

Animal Groups	Diet	Cholesterol	Phospho-lipid	Triglyceride	Beta-Lipo-proteins
Poor Responder (5)***	Stock Diet	64.0+3.3*	90.3+3.8	45.2+6.8	246+13
	High Chole-sterol Diet	87.0+2.9	94.4+3.4	47.4+6.0	262+10
		**		**	**
Normo Responder (9)	Stock Diet	68.8+2.6	102.1+3.0	47.1+5.1	254+12
	High Chole-sterol Diet	137.7+2.1	114.4+3.9	43.2+6.5	286+18
		**		**	**
Good Responder (6)	Stock Diet	67.2+4.2	101.3+4.9	48.9+9.8	238+10
	High Chole-Sterol Diet	191.3+8.9	139.5+6.7	50.4+7.1	323+20

(mg/100ml)

* Mean $\pm$ S.E. (mg/100 ml), ** Significant difference
between two groups ($p < 0.05$), ***Number of rats

TABLE II

Liver Cholesterol Content of Good and Poor
Responder Rats after Cholesterol Feeding

Animal Group	Low Cholesterol Diet		High Cholesterol Diet	
	Liver (mg/g)	Serum (mg/100 ml)	Liver (mg/g)	Serum (mg/100 ml)
Poor Responder (4)	1.9+0.17*	61.2+4.29	4.94+0.46	91.7+4.50
Good Responder (6)	2.05+0.09	72.5+3.30	4.78+0.36	173.3+17.0**

*Mean + S.E., **Statistically significant from poor responder group ($p < 0.01$).

Hepatic cholesterol content of good and poor responder rats is presented in Table II.   There was no significant difference between the hepatic cholesterol content of both animal groups when they were fed with a stock diet.   Although serum cholesterol level of good responder was markedly higher than that of poor responder after the feeding a high cholesterol diet for a week, the liver cholesterol content of both groups increased to the same degree.

An example of the breeding of normo and good responder rats within the respective groups is shown in Table III.   There was no significant difference in the serum cholesterol concentration between normo and good responder groups while a stock diet was given to these young rats.   However, after the feeding of a high cholesterol diet, the serum cholesterol concentrations in the offspring from the parents of good responders were significantly higher than those from the poor responders.   But there was not such a clear difference between poor and normo responder groups.

Table IV shows the serum cholesterol concentration of another group of hyperresponder rats who were inbred for 3 generations. The average sensitivity of serum cholesterol to oral cholesterol ingestion was not increased in these offspring.   However, the maximal serum cholesterol levels among these rats fed with a high cholesterol diet had the tendency to increase as indicated in the table. Estimate of heritability range of good responder was about 50 per cent.

The radioactivity of serum cholesterol at 1.5, 2.5 and 5 hours after oral administration of labeled cholesterol were not different between good and poor responder rats as shown in Table V.   These results suggest that the absorption of cholesterol from the intestine is not responsible for the sensitivity of the serum cholesterol

TABLE III

Inheritance of Response of Serum Cholesterol
to High Cholesterol Diet

Serum Cholesterol (mg/100 ml)

Animal Group		Parents	Offsprings		
Normo Responder	Male	154*(58)**	Male	(8)***118.3+6.1*(56.4+2.3)**	
		144 (55)			
	Female	139 (60)	Female	(10)	154.0+3.7 (69.6+2.5)
		129 (53)			
Good Responder	Male	210 (61)	Male	(6)	152.8+7.7 (54.2+0.5)
		196 (58)			
	Female	186 (63)	Female	(7)	183.3+8.1 (59.4+2.3)
		178 (56)			

*Serum cholesterol level after the feeding of high cholesterol
diet for 1 week and **that during the feeding of stock diet.
***Number of rats.   Serum cholesterol levels of the offspr-
ing from good responder rats significantlly higher than those
from poor responder rats after cholesterol feeding in both sexes.

TABLE IV

Serum Cholesterol Concentration of Good Responder Rats after
Cholesterol Administration after Repeated Inbreeding

Cholesterol Diet		Generations			
		0	1	2	3
Male	High	133*	120.6+7.1 (6)** (102 − 142)***	142.8+7.2 (11) (114 − 173)	149.0+11.1 (11) (111 − 223)
	Low	−	79.4+10.3	82.9+9.9	70.5+4.5
Female	High	131+2.5	203.3+17.2(7) (131 − 243)	168.6+7.2 (16) (101 − 213)	181.5+19.5 (8) (85 − 255)
	Low	−	81.0+5.5	74.9+6.3	68.8+3.7

*mg/100 ml, **Mean + S.E., Number in parenthesis represents the
number of rats. ***Range of serum cholesterol of rats.

TABLE V

Appearance of Radioactivity   in Peripheral Blood
after Oral Administration of 4-^{14}C Cholesterol

Time after Oral Administration (h)	Radioactivity in Serum (DPM/ml)		
	1.5	2.5	5.0
Poor Responder (5)*	219 + 78**	245 + 38	332 + 29
Good Responder (4)	205 + 42	216 + 16	325 + 5

*Number of rats, **Mean + S.E.

concentration to a high cholesterol diet.

In order to estimate the synthetic rate of cholesterol in the
liver, the liver slices from both groups were incubated with 1-^{14}C
sodium acetate in vitro.   TableVI indicates that the incorporation
of acetate into total lipids and cholesterol in the liver slices
are the same both in poor and good responder groups.   Therefore,
biosynthesis of cholesterol in the liver seems to be not different
between both groups.

TABLE VI

Incorporation of 1-^{14}C Acetate into Total Lipids and
Cholesterol in Rat Liver Slices in vitro

Animal Group	Incorporation of Acetate			
	Total Lipids		Cholesterol	
	($\times 10^4$DPM/g/h)	(n moles/g/h)	($\times 10^4$DPM/g/h)	(n moles/g/h)
Poor Responder (4)*	17.7+3.8**	80.5+17.0	8.3+2.1	37.5+9.0
Good Responder (4)	18.8+1.9	85.5+8.5	9.6+1.1	43.0+4.5

*Number of rats, **Mean + S.E., There was no significant
difference between two groups statistically in cholesterol as well as total lipid syntheses.

TABLE VII

Half Lives of 4-^{14}C Cholesterol in Good and Poor Responder Rats

Animal Group	Half Lives of Cholesterol (Days)	
	Low Cholesterol Diet	High Cholesterol Diet
Poor Responder	15.0±1.0*(5)** ⎤ p<0.05 p<0.01 ────8.4±0.5 (5) ⎤	
Good Responder	18.5±0.9 (5) ──── p<0.02 ─── 10.9±0.3 (6)	p<0.05

*Mean + S.E., **Number of rats

For the determination of the disappearance rate of cholesterol from peripheral blood, 4-^{14}C cholesterol dissolved in bovine serum albumin solution was injected intravenously in the poor and good responder rats who had been fed with a stock or high cholesterol diet.   The radioactivity in the plasma was determined at appropriate time intervals during 5-6 weeks.   Mean half life of the labeled cholesterol in the plasma of good responders was 18.5 days and that of poor responders was 15.0 days, when they were given a stock diet (Table VII).   After the feeding of a high cholesterol diet, the clearances of cholesterol in both groups were accelerated. In such a case, the half life of labeled cholesterol in good responders (10.9 days) was also longer than that of poor responders (8.4 days) as shown in Table VII.

TABLE VIII

Excretion of Bile and Radioactivity   from Bile Fistula of Rats after the Injection of Labeled Cholesterol

	Animal Group	Hours after Injection (h)		
		4	24	48
Bile	Poor Responder (6)*	3.4±0.7**	18.4±1.8	27.5±2.2
	Good Responder (4)	3.6±0.8	15.7±3.9	27.7±4.0
Counts	Poor Responder (6)	145.5±26.6**	513.6±42.2	769.2±53.2
	Good Responder (4)	115.4±15.5	345.4±47.8***	589.2±43.0***

*Number of rats, **Mean ± S.E. (ml/h or X10^{3}DPM)
***Significant difference between two groups

According to the calculation of two pool model analysis of
cholesterol turnover, the fractional. turnover rate of good responders was 15.8 per cent,and that of poor responders was 17.8 per cent.

Secretions of bile from the bile fistulae were almost the same
in both good and poor responder groups during the observed periods
as shown in Table VIII. However, the excretion of total radioactivity into the bile of good responders after the intravenous injection
of labeled cholesterol was less as compared with that of poor responders.

In order to examine the induction of cholesterol synthesis and
degradation in the liver, 2 ml per 100 g body weight of 50 per cent
glucose solution was ingested by a stomach tube to good and poor
responder rats fasted for 40 hours. At 0,3 and 5 hours after the
glucose administration 7α-hydroxylation of cholesterol was determined by the liver microsomes in vitro together with the estimation
of acetate incorporation into cholesterol in the liver slices (Table
IX).   After the glucose ingestion both cholesterol synthesis and
hydroxylation increased several fold.   Cholesterol synthesis in
both groups was low at the fasting time, and a significant difference was not found between the two groups. The increase of cholesterol synthesis by the glucose ingestion in good responders
almost the same as that in poor responders.   The hydroxylation
of cholesterol of hyperresponders at the fasting time was not different from that of hypo responders.   After the glucose administration, however, the increase of the former was lower than that of
hyporesponders at 3 hours after the treatment and seemed to delay

TABLE IX

Cholesterol Synthesis and 7α-Hydroxylation of Good and
Poor Responder Rats to Cholesterol Feeding

Hours after Glucose Ingestion	Cholesterol Synthesis (n moles/h/g)		
	0	3	5
Poor Responder	5.3 + 1.5*	24.2 + 2.8	28.3 $\pm$ 4.5
Good Responder	6.1 $\pm$ 1.7	26.3 $\pm$ 4.2	29.1 $\pm$ 6.8
	Cholesterol Hydroxylation (n moles/h/mg)		
Poor Responder	2.37 $\pm$ 0.25*	6.79 $\pm$ 0.38	7.28 $\pm$ 0.48
Good Responder	3.04 $\pm$ 0.28	4.38 $\pm$ 0.54**	6.35 $\pm$ 0.52

*Mean (3-4 animals) ± S.E., **significant difference
from poor responder group

TABLE X

Ratios of Specific Activities of Hepatic
and Serum Cholesterol

Hours after Injection		1.5	3	5
Animal Group		Ratio of Specific Activities		
Free	Poor Responder	0.46 ± 0.01*	0.62 ± 0.02	1.38 ± 0.12
	Good Responder	0.37 ± 0.02**	0.53 ± 0.02**	0.93 ± 0.01**
Total	Poor Responder	0.31 ± 0.07	0.42 ± 0.01	1.28 ± 0.12
	Good Responder	0.20 ± 0.02	0.32 ± 0.03	0.89 ± 0.15

*Mean ± S.E. (4 Animals), **Significantly different from
poor responder group.

as compared with the latter.   But 5 hours after the glucose, the
hydroxylation was almost identical in both groups.

    The ratio of specific activities of hepatic cholesterol to that
of serum cholesterol in hyperresponders were lower than that in poor
responders during the observed periods after the oral ingestion of
labeled cholesterol (Table X).   It probably indicates the impairment of the distribution rate of sterol to the liver from peripheral
circulation.

TABLE XI

Incorporation Rate of Acetate or Mevalonate into Cholesterol
in Hepatic Subcellular Fractions or Their Combinations

Incubation Systems	Incorporation of Acetate into Cholesterol	
	Young Rat	Old Rat
Mitochondria	0.1*	0.1
Microsomes	0.1·	0.1
Cytosol + Mitochondria	8.4	0.3
Cytosol + Microsomes	30.6 ± 4.8**	0.9 ± 0.6
Cytosol + Microsomes + Mitochondria	80.6 ± 10.1**	5.5 ± 1.5
	Incorporation of Mevalonate into Cholesterol	
Mitochondria	0.3	0.2
Microsomes	0.2	0.1
Cytosol + Mitochondria	10.4	5.4 ± 1.5
Cytosol + Microsome	39.7 ± 6.7**	18.0 ± 2.5
Cytosol + Microsomes + Mitochondria	47.9 ± 10.3**	13.5 ± 2.5

*n moles/h/system, **Significantly different from old rat.

TABLE XII

Aging Effect on Cholesterol 7α-Hydroxylation in Rat Liver

	Per Cent Conversion (%)	Net Hydroxylation (n moles/h/mg prot.)
Young Rat* (6)**	10.17±0.50***	6.25±0.32
	p<0.001	p<0.001
Old Rat* (3)	6.28±0.16	3.77±0.10

*1 and 6-7 months old, **Number of Rats, ***Mean ± S.E.

The effect of aging on cholesterol synthesis in hepatic micro-somes from acetate or mevalonate was examined in young rats aged about 1 month and adult rats aged 6-7 months (Table XI).   The incubation of a single subcellular fraction had no synthetic activi-ty of cholesterol in vitro.   But combined incubation systems of cytosol and microsomes showed remarkable synthetic activities from both acetate and mevalonate.   As shown in the table, cholesterol syntheses from acetate or mevalonate in these systems were decreased markedly in aged animals.

Cholesterol 7α-hydroxylase activity in the liver microsomes in vitro was also decreased in old rats as compared with   young rats (Table XII).   Therefore, both synthesis and degradation are de-creased in aged animals.

Some of the good and poor responder male rats were raised up to 15 months and their serum cholesterol was followed up.   The serum cholesterol concentration of hyperresponders was not different from that of poor responders at the age of 2 months, when they were fed with a stock diet as indicated in Table XIII.   However, at

TABLE XIII

Changes of Serum Cholesterol Levels by Aging

Animal Age		2	2	8	15
Diet		Stock	High Cholesterol	Stock	Stock
Poor Responder	(5)*	61.6±2.7**	87.0±2.9	72.4±3.4	78.9±3.3
			p<0.01	p<0.02	p<0.05
Good Responder	(5)	64.8±3.1	191.3±9.0	90.4±2.9	90.0±0.9

*Number of Rats, ** Mean ± S.E. (mg/100 ml)

TABLE XIV

Serum Lipid Levels of Good and Poor Responder Rats in Elderly Age

Animal Group	Cholesterol	Phospholipid	Triglyceride	Beta & Prebeta-Lipoproteins
Poor Responder	(5)*72.4+3.4	124.2+6.6	52.3+8.8	281+6.8
	⌐p<0.02	⌐p<0.01		⌐p <0.05
Good Responder	(5) 90.4+2.9	153.4+3.4	67.4+6.8	345+23.1

*Number of Rats, **Mean + S.E. (mg/100 ml).

8 months and 15 months, the former was significantly higher than
that of the latter.   This result suggests that the elevation of
serum cholesterol concentration of good responders to the course of
aging is larger than that of poor responders.   The concentrations
of serum phospholipid and dextran precipitable beta-lipoproteins
in good responders were also significantly higher than those in poor
responders in the older ages.   But the serum triglyceride concentration was not different between good and poor responder rats even
in this age (Table XIV).

DISCUSSION

        There have been many reports concerning the spontaneous hyper-
cholesterolemic animals or susceptible animals for dietary cholesterol.   Lofland et al. (33) reported the Squirrel monkey with genetic hypercholesterolemia and suggested that the cholesterol catabolism to bile acids was impaired in this monkey according to the
disappearance rate of labeled cholesterol or excretion of fecal bile
acids.   Cholesterol absorption, synthesis and fecal neutral sterol excretion were similar in the hyper- and normocholesterolemic
monkey.   Bell et al. (34) also demonstrated that the disappearance rate of labeled cholesterol from the peripheral circulation was
reduced in good responder pigeons to cholesterol load.   These
results suggested that the degradation of cholesterol decreases in
such hypercholesterolemic animals.   West and Roberts (35) showed
that hyporesponsive rabbits excreted more fecal steroids derived
from cholesterol than do hyperresponsive rabbits.   However, the
hyporesponsive rabbits stored more cholesterol ester in the liver.

        Adams et al. (36) also reported that Dutch rabbit kept lower
cholesterol levels on cholesterol feeding than New Zealand rabbits
and was resistant to formation of atheroma.   After cholesterol
feeding the liver cholesterol increased in the same degree in both
rabbit lines. They could not prove the acceleration of cholesterol
catabolism and biliary excretion of its metabolites in cholesterol

resistant Dutch rabbits.   Therefore, it was suggested that the
partition or balance of sterols between the liver and serum might
be affected.

In the present experiment, cholesterol transport into the liver
from serum seemed to be delayed in good responders, which might result in the reduction of bile acid synthesis and excretion.   In
our previous report, it was shown that the administration of anabolic
steroid with a high cholesterol diet markedly deposited cholesterol
in the liver (37).   It is suggested that the shift of cholesterol to the liver is accelerated by anabolic steroid, and serum cholesterol concentration decreases.   Some investigators explained the
hypolipidemic effect of unsaturated fatty acid by the change of the re-
distribution of lipid to the liver (38-39).   Therefore, one of
the mechanisms of hypocholesterolemic effect has been considered to
be stimulation of the shift of serum cholesterol.   It is not clear,
however, if a defect of transportation system of cholesterol is a primary event or not.   The possibility is not denied that some metabolic
disturbances may interfere with the distribution of cholesterol.

Recently, Goldstein and Brown (40, 41) demonstrated with the
cultured fibroblast from hypercholesterolemic patients that the receptor to serum low density lipoprotien was absent in the patients'
fibroblast, which led to the increase of hepatic cholesterol synthesis without the relation to a negative feedback control.   The
delay of cholesterol tranport to the liver might be concerned with
some defect of the receptor site of the hepatocytes.

There have been many reports investigating the lipid metabolism
of human primary hypercholesterolemia.   Miettinen et al.(42)
showed that the fecal excretion of bile acids was decreased in the
patients, and an inverse relationship was found between the serum
cholesterol and fecal bile acid excretion.   The turnover rate of
bile acids in such patients was prolonged, when compared with those
in hypercholesterolemia with the high triglyceride concentration
(43).   Therefore, they concluded that the decreased turnover
rate of cholesterol or bile acids was the primary cause of the disease.   However, Lewis and Myant (44), Nestel and Monger (45),
Grundy and Ahrens (46) and Samuel and Perl (47) reported that hypercholesterolemic patients did not differ from healthy controls
with the respect to the turnover rate of cholesterol or excretion
rate of fecal steroids.   In the cases of hypercholesterolemia with
hypertriglyceridemia, cholesterol or bile acid syntheses seemed to
be rather stimulated.

Langer et al.(48) demonstrated that the turnover rate of serum
low density lipoprotein in type II hyperlipidemia was decreased, judg-
ing from the disappearance rate of ^{131}I labeled low density lipoprotein from the peripheral circulation.   When labeled low density
lipoprotein from patients was infused into healthy volunteers,
the turnover rate was the same as that from normal persons.   On

the other hand, low density lipoprotein from normal subjects and that
from patients   were metabolized at the same slow rate from the circulation of the patients (49).   So, the defect seemed to be at
the side of the patient and not that of the lipoprotein.   Actually
amino acid composition of low density lipoprotein-apoprotein is not
different from healthy control and patient (50), though the lipid
composition is reported to be different (51,52).

Patton et al. (53) reported that the mean serum cholesterol
value of high cholesterol line of Racing Homer pigeons reached 405
mg/100 ml from the original population of 289 mg/100 ml by a passive
assortive mating.   Imai and Matsumura (54) tried to make a spontaneous hypercholesterolemic rat by repeated sibmating with good responder rat to cholesterol ingestion.   The progeny of both sexes became
progressively more susceptible to dietary hypercholesterolemia.
But their serum triglyceride concentrations were higher than those
of control animals.   Therefore, lipid metabolism in such rats
might be different from that of the present experiment.

Zucker and Zucker (55,56) demonstrated hereditary obesity in
a strain of rats.   The obese rats had high serum cholesterol concentrations as well as serum triglyceride.   It was reported that
the incorporation of labeled glucose and pyruvate into glyceride-
glycerol was enhanced in the adipose tissue of the obese rats (57).
Cholesterol synthesis in such rats may be accelerated as some type
of hyperlipidemias in human beings.   So, hypercholesterolemia derived from different etiologies are supposed also in animals.   In
the present experiment, good responders to a cholesterol diet do not
have high TG levels, and some similarity to the patient with primary
hypercholesterolemia is observed.   Therefore, the nature of hyperlipidemia in the rats in the present paper is rather similar to
mild hypercholesterolemia found in the aged men whose serum cholesterol levels are dependent on dietary cholesterol.

It was reported that severe atherosclerotic changes in the aortas were found in hypercholesterolemic monkeys, pigeons or rabbits.
Atherosclerosis, however, has not been produced in the rat, even
when a large amount of cholesterol was ingested.   Recently, it
was shown that the lesions were found in the spontaneous hyperten-
sive rats (SHR) fed cholesterol diet (58).   The combination of
some stress as cold or trauma was reported to induce the atherosclerotic changes in rats. (59,60).   Consequently, it may be possible that atherosclerosis is developed in rats, if hypercholesterolemic rats could be made artificially.   This might contribute to
atherosclerosis research for etiologic study and also to the prevention and treatment by   drugs or dietary regimens.

The increase of serum cholesterol concentration with age in
man has been well documented.   In the animals, however, consistent

results were not found in previous information.   Some investigators reported that serum cholesterol concentrations of animals did
not increase significantly with old age.   Others indicated an
increase of serum cholesterol levels in aged animals.   Weibust
(61) demonstrated that mean serum cholesterol levels in older
age groups were significantly higher than that in younger age
groups in some 8 strains of inbred mice.   This tendency was inci-
dent to the mice with high serum cholesterol concentrations in his
report.   In our present experiment, the elevation of serum cholesterol level in good responders by aging was more obvious   than that
in poor responders.

   It is considered that genetic defects in cholesterol metabolism
of   rats are masked when they are young and have high metabolic
activities, but are revealed by the impairment of cholesterol metabolism in the aging process.   If the animals have much more severe
hereditary retardation of cholesterol metabolism, they might show
hypercholesterolemia without the supplement of cholesterol even at
younger age.

ACKNOWLEDGEMENTS

   This work was supported by Research Grant from Aging Council
and Atherosclerosis in Japan.   The technical assistance of Miss
Kaori Hayashi and Miss Hiromi Kato is acknowledged.

REFERENCES

1. Cox,G.E.,C.B.Taylor and D.Patton. 1963. Origin of plasma cholesterol in man. Arch. Pathol. 76;60-88.

2. Dietchy,J.M. and J.D.Wilson. 1970. Regulation of cholesterol
   metabolism. New Engl. J. Med. 282:1128-1138 and 1179-1183.

3. Danielsson, H. and T.T.Tchen. 1970. Steroid metabolism. In:
   Metabolic Pathway II. Ed. by D.M. Greenberg, Academic Press, New
   York, pp. 117-168.

4. Taylor,C.B.,B.Mikkelson, J.A.Anderson, D.T.Forman and S.S.Choi.
   1965.Human serum cholesterol synthesis. Exp. Mol. Path. 4:
   480-488.

5. Gould,R.G. 1951. Lipid metabolism and atherosclerosis. Amer. J.
   Med. 11:209-227.

6. Taylor, C.B. and R.G.Gould. 1950. Effect of dietary cholesterol
   on rate of cholesterol synthesis in the intact animal measured

by means of radioactive carbon. Circulation 2:467-468.

7. Bhattathiry, E.P. and M.D. Siperstein. 1963. Feedback control of cholesterol synthesis in man. J. Clin. Invest. 42:1613-1618.

8. Wilson, J.D. 1962. Relation between dietary cholesterol and bile acid excretion in the rat. Am. J. Physiol. 203:1029-1037.

9. Beher, W.T., K.K. Casazza, M.E. Beher, A.M. Filus and J. Bertasius. 1970. Effect of cholesterol on bile acid metabolism in the rat. Proc. Soc. Exp. Biol. Med. 134:595-602.

10. Frantz, I.D. and B.T. Hinkelman. 1955. Acceleration of hepatic cholesterol synthesis by Triton WR 1339. J. Exp. Med. 101: 225-232.

11. Radding, C.M. and D. Steinberg. 1960. Studies on the synthesis and secretion of serum lipoproteins by rat liver slices. J.Clin Invest. 39:1560-1569.

12. Kandutsch, A.A. and S.E. Saucier. 1969. Prevention of cyclic and triton-induced increase in hydroxy methyl glutaryl coenzyme A reductase and sterol synthesis by puromycin. J.Biol. Chem. 244:2299-2305.

13. White, L.W. and H. Rudney.1970. Regulation of 3-hydroxy-3-methyl glutarate and mevalonate biosynthesis by rat liver homogenates. Effect of fasting, cholesterol feeding, and Triton administration. Biochemistry 9:2725-2731.

14. Yamamoto, R.S., L.B. Crittenden, L.Sokoloff and G.E. Jay Jr. 1963. Genetic variations in plasma lipid content in mice. J. Lipid Res. 4:413-418.

15. Bruell, J.H. 1963. Additive inheritance of serum cholesterol level in mice. Science 142:1664-1666.

16. Weibust, R.S. and G. Schlager, 1968. A genetic study of blood pressure, hematocrit and plasma cholesterol in aged mice. Life Sci. 7:(part II) 1111-1119.

17. Patton, N.M., R.V. Brown and C.C. Middleton. 1975. Atherosclerosis in familial lines of pigeons fed exogenous cholesterol. Atherosclerosis 21:147-154.

18. Wartman, A.M. and W.E. Conner. 1973. The cholesterol balance and turnover in genetically hypercholesterolemic pigeons. J. Lab. Clin. Med. 82:793-808.

19. Prichard, R.W., T.B. Clarkson, H.B. Lofland and H.D. Goodman. 1964. Pigeon atherosclerosis. Am. Heart J. 67:715-717.

20. Clarkson, T.B., H.B. Lofland,   B.C. Bullock and H.D. Goodman. 1971. Genetic control of plasma cholesterol. Studies on Squirrel monkeys. Arch. Pathol. 92:37-45.

21. Morris, M.D.and C.D. Fitch. 1968. Spontaneous hyperbeta-lipoproteinemia in the Rhesus monkey. Biochem. Med. 2:209-215.

22. Younger R.K., H.W. Scott, W.H. Butts and S.E. Stephenson Jr. 1969. Rapid production of experimental hypercholesterolemia and atherosclerosis in the rhesus monkey:comparison of five dietary regimens. J.Surg. Res. 9:263-271.

23. Thompson J.S. 1969.Atheromata in an inbred strain of mice. J. Atheroscler. Res. 10:113-122.

24. Stout, C. and M.E. Groover Jr. 1969. Spontaneous versus experimental atherosclerosis.Ann. N.Y. Acad. Sci. 162:89-98.

25. Dieterich R.A., W. Van Pelt and W. Galster. 1973. Diet-induced cholesterolemia and atherosclerosis in wild rodents. Athero-sclerosis 17:345-352.

26. Leffler, H.H. and C.H. McDougald. 1963. Estimation of cholesterol in serum. Am. J. Clin. Pathol. 39:311-315.

27. Haeflmayr, J. and R. Freed. 1966. Eine Methode Zur routin maessigen Bestimmung des Lipidphosphors und der Phosphatide. Med. Ernabr. 7:1-4.

28. Fletcher, M.J. 1968. A colorimetric method for estimating serum triglycerides. Clin. Chim. Acta.22:397-399.

29. Takeuchi, N. and Y. Yamamura. 1972. The effect of plasma-pheresis on cholesterol synthesis in the rat:Relationship to protein synthesis.   J. Lab. Clin. Med. 79:801-813.

30. Lowry, O.H., N.J. Rosenbrough, A.L. Farr and R.J. Randall. 1951. Protein measurement with the Folin phenol reagent. J.Biol. Chem. 193:265-276.

31. Sadahiro, R., N. Takeuchi, A. Kumagai and Y. Yamamura. 1970. Studies on cholesterol metabolism in experimental diabetic rat. End. Japon. 17:225-232.

32. Mitropoulos, K.A. and S. Balasubramaniam. 1972. Cholesterol 7 α-hydroxylase in rat liver microsomal preparations. Biochem. J. 128:1-9.

33. Lofland, H.B.,T.B.Clarkson,R.W.StClair and N.D.M.Lehner. 1972. Studies on the regulation of plasma cholesterol levels in Squirrel monkeys of two genotypes. J.Lipid Res. 13: 39-47.

34. Bell, F.P.,H.B.Lofland and T.B. Clarkson. 1970. Plasma cholesterol turnover and esterification in the pigeon. Lipids 5:153-155.

35. West C.E. and C.K.Roberts. 1974. Cholesterol metabolism in two strains of rabbits differing in their cholesterolemic response to dietary cholesterol. Biochem.Soc.Trans. 2:1275-1277.

36. Adams, W.C.,E.M.Gaman and A.S.Feigenbaum. 1972. Breed differences in the response of rabbits to atherogenic diet. Atherosclerosis 16:405-411.

37. Takeuchi, N.,M.Yamamoto, A.Kumagai and Y.Yamamura. 1970. Alterations of cholesterol metabolism induced by anabolic steroid administration to rat. Endocrinol. Japon. 17:195-202.

38. Lindstedt, S.,J.Avigan,D.S.Goodman,J.Sjoevall and D.Steinberg. 1965.The effect of dietary fat on the turnover of cholic acid and on the composition of the biliary bile acids in man. J. Clin. Invest.44:1754-1765.

39. Bieberdorf,F.A. and J.D.Wilson.1965. Studies on the mechanism of action of unsaturated fats on cholesterol metabolism in the rabbit. J.Clin. Invest. 44:1834-1844.

40. Goldstein,J.L. and M.S.Brown. 1974. Hyperlipidemia in coronary heart disease : a biochemical genetic approach. J. Lab. Clin. Med. 85:15-25.

41. Brown,M.S.,S.E.Dana and J.L.Goldstein. 1974. Regulation of 3-hydroxy-3-methylglutaryl Coenzyme A reductase activity in cultured human fibroblast. J.Biol. Chem.249:789-796.

42. Miettinen,T.A.,R.Pelkonen, E.A.Nikkilae and O.Heinonen. 1967. Low excretion of fecal bile acid in a family with hypercholesterolemia. Acta Med. Scand. 182:645-650.

43. Kottke, B.A. 1969. Differences in bile acid excretion, primary hypercholesterolemia compared to combined hypercholesterolemia and hypertriglyceridemia. Circulation 15:13-20.

44. Lewis,B. and N.B.Myant. 1967. Studies in the metabolism of cholesterol in subjects with normal plasma cholesterol levels and in patients with essential hypercholesterolemia.Clin.Sci. 32:201-213.

45. Nestel,P.J.and E.M.Monger.1967. Turnover of plasma esterified cholesterol in normocholesterolemic and hypercholesterolemic subjects and its relation to body fluid. J.Clin.Invest.46:967-974.

46. Grundy,S.M.and E.H.Ahrens. 1969. Mesurements of cholesterol turnover and synthesis and absorption in man carried out by isotope kinetic and sterol balance method. J.Lipid Res. 10:91-107.

47. Samuel,P.and W.Perl.1970. Long-term decay of serum cholesterol radioactivity,body cholesterol metabolism in normals and patients with hyperlipoproteinemia and atherosclerosis. J.Clin.Invest. 49:346-357.

48. Langer ,T.,W.Stroler and R.I.Levy.1972. The metabolism of low density lipoprotein in familial type II hyperlipoproteinemia. J.Clin.Invest.51:1528-1536.

49. Simons,L.A.,D.Reichl,N.B.Myant and M.Mancini, 1975. The metabolism of the apoprotein of plasma low density lipoprotein in familial hyperbetalipoproteinaemia in the homozygous form. Atherosclerosis 21:283-298.

50. Gotto,A.M,W.V.Brown,R.I.Levy,M.E.Biᴣrnbaumer and D.S.Fredrickson, 1972. Evidence for the identity of the major apoprotein in low density and very low density lipoproteins in normal subjects and patients with familial hyperlipoproteinemia. J.Clin.Invest. 51: 1486-1496.

51. Slack,J.and G.L.Mills. 1970. Anomalous low density lipoproteins in familial hyperlipoproteinemia. Clin.Chim.Acta 29:15-25.

52. Ruderman,N.B.,A.L.Jones,R.M.Krause and E.Shafrir. 1970. A biochemical and morphologic study of very low density lipoproteins in carbohydrate-induced hypertriglyceridemia. J.Clin.Invest. 50:1355-1368

53. Patton,N.M.,R.V.Brown and C.C.Middleton, 1974. Familial cholesterolemia in pigeons. Atherosclerosis 19:308-314.

54. Imai,Y.and H.Matsumura. 1973. Genetic studies on induced and spontaneous hypercholesterolemia in rats. Atherosclerosis 18: 59-64.

55. Zucker,L.M.and T.F.Zucker. 1961. Fatty a new mutation in the rat. J.Hered. 52:295-278.

56. Zucker,T.F.and L.M.Zucker. 1962. Hereditary obesity in the rat associated with high serum fat and cholesterol. Proc. Soc. Exp. Biol. Med. 110:165-171.

57. Bray,G.A. 1968. Lipogenesis from glucose and pyruvate in fat cells from genetically obese rats. J.Lipid Res. 9:681-686.

58. Uchida, K. personal communication.

59. Sellers, E.A.and D.G.Baker. 1960. Coronary atherosclerosis in rats exposed to cold. Canad.Med. Ass. J. 83:6-13.

60. Bondjers,G.and T. Bjoernheden. 1970. Experimental atherosclerosis induced by mechanical trauma in rats. Atherosclerosis 12:301-306.

61. Weibust, R.S. 1973. Inheritance of plasma cholesterol levels in mice. Genetics 73:303-312.

IMPORTANCE OF SEX AND ESTROGENS IN AMELIORATION OF LETHAL CIRCULATORY STRESS REACTIONS: RELATIONSHIP TO MICROCIRCULATORY AND RETICULOENDOTHELIAL SYSTEM FUNCTION

Burton M. Altura

Department of Physiology, S.U.N.Y. Downstate Medical Center

450 Clarkson Avenue, Brooklyn, New York 11203

Recently, sex hormones have been shown to alter the concentration of elastin and collagen in the vascular walls of chickens (1) and rats (2, 3). Administration of estrogen has also been reported to result in a decrease in mucopolysaccharide content (4) as well as to decrease oxygen consumption of the vascular wall (5). It has been postulated by a number of investigators that these changes may be important in the development, and amelioration, of atherosclerotic lesions (6-8). The influence of sex and sex hormones on vascular reactivity has not, however, been systemically investigated. Furthermore, since injury (and inflammation) is thought to act as a potent stimulus for initiation of development of atherosclerotic lesions (8-12), it would be important to determine whether sex, or estrogen administration, can influence a mammal's reaction to a systemic injury which has as its target the peripheral vascular system.

With these points in mind, the present study was designed to determine whether sex and administration of estrogen (acutely and in multiple low doses) can influence: a) survival of rats (male and female) subjected to lethal forms of circulatory trauma; b) reactivity of rat splanchnic microvessels to constrictor catecholamines, neurohypophyseal hormones and other selected vasoactive hormones and drugs; and c) the tone of splanchnic vessels of rats subjected to lethal forms of circulatory trauma. In addition, since macrophages are thought to play a role in clearing the blood-vascular system of lipids (13-15), and may be important in the origin of foam cells (16-18), experiments were designed with male and female rats to determine whether sex and administration of estrogen (acutely and in multiple low doses) can influence the phagocytic function of the reticuloendothelial system (RES). In addition, these experiments should enable one to determine whether RES function is directly linked with microcirculatory integrity (19-21), sex hormones (22, 22a) and an organism's response to lethal circu-

289

latory stress (20, 23-27).

METHODS

Trauma Models and Survival Studies in Male and Female Rats

Different degrees of bowel ischemia shock were induced in lightly anesthetized (Nembutal, 3 mg/100g i.m., Abbot Labs.) untreated inbred male
and female Wistar strain rats (150 ± 20 g), and male Wistar rats pretreated
with either a single, acute dose, or multiple doses, of 17- β-estradiol benzoate
(Sigma Chemical Co., St. Louis, Mo.), administered s.c. in sesame oil,by a
temporary occlusion of the superior mesenteric artery, similar to that described
previously (20, 21). In other experiments, lightly anesthetized (Nembutal, 3mg/
100g) untreated male and female Wistar rats (150 ± 20g) and male Wistar rats
pretreated with estradiol, as above, were subjected to 400, 600 or 800 revolutions of Noble-Collip drum trauma as described previously (23). All animals
were observed for 7 days for survival. The statistical validity of the survival
data was assessed by means of the Chi-Square test. Arterial blood pressure was
carefully monitored in selected animals (controls and estradiol-treated) before
and after bowel ischemia and drum trauma. Bowel ischemia and drum trauma
were selected as animal trauma models because both forms of circulatory stress
are associated with a rapid onset of considerable microvascular pathology,espe-
cially to vascular walls (28, 29).

Microcirculatory Studies in Normal Animals (Untreated and Estradiol-treated) and Animals Subjected to Circulatory Trauma

Mesenteries of Nembutal (3 mg/100 g) anesthetized male and female rats
(untreated, estradiol-treated)were exteriorized for direct microscopic observation of arterioles, venules, etc. and kept under physiologic conditions according to procedures described previously (21). Measurements for quantitative
changes in microvascular lumen sizes were made before (control) and after topical application of graded doses (6-12 in number; 0.1 ml volume) of epinephrine (Adrenalin hydrochloride, Parke, Davis and Co., Detroit, Mich.), norepinephrine (norepinephrine bitartrate, Levophed, Winthrop Labs., New York,
N.Y.), dopamine hydrochloride (Mann Research Labs., New York, N.Y.),
synthetic [8-lysine]-vasopressin (Sandoz Ltd., Hanover, N.J., approximate
rat pressor assay = 270 I U/mg), synthetic oxytocin (Sandoz, preservative free,
400 I U/ml), serotonin creatinine sulfate (Nutritional Biochemicals Corp.,
Cleveland, Ohio) and angiotensin II amide (Ciba Pharmaceutical Co., Summit,
N.J.).Only one type of drug agonist was utilized with any one mesenteric
preparation. In vivo microscopic observations for discrete drug effects were
made at magnifications up to approximately 4000 times using an image-splitting
television microscope recording system (30). Such a system has recently been

effectively used to make rapid in vivo micrometric measurements, from which
complete log dose-response curves have been constructed for drug and agonist
effects on various kinds of muscular microvessels (e.g., precapillary sphincters,
metarterioles, arterioles and venules)(21,31-35). In other experiments, we used
the image-splitting television microscope recording system to determine the influence of sex and estradiol-treatment on the tone, i.e. diameters, of the microscopic capacitance vessels, i.e. the muscular venules, of rats subjected to bowel
ischemia since these vessels are thought to dysfunction in states of severe circulatory stress (36). Means and S.E.M.'s of all paired doses, and time intervals, were calculated and compared for statistical significance by appropriate
means: Student's t test or analysis of variance.

RES Phagocytic Index

The procedure in these experiments essentially consisted of determining
RES phagocytic indices (Kvalues) (20, 21, 23, 24) in four different groups of
animals: I) normal control inbred male and female Wistar strain rats (150 + 20g);
II) male Wistar rats pretreated every 12 hrs with 10, 100 or 1000 µg/kg body wt.
of 17-β-estradiol s.c. for either one or three days; III) untreated male Wistar
rats subjected to bowel ischemia (i.e. a 20 min temporary occlusion of the
superior mesenteric artery) or Noble-Collip drum trauma (400 revolutions at
40 rpm); and IV) male rats pretreated with single, acute massive doses of 17-
β-estradiol s.c. (i.e. 1.0 or 10 mg/kg) either 2 or 8 hours prior to bowel ischemia or Noble-Collip drum trauma as in Group III. The K values in Groups III
and IV were obtained three hours after bowel ischemia and drum trauma. Phagocytic indices were determined by measuring the rate of clearance of carbon
(4 mg in calf skin gelatin per 100 g body wt. (20, 21, 23, 24). The colloidal carbon utilized in these studies was Pelikan C11/1431a (Gunther-Wagner, Hann-
over, Germany). Phagocytic indices were calculated:

$$K = \frac{\log_{10} C_1 - \log_{10} C_2}{t_2 - t_1}$$

where K is the phagocytic index and C_1 and C_2 are the colloidal carbon concentrations in mg per 100 ml of blood at t_2 and t_1 . Means and S.E.M.'s were
calculated and compared for statistical significance by Student's t test.

RESULTS

Sex as a Factor in Survival of Rats Subjected to Bowel Ischemia and Trauma

Tables I and II demonstrate that as either the period of superior mesenteric
occlusion becomes longer in duration or as the number of drum rotations are increased, there is a graded decrease in survival in both male and female rats.
In addition, these two Tables indicate that the inbred female rats are signifi-

cantly more resistant to both the bowel ischemia and the drum trauma than are
the corresponding inbred male rats.

Influence of Estrogen Treatment on Resistance of Male Rats to Bowel Ischemia and Trauma.

Table III indicates that male rats pretreated with single, acute massive
doses of 17-β-estradiol (1 or 10 mg/kg), at least eight hours prior to being subjected to circulatory stress, but not two hours before stress, are significantly
more resistant to bowel ischemia and drum trauma than are untreated control
male rats. In addition, the data in Table III demonstrate that the greater the
pretreatment dose of 17-β-estradiol, the more resistant the male rats are to
bowel ischemia and trauma.

Table IV indicates that if the estradiol is given in multiple doses (i.e.,
one dose every 12 hours for a duration of three days) instead of a single, massive
dose (Table III), a dose of as little as 10 μg/kg of body wt.(or in other words a
total dose of 60 μg/kg) can effectively enhance resistance of male rats to bowel
ischemia and trauma. It is of some interest to note that a dose of one mg/kg
twice a day for three days results in inducing a complete resistance (i.e. 100%
survival) to both forms of lethal circulatory stress.

TABLE 1

Sex as a Factor in Survival of Inbred Rats Subjected to Bowel Ischemia

Duration of Occlusion (min) and Sex	Survivors/Total Rats	Survival (%)
20 minutes		
Male	10/25	40
Female	17/20	85*
45 minutes		
Male	2/20	10
Female	12/20	60*
75 minutes		
Male	0/20	0
Female	4/20	20*

* Significantly different from paired male animals (P< 0.02)

TABLE II

Sex as a Factor in Survival of Inbred Rats Subjected to Noble-Collip Drum Trauma

No. Revolutions in Drum and Sex	Survivors/Total Rats	% Survival
400 revolutions		
Male	8/16	50
Female	16/16	100*
600 revolutions		
Male	4/20	20
Female	15/20	75*
800 revolutions		
Male	0/20	0*
Female	4/20	20*

*Significantly different from paired male animals (P<0.02)

RES Phagocytic Function in Male and Female Rats and Male Rats Pretreated with Estrogen

Table V indicates that unpretreated, control inbred Wistar strain female rats have a greater ability to clear colloidal carbon particles from the bloodstream than inbred male rats of the same strain. In addition, the data in Table V indicate that when estradiol is given to male rats in the same multiple dose   regimens, which we have shown will enhance survival after lethal circulatory stress (Table IV), RES phagocytic activity is enhanced by at least 100% over control levels.

The data in Table VI indicate that when male rats are pretreated, at least eight hours before circulatory shock and trauma, with single acute massive doses of estradiol(in regimens which protect animals against circulatory stress-Table III) the usual early RES phagocytic depression seen in untreated control males (20, 23, 24) does not become manifest.

TABLE III

Influence of Acute Pharmacologic Doses of 17-β-Estradiol on Survival
of Inbred Male Rats Subjected to Bowel Ischemia and Noble-Collip
Drum Trauma

Group and Time of Estradiol Pretreatment	Dose (mg/kg)	Survivors/Total	% Survival
Bowel Ischemia (BI)			
Controls	0	10/22	45
BI + Estradiol			
– 2hr	1	13/22	59
	10	14/22	64
– 8hr	1	16/22	73*
	10	19/22	86*
Drum Trauma (DT)			
Controls	0	10/20	50
DT + Estradiol			
– 2hr	1	12/20	60
	10	13/20	65
– 8hr	1	15/20	75*
	10	19/20	95*

Bowel ischemia was induced by a 20 min temporary occlusion of the superior
mesenteric artery. Noble-Collip drum trauma was produced using 400 revolutions.
* Significantly different from untreated controls ($P < 0.02$)

Sex as a Factor in Responsiveness of Arterioles to Vasoactive Agents

Figure 1 summarizes some of the data we obtained when various constrict-
or adrenergic amines were applied topically to mesenteric arterioles in female and male rats. It can be readily seen that the log dose-response curves
for both epinephrine and norepinephrine in female rats are significantly shifted
7- and 4-fold, respectively, to the left of those obtained in untreated male
rats, while those for dopamine and phenylephrine in female versus male rats do
not exhibit similar differences. Since the dose-response curves for constrictions
induced by dopamine or phenylephrine were not affected by a difference in

TABLE IV

Influence of Multiple Doses (Given Every 12 Hours) of 17-β-Estradiol
on Survival of Inbred Male Rats Subjected to Bowel Ischemia and
Noble–Collip Drum Trauma

Group and Duration of Pretreatment (days)	Dose (μg/kg)	Survivors/Total	% Survival
Bowel Ischemia (BI)			
Controls	0	10/25	40
BI + Estradiol			
1 day	10	10/22	45
	100	13/22	59
	1000	17/22	77*
3 days	10	15/22	68*
	100	21/22	96*
	1000	22/22	100*
Drum Trauma (DT)			
Controls	0	12/25	48
DT + Estradiol			
1 day	10	11/22	50
	100	14/22	64
	1000	18/22	82*
3 days	10	16/22	73*
	100	20/22	91*
	1000	22/22	100*

Bowel ischemia was induced by a 20 min temporary occlusion of the superior mesenteric artery. Noble–Collip drum trauma was produced by 400 revolutions at 40 rpm.
*Significantly different from untreated controls ($P < 0.02$)

sex, we naturally wondered whether: 1) the sex-linked differences were specific for the constrictor catecholamines epinephrine and norepinephrine; and 2) would exogenous administration of sex hormones, to male and female animals, alter reactivity to catecholamines and/or other vasoactive constrictor agents.

Figure 2 indicates that concentration–effect curves for the neurohypophyseal hormone-induced arteriolar vasoconstrictions in female rats are displaced

TABLE V

RES Phagocytic Indices (K Values) in Untreated Male and Female
Rats and Male Rats Pretreated (Every 12 Hours) with 17-β-Estradiol

Sex and Treatment- Duration and Dose (μg/kg)	N	K ± S.E.M.
Controls		
Males	25	0.040 ± 0.002
Females	25	0.049 ± 0.002*
Pretreatment w/Estradiol		
Males		
I day (10)	12	0.040 ± 0.003
(100)	12	0.048 ± 0.004
(1000)	12	0.056 ± 0.004*
3 days (10)	12	0.082 ± 0.008*
(100)	12	0.085 ± 0.005*
(1000)	12	0.090 ± 0.010*

Test dose of colloidal carbon in calf-skin gelatin = 4 mg/100g body wt.
*Significantly different from untreated, control males ($P < 0.01$)

in a parallel manner to the left of those obtained in male animals, similar to
that for epinephrine and norepinephrine. It is of some interest to note that the
dose-response curves for oxytocin, in female rats, are displaced 14-fold to the
left of those in male animals, while those for vasopressin are displaced six-fold.
Sex-linked differences were not observed on mesenteric arterioles with regards
to other vasoconstrictors such as serotonin and angiotensin (37).

Influence of Estrogen Pretreatment of Male Rats on Reactivity of Arterioles to Vasoactive Hormones

Figure 3 indicates that pretreatment of male Wistar rats with a single
dose of 17-β-estradiol (10 μg/100g body wt. 18-24 hours prior to observation)
results in a significant enhancement of the vasoconstrictor actions of both
epinephrine and norepinephrine. Although the concentration-effect curves are
displaced in a parallel manner only two-fold in the case of epinephrine, there
is over a six-fold left-ward shift for norepinephrine. It should be noted that

TABLE VI

INFLUENCE OF ACUTE PHARMACOLOGIC DOSES OF 17-β-ESTRA-
DIOL ON RES PHAGOCYTIC INDICES OF MALE RATS SUBJECTED
TO BOWEL ISCHEMIA AND NOBLE-COLLIP DRUM TRAUMA

Group and Time of Estradiol Pretreatment	N	Dose (mg/kg)	$K \pm S.E.M.$
Controls	20	0	0.038 ± 0.002
Bowel Ischemia (BI)			
BI Controls	12	0	$0.020 \pm 0.004*$
BI + Estradiol			
– 2 hr	10	1	$0.026 \pm 0.004*$
	12	10	$0.022 \pm 0.004*$
– 8 hr	12	1	0.038 ± 0.006
	10	10	0.042 ± 0.006
Drum Trauma (DT)			
DT Controls	14	0	$0.010 \pm 0.002*$
DT + Estradiol			
– 2 hr	12	1	$0.014 \pm 0.004*$
	12	10	$0.016 \pm 0.004*$
– 8 hr	12	1	0.034 ± 0.004
	12	10	0.040 ± 0.006

Test dose of colloidal carbon in calf-skin gelatin = 4 mg/100 g body wt. K
values were obtained 3 hrs after bowel ischemia (20 min. occlusion of superior mesenteric artery) and drum trauma (400 revolutions at 40 rpm).
*Significantly different from unshocked controls ($P < 0.01$).

the maximum response to norepinephrine is also potentiated in the estrogen-
treated male animals.

Figure 4 indicates that pretreatment of male rats with single, low doses
of estradiol (10 μg/100g body wt. 18-24 hours prior to observation) results in
a significant potentiation of the vasoconstrictor actions of vasopressin and oxytocin as well. Although not shown, a similar estrogenic pretreatment regimen
fails to alter either the concentration-effect curves or the maximum lumen
narrowings to either angiotensin or serotonin (37). In addition, it should be

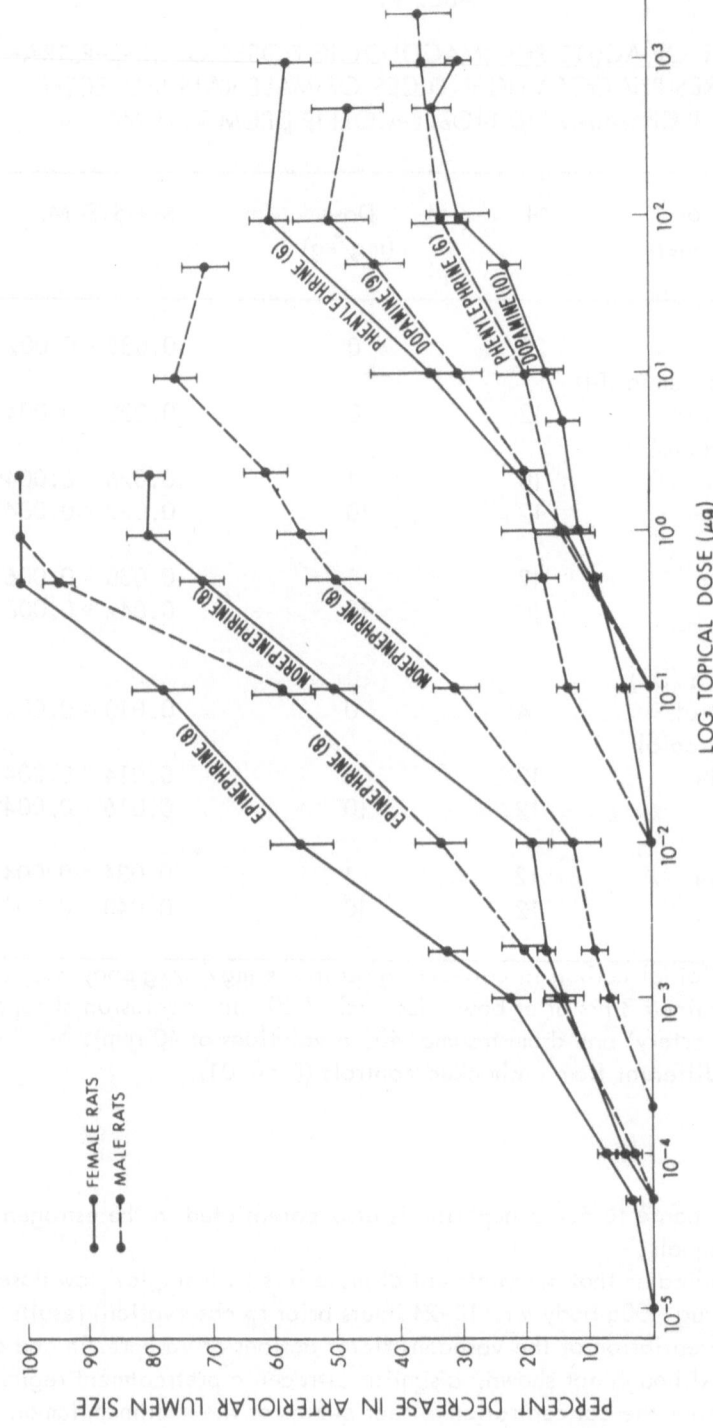

Fig. 1.   Graded contractile responses of mesenteric arterioles in untreated male and female rats to topically applied adrenergic amines. Numbers in parentheses = N. (From reference 38.)

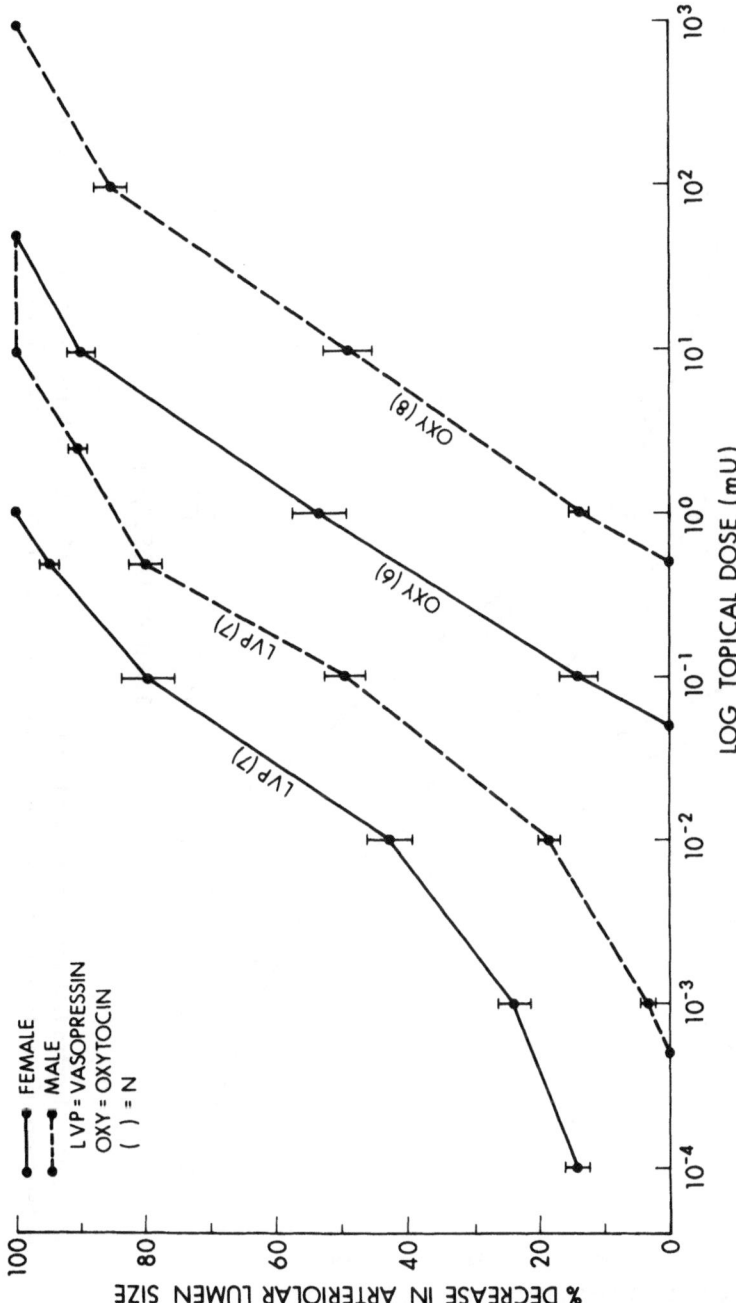

Fig. 2. Graded contractile responses of mesenteric arterioles in untreated male and female rats to lysine–vaso-pressin and oxytocin. (From reference 37.)

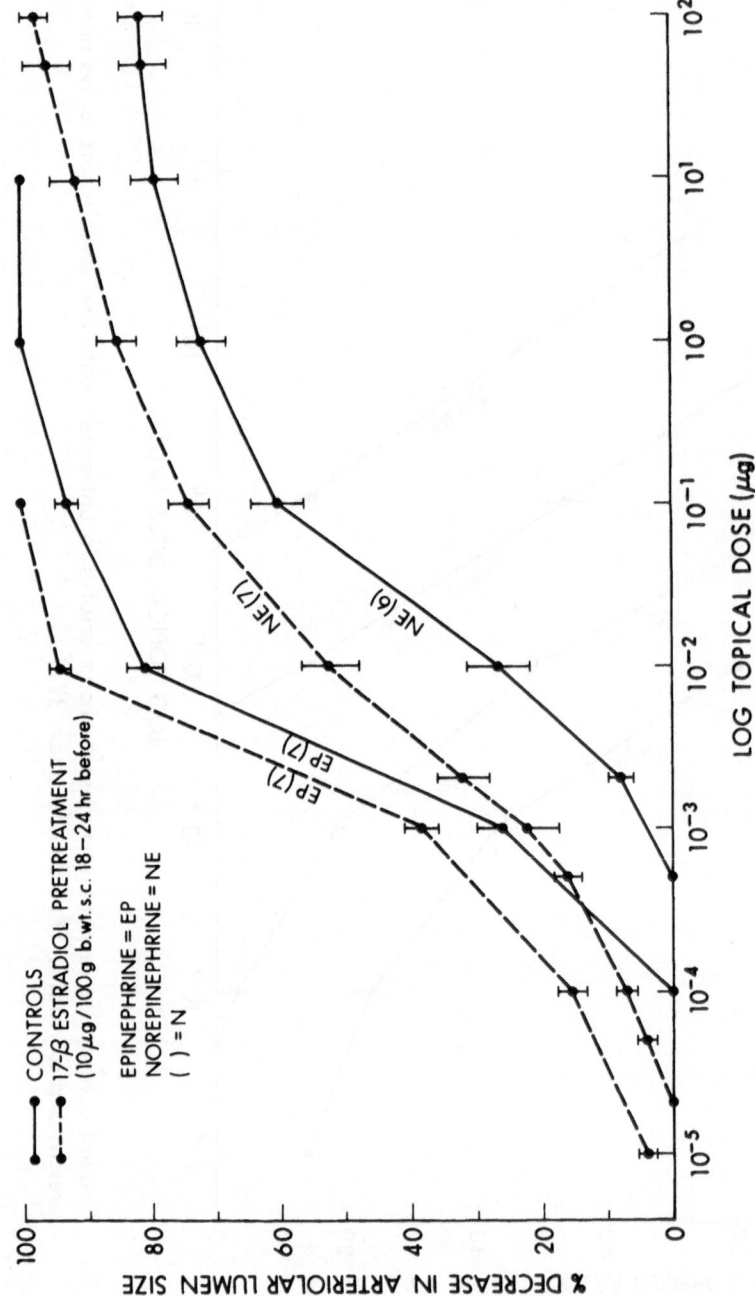

Fig. 3.   Influence of estradiol pretreatment of male rats, 18 to 24 hours before observation, on reactivity of mesenteric arterioles to epinephrine and norepinephrine. (From reference 37.)

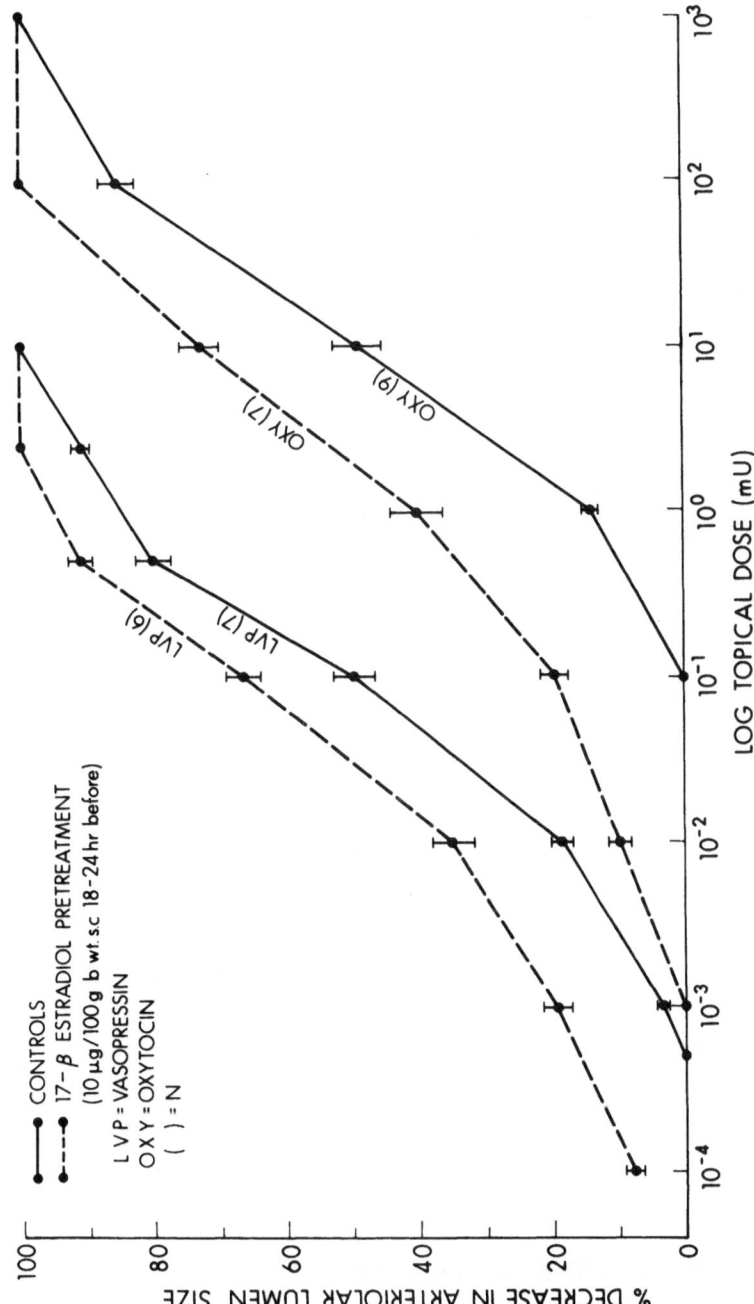

Fig. 4.   Influence of estradiol pretreatment of male rats on reactivity of mesenteric arterioles to vasopressin and oxytocin. (From reference 37.)

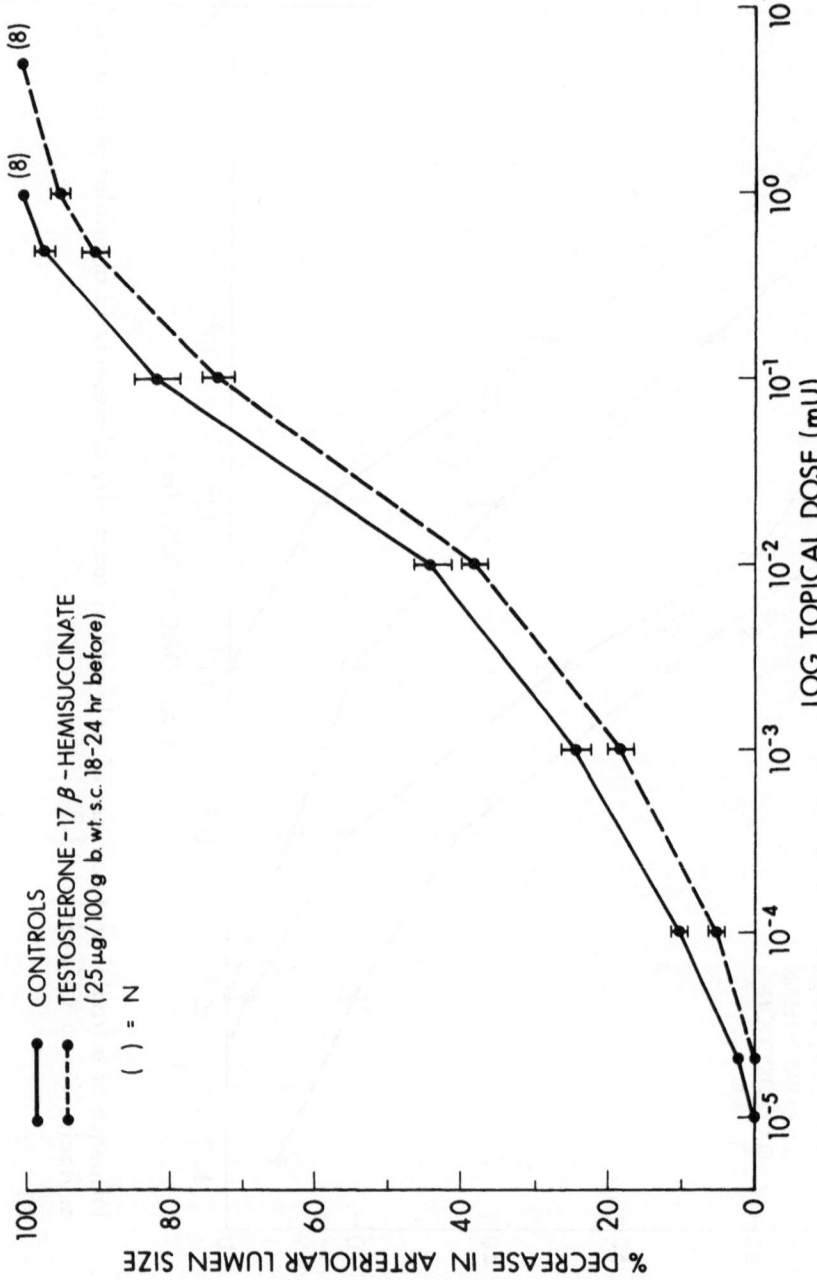

Fig. 5.   Influence of testosterone pretreatment of female rats on reactivity of mesenteric arterioles to vasopressin.

TABLE VII

MEAN ARTERIAL BLOOD PRESSURE 30 AND 60 MIN AFTER BOWEL ISCHEMIA SHOCK IN UNTREATED MALE AND FEMALE RATS AND MALE RATS PRETREATED WITH TWO DOSES OF 17-β-ESTRADIOL EVERY 12 HRS FOR THREE DAYS

Sex and Estradiol Treatment (µg/kg)	Blood Pressure (mm Hg ± S.E.M.)		
	Before Bowel Ischemia	30 min post BI	60 min post BI
Controls			
Males	110 ± 8.2	80 ± 6	64 ± 8
Females	120 ± 8.6	100 ± 4*	88 ± 4*
Pretreatment w/Estradiol			
Males (100)	114 ± 9.6	100 ± 8	82 ± 6
(1000)	112 ± 6.4	106 ± 6*	90 ± 6*

All groups were subjected to a 20 min temporary occlusion of the superior mesenteric artery. N = 6 - 12 for each group.
*Significantly different from paired untreated, control males (P<0.02).

pointed out that similar estrogenic pretreatment in male Wistar rats also enhanced, selectively, the constrictor actions of the catecholamines and neurohypophyseal hormones on metarterioles as well as on precapillary sphincters.

Influence of Androgen Pretreatment of Female Rats on Reactivity of Microvessels to Vasoactive Hormones

In view of the above experiments, we directed our attentions to pretreatment of female rats with androgens. Figure 5 demonstrates that pretreatment of female Wistar rats with a single dose of 25 µg/100g body wt. of testosterone (18-24 hours prior to microscopic observation) inhibited rather than potentiated the constrictor action of neurohypophyseal hormones. Although not shown, similar pretreatment regimens with testosterone in female rats resulted in an attenuation or rightward shift of the dose-response curves for epinephrine and norepinephrine as well.

Other preliminary experiments indicate that single, low pretreatment doses of estradiol tend to oppose the vasodilator actions of histamine and certain prostaglandin compounds, while low doses of testosterone tend to enhance (or potentiate) the actions of these vasodilator compounds in the mesenteric microvessels.

Blood Pressure Responses of Male and Female Rats, and Male Rats Pretreated with Estradiol Before and After Lethal Circulatory Stress

In view of the above findings, demonstrating sex influences in resistance
of animals to lethal circulatory stress, the RES, and vascular reactivity, it
was of interest to determine whether or not there was a differential response of
the blood pressure in the untreated males and females, as well as the estradiol-
treated males, when the rats were subjected to lethal circulatory stress. Table
VII indicates the femoral arterial blood pressure measurements that were obtained in untreated males and females as well as in males given estradiol in
multiple doses (i.e., one dose every 12 hours for a duration of three days) before and after being subjected to lethal bowel ischemia. As can be see in
Table VII, there were no significant differences in the mean control blood
pressures in either of the different groups of rats. We did, however, note
several differences post-trauma. The untreated females as well as the estradiol-treated males showed significantly higher blood pressures 30 minutes as
well as 60 minutes post-trauma. There is, thus, some relationship of the blood
pressure response to the increased susceptibility of the untreated inbred males
to the lethal effects of bowel ischemia.

Sex, Estrogen Treatment and Tone of Microscopic Capacitance Vessels of Rats Subjected to Lethal Circulatory Stress

Considerable evidence has accumulated to suggest that in the late stages
of circulatory shock and trauma, the small muscular venules in the splanchnic
vasculature dilate resulting in a pooling and sequestration of blood in the capacitance side of the circulation (see ref. 36 for review). In view of the latter,
and the above findings, we thought it might be useful to determine whether or
not sex hormones could influence the dilatory response of splanchnic capacitance vessels in the late stages of lethal circulatory stress. The data in Table
VIII tend to indicate that, at least with respect to rats subjected to bowel
ischemia, sex and sex hormones may be important factors in the response of
the capacitance vessels late in circulatory trauma. For example, the untreated
females as well as the estradiol-treated males exhibit significantly less venular
dilation than untreated male rats.

DISCUSSION

It is generally thought that female mammals are more resistant to a number
of diseases and stresses than are male mammals (39, 40). Very little, if any, systematic investigation has, however, been made in regard to peripheral circulatory diseases such as hypertension, atherosclerosis and circulatory shock syn-

TABLE VIII

INFLUENCE OF SEX AND ESTROGENS ON TONE OF MESENTERIC MICROSCOPIC MUSCULAR VENULES OF RATS SUBJECTED TO LETHAL BOWEL ISCHEMIA

Group and Estradiol Pretreatment (µg/kg)	Venular Lumen Size (µ ± S.E.M.)		
	Before Shock	90 min. post shock	% Increase in Lumen
Controls			
Males	37.4 ± 3.0	49.5 ± 3.7	32
Females	40.2 ± 2.8	46.4 ± 3.2	15*
Pretreatment w/Estradiol			
Males (100)	38.8 ± 2.8	46.3 ± 3.3	19*
(1000)	40.4 ± 3.2	47.1 ± 2.9	16*

All animals were subjected to a 45 min temporary occlusion of the superior mesenteric artery. N = 6-9 for each group. Estradiol was given 2 x/day for a duration of three days.
*Significantly different from untreated, male controls (P < 0.03).

dromes. In this regard, the present studies clearly demonstrate that inbred female rats are more resistant to the lethal effects of circulatory stresses than are inbred male animals of the same strain. The fact that pretreatment of male rats with either acute, single massive doses or multiple low doses of 17-β-estradiol can effectively enhance resistance to at least two different forms of lethal circulatory stresses suggests to us that female sex hormones may be primarily responsible for the greater resistance of the inbred female rats.

Several findings in the present report, when taken in concert with previous findings, lead us to believe that the sexual differences in resistance to circulatory stress and trauma may be a reflection of the direct (or indirect) actions of sex hormones on the RES and walls (smooth muscle cells) of peripheral blood vessels.

In this context, it is of interest to note that not only can sex hormones influence RES clearance of particulate matter (22; present findings), but such hormones have been shown to enhance clearance of bacterial and viral organisms from the blood stream (41) as well as to result in raised serum level of gamma-globulin and increase protection of experimental animals against virulent infection (41). These factors may be quite important in the observed

differential resistance of male and female animals to bowel ischemia and trauma for several reasons: (a) Retention (or improper clearance) of pathogenic
bacteria is known to exacerbate mortality in circulatory stress and trauma (18,
27, 42, 43). b) Female mice have been demonstrated to clear bacterial micro-
organisms at a more rapid rate than male mice of the same strain (22, 44); female rats are more resistant than male rats of the same strain to circulatory
stress (present findings). Furthermore, (c) RES function is known to play not
only an important role in resistance to the circulatory stresses used here (19, 20,
21, 23, 27, 45), as well as to circulatory stress in general (19, 20, 21, 23-27),
and is shown here more active in females than males of the same strain, but
also can be enhanced by administration of estrogens (present findings, refs.
22, 41, 45). Moreover, the many vasoactive and toxic substances that are lib-
erated by circulatory stress (for recent review see ref. 46), including endotoxin,
toxic peptides and lysosomal enzymes, might all act in concert on the RES
causing a deleterious (or cytotoxic) effect on the RE cells thus lowering their
potential capacity for phagocytosis and detoxification. Enhanced RES function
of female animals (and estradiol-treated males) could result in neutralization
of these toxins. Although the present data do not directly indicate that estrogenic hormones can bring this about, our findings do demonstrate that such
sex steroids can result in not only a restoration of normal RES function but also
hyperactive function of this system within   8-72 hours after systemic administration. In addition, it should be mentioned that estradiol pretreatment has
been reported to significantly decrease serum acid phosphatase (a measure of
lysosomal membrane rupture)activity in male rats subjected to circulatory shock
(47). The latter findings would support the idea that RE (Kupffer cells) in the
presence of estrogen would have better phagocytic capabilities.

The actions of estrogenic hormones on the walls of blood vessels could
also be invoked to explain the present findings. Resistance or tolerance to
circulatory stress and trauma could generally be attributed to a stability in
vascular smooth muscle cell responsiveness to circulatory vasoactive substances
and/or autonomic nervous system stimuli. Both the depression in blood pressure
(Table VII) and the tendency of microscopic capacitance vessels to undergo
marked vasodilation (Table VIII) in the inbred, untreated Wistar males subjected
to circulatory stress and trauma could be used as support for the latter hypothesis.
The fact that females (Figs. 1 and 2) and estradiol -treated males (Figs. 3 and
4) sustain a more reactive microvasculature than is found in untreated males or
females treated with androgen (Fig. 5) only lends additional support to the
idea that sex hormone interactions with walls of peripheral blood vessels are
probably important in resistance of mammals to lethal circulatory stress.

Overall, these findings could be used to suggest that sex and sex hormones
may not only play important roles in control of macrophage function, peripheral
blood flow and reactivity of vascular smooth muscle, but may be important factors in the amelioration of an organism's reaction to systemic vascular stress.
Although specific information on atherosclerosis has not as yet been acquired,

the present findings, when viewed in light of certain information in the literature, could be used to suggest that sex hormonal influences on systemic macrophage function and vascular smooth muscle cells may be important in the development, and amelioration , of atherosclerotic lesions in vessel walls:

1. Macrophages of the RES play a role in clearing the blood-vascular
system of lipids (13-15) and may be important in the evolution of certain
types of foam cells (16-18). In addition, oral ingestion of many lipids can
depress RES phagocytic activity in animals and man (48, 49). Tonic stimulation
by estrogens (in female mammals) of RES functions could, thus, possibly account
for the low incidence of vascular lesions in female mammals.

2. Altered vascular smooth muscle cells are thought to play important
roles in the etiology of atherosclerotic lesions (2, 3, 9-12, 17, 50). The increased elastin, collagen and mucopolysaccharides seen in atheromatous lesions are thought to be fabricated by deranged vascular smooth muscle cells
(8, 10, 17, 51). Estrogens can alter the concentration of these substances in
vascular walls (1-4). Tonic stimulation of vascular smooth muscle by estrogens
(in female mammals) could result in stabilization of the membranes and metabolism of these cells, thus resulting in a low incidence of vascular lesions in females.

3. Ageing not only results in depressed RES macrophage functions (14, 15,
18, 51) and vascular smooth muscle responsiveness (43, 52, 53) but high inci-
dences of atherosclerotic lesions. By the time women reach menopause (i.e.,
incur a loss of circulating estrogens) the incidence and distribution of atherosclerotic lesions approximates that of males of the same age (54). A loss in
macrophage functions and vascular smooth muscle viability on ageing in males,
as well as in menopausal women, could be expected to act synergistically with
one another and result in: a) decreased clearing of the blood-vascular system
of lipids; and b) a susceptibility of vascular smooth muscle cells to injury.
The consequence of these events could be the high incidence of atherosclerotic
lesions found in older men and women.

ACKNOWLEDGEMENTS

The author is grateful for the excellent technical assistance provided by
D. Dyce, C. Parillo, J. Hanely, R.W. Burton and Y. Waldemar throughout
these studies. The studies reported herein were supported by Research Grants
HL-12426, HL-18002, HL-18015 and MH-26236 from the U.S. Public Health
Service.

REFERENCES

1.   Cembrano, J., M. Lillo, L. Val and J. Mardones. 1960. Influence of sex

differences and hormones on elastin and collagen in aorta of chickens. Circ. Res. 8 : 527-529.

2.   Wolinsky, H. 1972. Effects of estrogen and progestogen on the response of the male rat aorta to hypertension. Circ. Res. 30 : 341 - 349.

3.   Wolinsky, H. 1972. Effects of androgen on the male rat aorta. J.Clin. Invest. 51 : 2552-2555.

4.   Priest, R.E., R.M. Koplitz and E.P.Benditt. 1960. Estradiol reduces incorporation of radioactive sulfate into cartilage and aortas of rats. J. Exp. Med. 112 : 225-236.

5.   Malinow, M.R., J.A. Moguilevsky and L. Gershenson. 1964. Cyclic changes in the O_2 consumption of the aorta in female rats. Circ. Res. 14: 364-366.

6.   Stamler, H. 1963. Relationship of sex and gonadol hormones to athero-sclerosis. In Atherosclerosis and Its Origin, ed. by M. Sandler and G.H. Bourne, Academic Press, New York, pp. 231-262.

7.   Pick, R.,G.B. Clarke and L.N. Katz. 1968. Estrogen and atherosclerosis In Progress in Biochemistry and Pharmacology; Recent Advances in Atheroscle-rosis, vol 4, ed. by C.J. Miras, A.N. Howard and R. Paoletti, S.Karger, New York, pp. 354-362.

8.   Wolinsky, H. 1973. Mesenchymal response of the blood vessel wall. A potential avenue for understanding amd treating atherosclerosis. Circ.Res. 32 : 543-549.

9.   Fry, D.L. 1973. Responses of the arterial wall to certain physical factors. In Atherogenesis: Initiating Factors, Ciba Foundation Symposium 12,   ed.   by R. Porter and J. Knight, Elsevier, Amsterdam, pp.93-100.

10.   Ross, R. and J.A. Glomset.1973. Atherosclerosis and the, arterial smooth muscle cell. Science 180 : 1332-1339.

11.   Harker, L.A., S.J. Slichter, C.R. Scott and R. Ross. 1974. Homocys-tinemia: Vascular injury and arterial thrombosis. N. Engl. J. Med. 291 : 537-543.

12.   Wolinsky, H.,S. Goldfischer, M. Daly, L.E. Kasak and B. Coltoff-Schiller. 1975. Arterial lysosomes and connective tissue in primate athero-sclerosis and hypertension. Circ.Res. 36 : 553-561.

13.   Day. A.J. 1964. The macrophage system, lipid metabolism and athero-sclerosis. J. Atheroscler. Res. 4 : 117-130.

14.   Stuart, A.E. 1970. The Reticuloendothelial System. Livingstone, Edin-burgh.

15.   Vernon-Roberts, B. 1972. The Macrophage. Cambridge University Press, Cambridge.

16.   French, J.E. 1966. Atherosclerosis in relation to the structure and func-tion of the arterial intima, with special reference to the endothelium. Intern. Rev. Exp. Pathol. 5 : 253-353.

17.   Geer, J.C. and M.D. Haust. 1972. Smooth Muscle Cells in Atheroscle-rosis. S. Karger, Basel.

18.   Carr, I. 1973. The Macrophage. A Review of Ultrastructure and Func-tion. Academic Press, New York.

19.   Zweifach, B.W. 1958. Microcirculatory derangements as a basis for the lethal manifestations of experimental shock. Brit. J. Anaesthesia 30 :466-484.

20.   Altura, B.M. and S.G. Hershey. 1971. Acute intestinal ischemia shock and reticuloendothelial system function. J. Reticuloendothelial Soc. 10: 361-371.

21.   Altura, B.M. and B.T. Altura. 1974. Peripheral vascular actions of glucocorticoids and their relationship to protection in circulatory shock . J. Pharmacol. Exp. Ther. 190 : 300-315.

22.   Nicol, T., B. Vernon-Roberts and D.C. Quantock. 1965. The influence of various hormones on the reticulo-endothelial system: endocrine control of body defence. J. Endocrinol. 33 : 365-383.

22a. Halevy, S. and B.M. Altura. 1974. Genetic factors influencing resis-tance to trauma. Circulatory Shock 1: 287-293.

23.   Altura, B.M. and S.G. Hershey. 1968. RES phagocytic function in trauma and adaptation to experimental shock . Am. J. Physiol. 215 : 1414-1419.

24.   Altura, B.M. and S.G.Hershey. 1972. Sequential changes in reticu-loendothelial system function after acute hemorrhage. Proc. Soc. Exp. Biol. Med. 139 : 935-939.

25. Schildt, B., I. Gertz and L. Wide. 1974. Differentiated reticuloendo-thelial system (RES) function in some critical surgical conditions. Acta Chir. Scand. 140 : 611-617.

26. Altura, B.M. and S.G. Hershey. 1973. Reticuloendothelial function in experimental injury and tolerance to shock. Advan. Exp. Med. Biol. 33 : 545-569.

27. Sabo, T.M. 1975. Reticuloendothelial systemic host defense after sur-gery and traumatic shock. Circulatory Shock 2 : 91-108.

28. Chambers, R., B.W. Zweifach and B.E. Lowenstein. 1944. Circulatory reactions of rats traumatized in the Noble-Collip Drum. Am. J. Physiol. 139 : 123-128.

29. Altura, B.M., S.G. Hershey and V.D.B. Mazzia. 1966. Microcircu-latory approach to vasopressor therapy in intestinal ischemic (SMA) shock. Am. J. Surgery 111 : 186-192.

30. Baez, S. 1966. Recording of microvascular dimensions with an image-splitter television microscope. J. Appl. Physiol. 211 : 299-301

31. Altura, B.M. 1971. Chemical and humoral regulation of blood flow through the precapillary sphincter. Microvas. Res. 3 : 361-384.

32. Altura, B.M. 1972. Can metarteriolar vessels occlude their lumens in response to vasoactive substances? Proc. Soc. Exp. Biol. Med. 140 : 1270-1274.

33. Altura, B.M. 1973. Selective microvascular constrictor actions of some neurohypophyseal peptides. Eur. J. Pharmacol. 24 : 49-60.

34. Altura, B.M. 1975. Dose-response relationships for arginine vasopressin and synthetic analogues on three types of rat blood vessels: Possible evidence for regional differences in vasopressin receptor sites within a mammal. J. Pharmacol. Exp. Ther. 193 : 413-423.

35. Altura, B.M. 1975. Pharmacologic effects of alpha-methylDOPA, alpha-methylnorepinephrine and octopamine on rat arteriolar, arterial and terminal vascular smooth muscle. Cir. Res. 36 (suppl. I): I-233-I-240.

36. Hershey, S.G. and B.M. Altura 1973. Vasopressors in low-flow states. In Pharmacology of Adjuvant Drugs, ed. by H.L. Zauder, F.A.Davis Co., Philadelphia, pp. 31-76.

37.   Altura, B.M. 1975. Sex and estrogens and responsiveness of terminal arterioles to neurohypophyseal hormones and catecholamines. J. Pharmacol. Exp. Ther. 193 : 403–412.

38.   Altura, B.M. 1972. Sex as a factor influencing the responsiveness of arterioles to catecholamines. Eur. J. Pharmacol. 20 : 261–265.

39.   Hamilton, J.B. 1948. The role of testicular secretions as indicated by the effects of castration in man and by studies of pathological conditions and the short lifespan associated with maleness. Rec. Progr. Hormone Res. 3 : 257–312.

40.   Zarrow, M.X. and M.E. Denison. 1956. Sexual differences in the survival time of rats exposed to a low ambient temperature. Am. J. Physiol. 186 : 216–218.

41.   Nicol, T., D.L.J. Bilbey, L.M. Charles, J.L. Cordingley and B. Vernon-Roberts. 1964. Oestrogen: the natural stimulant of body defence. J. Endocrinol. 30 : 277–291.

42.   Smith, L.L. and U.P. Vergut. 1964. The liver and shock. Progr. Surg. 4 : 55–107.

43.   Hruza, Z. 1971. Resistance to Trauma . Thomas, Springfield.

44.   Nicol, T. and L.J. Bilbey. 1960. The effect of various steroids on the phagocytic activity of the reticuloendothelial system. In Reticuloendothelial Structure and Function, ed. by J.H. Heller, Ronald Press, New York, pp.301–320.

45.   Altura, B.M. and S.G. Hershey. 1970. Effects of glyceryl trioleate on the reticuloendothelial system and survival after experimental shock. J. Pharmacol. Exp. Ther. 175 : 555–564.

46.   Lefer, A.M. 1973. Blood-borne humoral factors in the pathophysiology of circulatory shock . Circ.Res. 32 : 129–139.

47.   Ramazotto, L.J., R. Carlin and R. Engstrom. 1973. Serum acid phosphatase activity during hemorrhagic shock. Life Sciences 12 : 563–573.

48.   Berken, A. and B. Benacerraf. 1968. Depression of reticuloendothelial system phagocytic function by ingested lipids. Proc. Soc. Exp. Biol. Med. 128 : 793–795.

49.   Berken, A. and A.A. Sherman .1972. Reticuloendothelial system depression in man after olive oil ingestion. Proc. Soc. Exp. Biol. Med. 141: 656-658.

50.   Wissler, R.W. 1968. The arterial medial cell, smooth muscle cell or multifunctional mesenchyme? J. Atherosclerosis Res: 8 : 201-213.

51.   Benacerraf, B. 1958. Quantitative aspects of phagocytosis. In Liver Function, ed. by R. Brauer. A.I.B.S., Washington, pp. 205-227.

52.   Fleisch, J.H., H. Mailing and B.B. Brodie. 1970. Beta-receptor activity in aorta: variations with age and species. Circ.Res. 26 : 151-162.

53.   Ericsson, E. and L. Lundholm . 1975. Adrenergic β-receptor activity and cyclic AMP metabolism in vascular smooth muscle; variations with age. Mechanisms of Ageing and Development 4 : 1-6.

54.   Walton, K.W. 1969. The biology of atherosclerosis. In The Biological Basis of Medicine, vol.6, ed. by E.E. Bittar and N. Bittar. Academic Press, New York, pp. 193-233.

INBRED MICE AND THEIR HYBRIDS AS AN ANIMAL MODEL FOR

ATHEROSCLEROSIS RESEARCH

A. Roberts and J.S. Thompson

Department of Anatomy

University of Toronto

This study was undertaken to determine if there are genetic factors in mice that influence the development of fatty deposits in the wall of the aortic sinus and the control of serum total cholesterol levels. The relationship of these two phenomena to each other was also studied.

In 1969 (1), it was shown that the male C57BL/6J inbred mouse was a suitable animal in which to produce consistent atheromatous lesions in the wall of the aortic sinus. Lesions were produced by placing the animals on a high-fat, high-cholesterol diet containing 30 per cent cocoa butter, 5 per cent cholesterol and 30 per cent protein in the form of casein. The animals were introduced to this diet at six weeks of age. Initially for a period of three days a mixture of 70 per cent high-fat, high-cholesterol diet and 30 per cent regular Purina laboratory chow was used to introduce the animal to the diet; then a mixture of 80 per cent diet and 20 per cent chow was given for three days. Finally the experimental animals were continued on a mixture of 90 per cent diet and 10 per cent chow for the duration of the experiment. It was found that by introducing the high-fat, high-cholesterol diet in this way the mice accepted and tolerated the diet with relatively few deaths before the time of sacrifice.

In the hope of finding two inbred strains that differed markedly in their response to the high-fat, high-cholesterol diet, male mice of 13 inbred strains were investigated by dividing animals of each strain into an experimental group, starting on the high-fat, high-cholesterol diet at six weeks of age, and a corresponding control group continued on the regular laboratory diet. The first ten in the following list of 13 strains tolerated the high-fat, high-cholesterol

313

diet well enough so that meaningful results could be obtained.

1.	CBA/J	6.	C57BL/6J	10.	C57L/J
2.	BALB/cJ	7.	SWR/J	11.	C58/J
3.	C3H/HeJ	8.	C57BL/10J	12.	A/J
4.	A/HeJ	9.	C57BR/cdJ	13.	129/J
5.	DBA/1J				

Two strains were selected that showed marked differences in their reaction to the high-fat, high-cholesterol diet. Male mice of the C57BR/cdJ strain subjected to the diet developed large lesions with many foam cells while the corresponding CBA/J male mice developed smaller lesions with very few foam cells. The corresponding control mice of both strains developed small lesions very slowly. The C57BR/cdJ strain was selected as the P_1 parent strain and the CBA/J strain as the P_2 parent strain for further crossbreeding and backcrossing studies.

The two parent strains were also investigated to determine if their serum total cholesterol levels could be related to the size of lesion and total number of foam cells in the wall of the aortic sinus. The C57BR/cdJ (P_1) and CBA/J (P_2) strains were compared by dividing male mice of each strain into a control group, continued on the regular laboratory chow, and an experimental group fed the high-fat, high-cholesterol diet starting at 10 weeks of age. Each animal was identified by coded ear punches and weighed at 10 weeks and weighed again at the time of sacrifice. The experimental animals with corresponding controls were sacrificed at intervals of 3, 5, 10 and 15 weeks after commencement of the diet in sample sizes of approximately 15 to 20 mice for each experimental and each control group using intraperitoneal sodium pentobarbital anaesthesia. Blood was removed from the inferior vena cava, and the serum total cholesterol level was determined using the Technicon Auto-Analyser method N-24a at the Wellesley Hospital laboratory, Toronto. Immediately following removal of the blood from the inferior vena cava, the heart and ascending aorta were removed for sectioning. The sections through the area of the aortic sinus were cut with a freezing microtome and stained with oil red O and counterstained with haematoxylin and light green. It was found that the aortic sinus wall, where the aortic valves attach, consistently showed the largest lesions. Therefore only sections that contained a portion of the attachment(s) of the aortic valves to the sinus wall were considered, and usually 10 of the 21 sections from each heart fulfilled this criterion. From the 10 sections one section was selected that showed the highest total number of foam cells and the largest single lesion.

The following two parameters plus total serum cholesterol were chosen for study:

1. The total number of foam cells in each section. Each
    section was classified into one of four categories:
    a) No foam cells.
    b) One to four.
    c) Five to fifteen.
    d) More than fifteen foam cells.
    A foam cell was considered to be a cell in which there
    were sufficient fat droplets to make the cytoplasm of the
    cell bulge. More than 15 foam cells in a section were
    usually difficult to count individually as the nuclear
    and cell boundaries could not be clearly identified.

2. The size of the largest single lesion in the section.
    Again each section was classified into one of four
    categories:
    a) No lesion.
    b) Occupying less than 1/8 of the aortic sinus wall
        between the attachment of two adjacent valve cusps.
    c) Occupying 1/8 to 1/4 of the aortic sinus wall.
    d) Occupying more than 1/4 of the aortic sinus wall.

Fortran computer programs were developed to determine the value
of chi square used in comparing any two groups for the size of the
single largest lesion and total number of foam cells and to perform
the t prime (t^1) test which was used for determining the significance
of differences between the mean total cholesterol levels of any two
groups. The results obtained in making comparisons between different
groups of mice were considered to be significant when $p < 0.05$.

Initially the mean serum total cholesterol levels were from
pooled samples of blood obtained from two to five mice. With time
the skill of the operators improved so that enough blood for a
single total cholesterol determination could be obtained from an
individual mouse. To allow use of a blood sample obtained from a
single mouse, both parental series were repeated using sample sizes
of approximately 15 mice for each experimental and each control
group after the experimental mice had been on the 90 per cent high-
fat diet for 3, 5, 10 and 15 weeks.

Figure 1 illustrates the mean serum total cholesterol levels
of both parent strains for individual and pooled samples on the
high-fat and regular diets. The mean serum total cholesterol levels
for both pooled and individual samples of the C57BR/cdJ (P_1) strain
were significantly higher for the experimental animals than for
their corresponding controls throughout the 15 weeks. The mean
serum total cholesterol levels for the pooled samples from
experimental CBA/J (P_2) strain were significantly higher than the
controls at 3, 5 and 10 weeks, and for individual samples the
experimental were significantly higher than the control throughout
the 15 weeks on the diet. The C57BR/cdJ had significantly higher

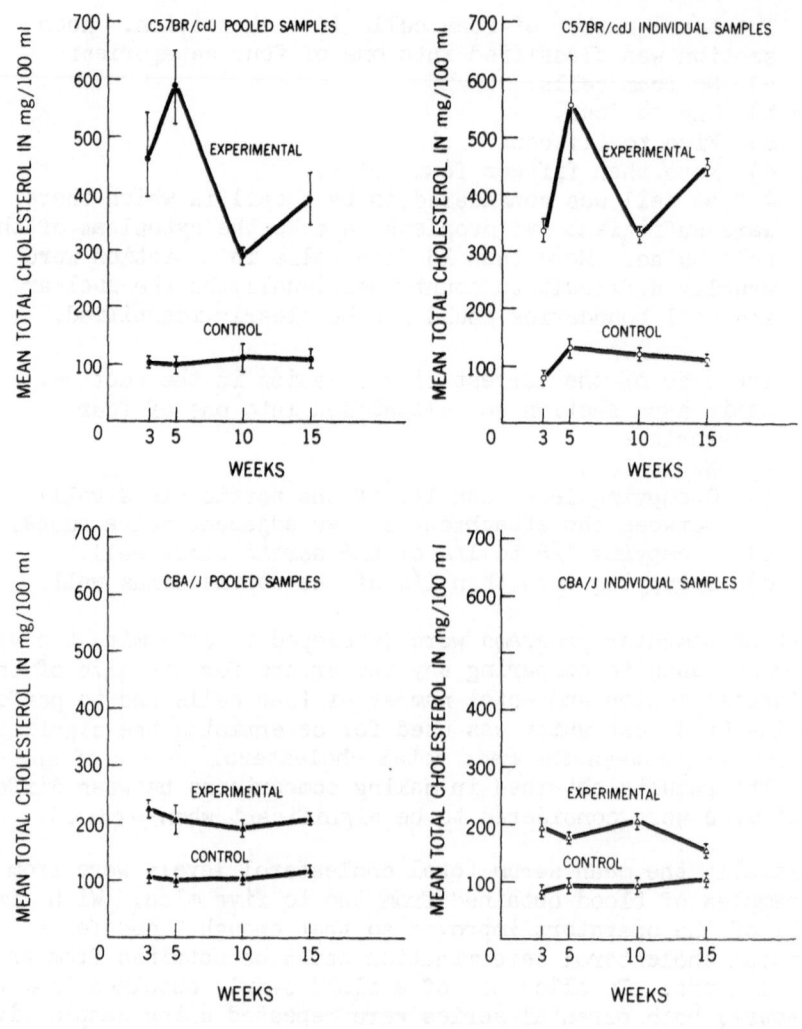

FIGURE 1

Mean serum total cholesterol levels of the parent strains from
individual or pooled samples on the high-fat and regular diets.
(Mean ± 1 S.E.)

levels than the CBA/J throughout the 15 weeks on the high-fat,
high-cholesterol diet for both pooled and individual samples. The
experimental C57BR/cdJ (P_1) strain showed an elevated mean serum
total cholesterol level at 3 weeks, this rose higher at 5 weeks,
decreased at 10 weeks and rose again at 15 weeks for both the
individual and pooled samples while their corresponding controls

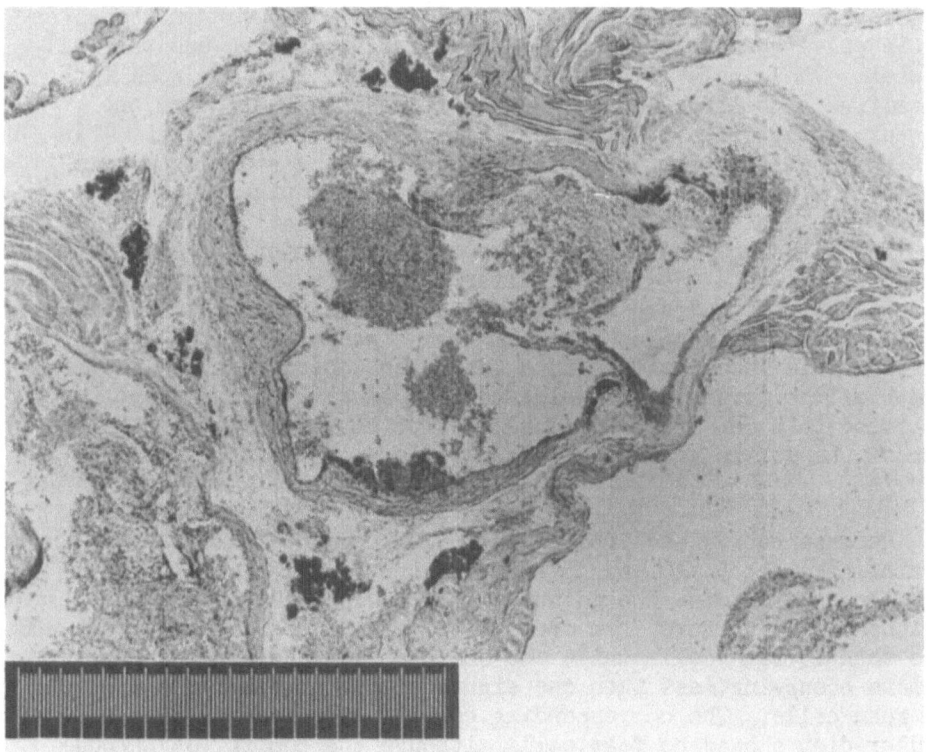

FIGURE 2

Cross-section of the wall of the ascending aorta of the C57BR/cdJ
(P_1) strain after three weeks on the 90 per cent high-fat, high-
cholesterol diet. An atheromatous deposit occupies more than one
quarter of the sinus wall between the attachment of adjacent valve
cusps. The whole scale in the lower left corner represents one
millimeter.

remained in the range of about 100 mg per 100 ml throughout the
experiment. There is no apparent explanation for the decrease in
mean serum total cholesterol levels at 10 weeks on the high-fat,
high-cholesterol diet and the subsequent rise at 15 weeks. In a
third series of parent strains, which have not been included because
the sections from the hearts have not been examined, the experimental
C57BR/cdJ mice also showed a decrease in serum total cholesterol
levels at 10 weeks and a rise again at 15 weeks.

Figure 2 is a photograph of a cross-section of the wall of the
ascending aorta of the C57BR/cdJ (P_1) strain after 3 weeks on the

90 per cent high-fat, high-cholesterol diet. The section shows the
aortic valve cusps attaching to the wall of the aorta and the wall
between. The single largest lesion in the aortic sinus wall is
classified as a large lesion because it occupies more than one
quarter of the sinus wall between two adjacent valve cusps. This
section shows more than 15 foam cells. The dark staining material
outside the wall of the aorta is normal adipose tissue.

Figure 3 is a photograph of a cross-section of the ascending
aorta of the CBA/J (P_2) strain after 3 weeks on the high-fat, high-
cholesterol diet. There is a slight deposit of fat, that is difficult to see in the photograph, in the attachment of the aortic
valves. This is classified as a lesion that occupies less than one
eighth of the aortic sinus wall, and no foam cells are present. It
was found that fat droplets usually first appeared in the attachment of the aortic valve cusp or at the opening of the coronary
arteries.

Representative sections of the C57BR/cdJ and CBA/J parent
strains taken at 5, 10 and 15 weeks on the 90 per cent high-fat,
high-cholesterol diet showed that C57BR/cdJ strain usually had large
lesions occupying more than one quarter of the aortic sinus wall and
more than 15 foam cells, while the CBA/J strain usually had small
lesions occupying less than one eighth of the aortic sinus wall and
few foam cells. The corresponding control mice continued on the
regular diet showed no foam cells, although the control C57BR/cdJ
strain had significantly larger lesions at 3, 5 and 15 weeks than
the corresponding CBA/J strain.

In order to determine if there was a parental influence on the
development of lesions and serum total cholesterol levels, the two
parent strains were reciprocally crossbred to produce two series of
F_1 offspring -- one with a C57BR/cdJ mother and the other with a
CBA/J mother. The two F_1 series were reciprocally crossbred to each
other to produce four series of F_2 offspring. The two F_1 series
were backcrossed to each parent strain to produce four series of B_1
mice (P_1 x F_1 = B_1) and four series of B_2 mice (P_2 x F_1 = B_2). The
F_1, F_2, B_1 and B_2 generations were examined as the parent strains
had been by dividing each series into experimental groups, starting
on the high-fat, high-cholesterol diet at 10 weeks of age, and their
corresponding controls, continued on the regular laboratory diet.
The mice were tagged and weighed at 10 weeks of age and weighed
again at the time of sacrifice when blood was removed from the
inferior vena cava for serum total cholesterol determination, and the
heart was removed for sectioning through the area of the aortic sinus
wall. No dominant maternal or paternal influence could be
demonstrated in the experimental and control groups of the F_1, F_2,
B_1 and B_2 generations for the three parameters of total number of
foam cells, size of the largest single lesion and mean serum total
cholesterol levels.

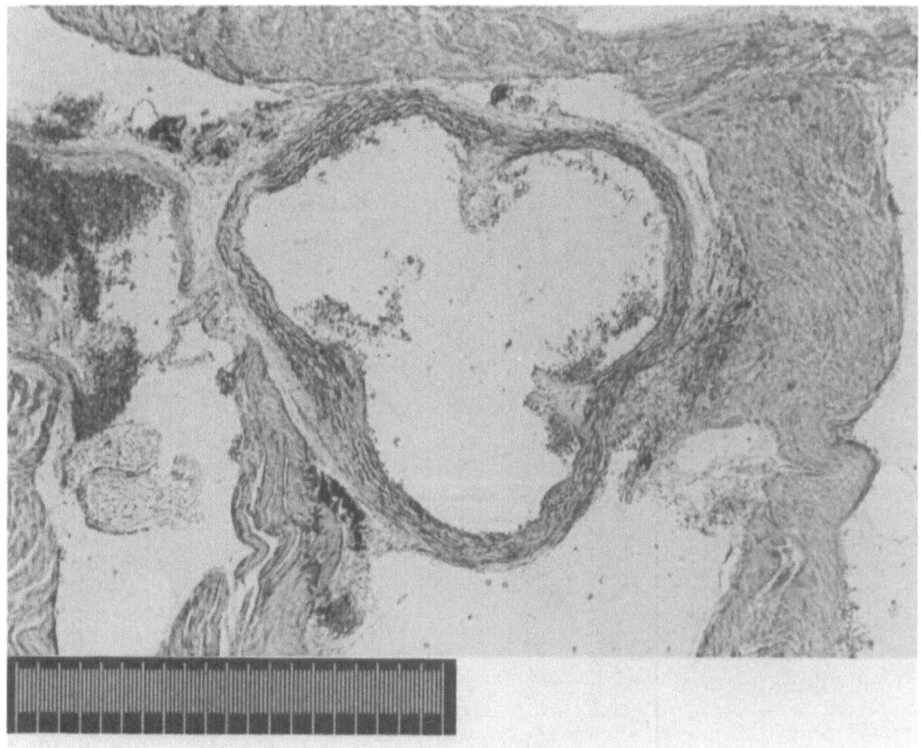

FIGURE 3

Cross—section of the wall of the ascending aorta of the CBA/J (P_2)
strain after three weeks on the 90 per cent high—fat, high—
cholesterol diet. Slight deposits of fat that are present in the
attachments of the aortic valves to the sinus wall are not seen
clearly in the photograph. The whole scale in the lower left
corner represents one millimeter.

    Figure 4 shows that the mean serum total cholesterol levels of
the F_1 and F_2 generations fall between those of the parent strains
throughout the 15 weeks on the high—fat, high—cholesterol diet. The
C57BR/cdJ (P_1) strain had significantly higher values than the F_1,
F_2 and CBA/J mice throughout the experiment,except at three weeks
when the C57BR/cdJ strain was not significantly higher than the F_2
generation. The F_2 generation had higher mean serum total
cholesterol levels than the F_1 generation throughout, but had only
significantly higher values ($p < 0.01$) at 3 and 15 weeks. The F_1

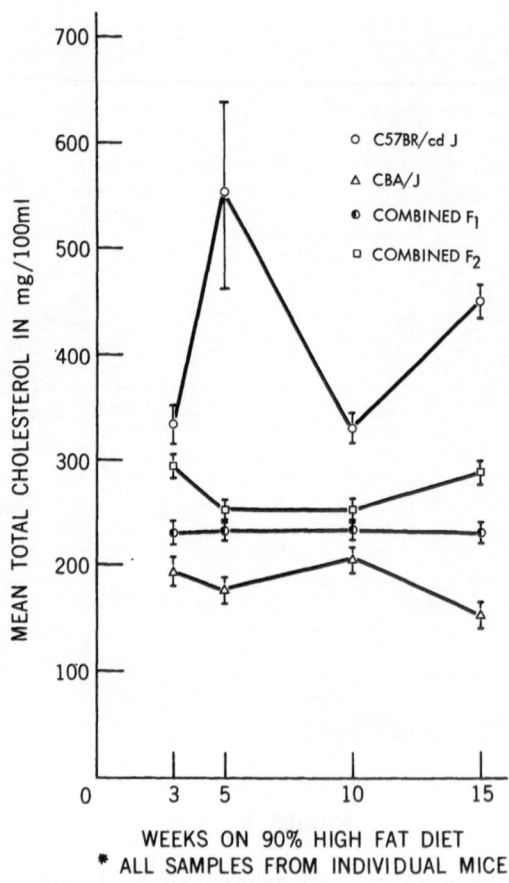

FIGURE 4

Mean serum total cholesterol levels of the C57BR/cdJ, CBA/J, F_1 and F_2 mice on the high-fat, high-cholesterol diet. (Mean ± 1 S.E.)

generation was closer to, but had significantly higher mean serum total cholesterol levels than, the CBA/J (P_2) strain throughout the 15 weeks.

Figure 5 shows that the mean serum total cholesterol levels of the two backcross generations fall between those of the two parent strains on the high-fat, high-cholesterol diet. Again the C57BR/cdJ strain had significantly higher mean serum total cholesterol values than the B_1, B_2 and CBA/J mice, except at three weeks when the C57BR/cdJ strain was not significantly higher than the B_1 generation. The B_1 generation had significantly higher mean serum total

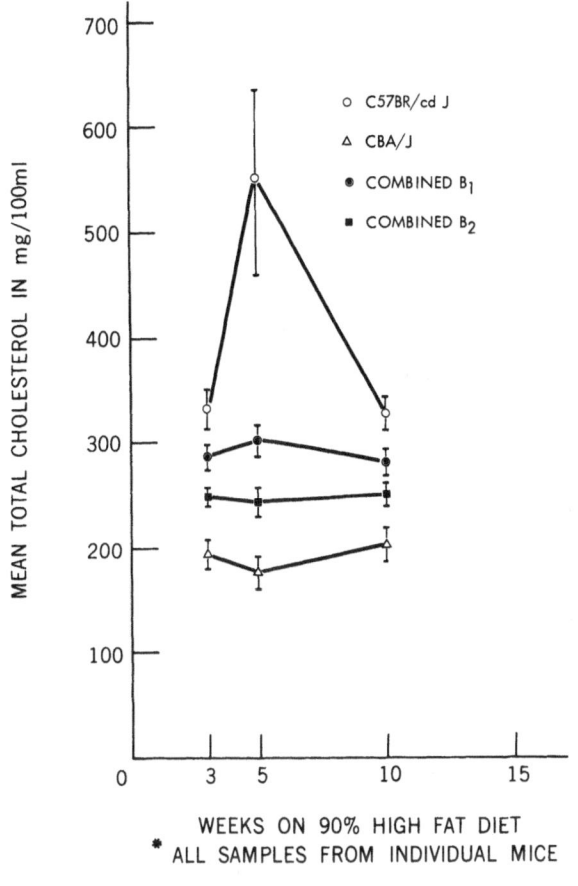

FIGURE 5

Mean serum total cholesterol levels of the C57BR/cdJ, CBA/J, B_1 and
B_2 mice on the high-fat, high-cholesterol diet. (Mean $\pm$ 1 S.E.)

cholesterol levels than the B_2 and CBA/J, while the B_2 had significantly higher levels than the CBA/J throughout the experiment.   The
B_1 generation is closer to the C57BR/cdJ (P_1) strain and the B_2
generation is closer to the CBA/J (P_2) strain.

     Figure 6 demonstrates the relative closeness for mean serum to-
tal cholesterol levels of the control groups of the two parent
strains and the F_1, F_2, B_1 and B_2 generations that were continued on
the regular laboratory diet. The range for the control mice for the
six groups lies between 79 and 143 mg per 100 ml. Interestingly,
the C57BR/cdJ control mice had significantly higher mean serum total
cholesterol levels than the CBA/J mice at 5 and 10 weeks.

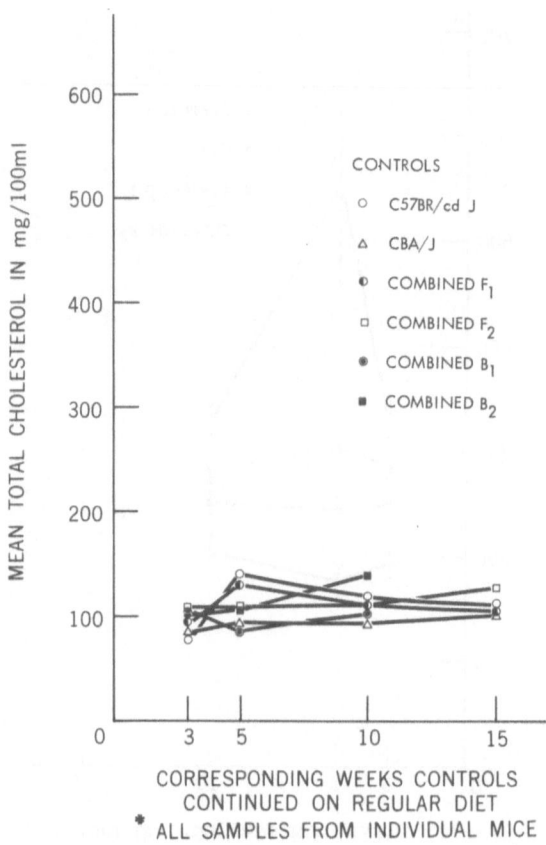

FIGURE 6

Mean serum total cholesterol levels of the controls of the
C57BR/cdJ, CBA/J, F_1, F_2, B_1 and B_2 mice continued on the regular
laboratory diet. (Mean $\pm$ 1 S.E.)

COMPARISON OF THE PARENT STRAINS AND THE
F_1, F_2, B_1 AND B_2 GENERATIONS

For the three parameters of total number of foam cells, size
of the largest lesion and mean serum total cholesterol levels the
C57BR/cdJ (P_1) strain had significantly higher values than the
CBA/J (P_2) strain on the high-fat, high-cholesterol diet throughout
the 15 weeks. On comparing the control mice of the two parent
strains, the C57BR/cdJ had significantly higher values than the
CBA/J at 3, 5 and 15 weeks for size of the largest lesion and at 5
and 10 weeks for mean serum total cholesterol levels. Both the

C57BR/cdJ and CBA/J strains on the high-fat diet had significantly higher values for all three parameters than their corresponding controls.

The two series of the F_1 generation (one with the C57BR/cdJ mother and the other with the CBA/J mother) showed no significant differences when corresponding groups were compared by pairs (experimental versus experimental and control versus control) except for the two control groups at the 10 week interval. Thus the mother and father appear to exert an equal influence, and the two F_1 series were combined into single experimental and control populations. On the high-fat diet the F_1 generation fell between the two parent strains for total number of foam cells and mean serum total cholesterol levels, but were closer to the CBA/J (P_2) strain. However, the F_1 generation on the high-fat diet had lower values for size of the largest lesion than did the CBA/J strain. The F_1 on the high-fat diet had significantly higher values than the control F_1 for all three parameters throughout the 15 weeks.

The two series of the F_1 generation were reciprocally crossbred to produce four series of the F_2 generation. The four series were compared with each other by pairs — the experimental group of one series compared with the experimental group of another series, and the control group of one series compared with the control group of another series for corresponding weekly intervals (3, 5, 10 and 15 weeks). There was no significant difference for total number of foam cells and size of the largest single lesion and only a few significant differences for the parameter of mean serum total cholesterol levels, thus indicating that the mother and father exert an equal influence, and the four series were combined into experimental and control F_2 populations. The experimental F_2 had significantly higher values than the control F_2 for all three parameters. On the high-fat diet the F_2 generation fell between the two parent strains, and for all three parameters the C57BR/cdJ strain had significantly higher values than the F_2 generation, except at the third week for mean serum total cholesterol levels when the C57BR/cdJ was not significantly higher than the F_2 generation. For all three parameters the experimental F_2 had significantly higher values than the experimental CBA/J strain except for the occasional group. The experimental F_2 on the high-fat diet had significantly higher values than the experimental F_1 for size of the largest lesion throughout the experiment, for total number of foam cells at 3 and 5 weeks and for mean serum total cholesterol levels at 3 and 15 weeks.

The two series of the F_1 generation were reciprocally backcrossed to each parent strain producing four series of the B_1 generation and four series of the B_2 generation. Again the mother and father exert an equal influence because there were no significant differences between the four series of the B_1 generation and also between the four series of the B_2 generation for each of the three

parameters when compared with each other (experimental versus
experimental and control versus control) at 3, 5 and 10 weeks. The
four series of the B_1 generation were combined into experimental and
control populations as were the four series of the B_2 generation.

On the high-fat, high-cholesterol diet the B_1 had values closer
to the C57BR/cdJ (P_1) strain and the B_2 had values closer to the
CBA/J (P_2) strain for all three parameters. The B_1 generation had
significantly higher values than the B_2 generation for the parameters of total number of foam cells and mean serum total cholesterol
level throughout the experiment, and the B_1 had significantly larger
lesions at the third and tenth weeks. The F_2 generation always fell
between the two backcross generations, while the F_1 generation fell
below the two backcross generations for the three parameters.

There were no significant differences between the controls of
the P_1, P_2, F_1, F_2, B_1 and B_2 populations for the parameter of total
number of foam cells. For the parameter of the size of the largest
single lesion the control C57BR/cdJ (P_1) strain at 3, 5 and 15 weeks
and the control F_2, B_1 and B_2 generations at 3 and 5 weeks had significantly higher values than the control CBA/J (P_2) strain.
For the parameter of mean serum cholesterol levels the control mice
of the C57BR/cdJ strain had significantly higher values at 5 and 10
weeks, and the control mice of the F_1, F_2 and B_2 generations had
significantly higher values at 3, 5 and 10 weeks, than the CBA/J
control mice.

Figure 7 arranges the two parent strains and the F_1, F_2, B_1 and
B_2 generations on the high-fat, high-cholesterol diet from the lowest
value to the highest value for the three parameters of:

1. total number of foam cells
2. size of the single largest lesion
3. mean serum total cholesterol levels

The C57BR/cdJ and CBA/J parent strains and the F_1, F_2, B_1 and
B_2 generations were compared with each other by pairs, and it was
found that most populations differed significantly from each other
at the $p < 0.01$ level of confidence. Thus a distance equal to or
greater than "a" indicates that the upper population in Figure 7
had significantly higher values at the 99% level of confidence at
all weeks than a lower population. In the parameters of total number
of foam cells and size of the largest lesion the C57BR/cdJ (P_1)
strain had significantly higher values at all weeks than any of the
other populations. The distance "b" indicates that there was a significant difference at the 99% level of confidence between two populations in two out of three or three out of four comparisons after
3, 5, 10 and 15 weeks on the high-fat diet. The distances "c" and
"d" indicate a significant difference in two out of four and one
out of four of the weekly intervals, respectively.

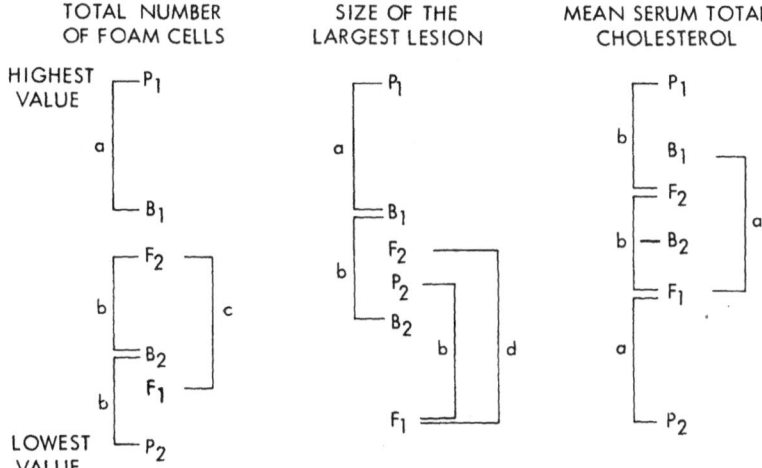

ᵃ p < 0.01 IN 100% OF THE WEEKLY INTERVALS (3,5,10,15)
ᵇ p < 0.01 IN 67 TO 75% OF THE WEEKLY INTERVALS
ᶜ p < 0.01 IN 50% OF THE WEEKLY INTERVALS
ᵈ p < 0.01 IN 25% OF THE WEEKLY INTERVALS

* p <0.01 in 100% of the weekly intervals between any two groups separated by the distance ⩾ a, except in the cases designated by b, c and d.

FIGURE 7

Arrangement of the C57BR/cdJ, CBA/J, F_1, F_2, B_1 and B_2 mice on the high-fat, high-cholesterol diet from the lowest value to the highest value for the three parameters of total number of foam cells, size of the largest single lesion and mean serum total cholesterol.

Figure 7 indicates that the C57BR/cdJ (P_1) strain always had the highest values for all three parameters while the CBA/J (P_2) strain had the lowest values for the total number of foam cells and mean serum total cholesterol levels. For the two parameters of total number of foam cells and mean serum total cholesterol levels the order is $P_1 > B_1 > F_2 > B_2 > F_1 > P_2$, while for the size of largest lesion this order is changed so that P_2 falls between the F_2 and B_2 and $P_1 > B_1 > F_2 > P_2 > B_2 > F_1$.

If this were a simple genetic model based upon a single gene we would expect the following: $P_1 > B_1 > F_1$, $F_2 > B_2 > P_2$, but in our experiments B_2 is always greater than F_1 for the three parameters.

TABLE I

TYPE OF INHERITANCE INVOLVED IN RESPONSE TO THE
HIGH-FAT DIET

Generation	Predicted Results Based On The Single Gene Hypothesis		Experimental Results Obtained
	Dominance	Co-dominance	
F_1	$F_1 = P_1$ or P_2	F_1 Midway Between P_1 & P_2	(a) F_1 Closer to P_2 (b) Wide Range of Values Within Each Series of F_1

F_2	3:1 Ratio	1:2:1 Ratio	(a) Variance of F_2 Larger Than Variance of F_1 For Mean Cholesterols
			 (b) Within Each Series of F_2
			   i) Wide Range of Values
			   ii) No Discernible Ratio

B_1 and B_2	Parents Dominant 4:0 Ratio
	 Parents Recessive 1:1 Ratio
		1:1 Ratio	(a) Within Each Series of B_1 and B_2
			   i) Wide Range of Values
			   ii) No Discernible Ratio

Table 1 is a comparison of the results predicted on the basis of a single gene hypothesis (either dominant-recessive or co-dominant genes for the two parent strains) and the actual experimental results obtained. The experimental results indicate a multifactorial (polygenic) system of inheritance for the following reasons:

1. The F_1 generation was closer to the CBA/J (P_2) strain for all three parameters.
2. The variance of the F_2 was larger than the variance of the F_1 for mean serum total cholesterol levels throughout the experiment on the high-fat diet.
3. There was a wide range of values within each of the two series of the F_1, within each of the four series of the F_2, within each of the four series of the B_1 and within each of the four series of the B_2 generations. This is to be expected in multifactorial inheritance.

4. There were no discernible ratios within any of the F_1, F_2, B_1 and B_2 generations, although in single factor inheritance there should be.

CONCLUSIONS

1. The inbred strain of mouse is a relatively inexpensive and easily controlled animal that produces consistent results within each of the P_1, P_2, F_1, F_2, B_1 and B_2 generations.
2. The mother and father exert an equal influence on the development of fatty deposits in the aortic sinus wall and on serum total cholesterol levels.
3. Different strains of inbred mice react to the high-fat, high-cholesterol diet in different ways.
4. The control mice of the CBA/J (P_2) strain had significantly lower values of serum total cholesterol and size of the largest lesion at some weeks than the control mice of the C57BR/cdJ and F_1, F_2, B_1 and B_2 generations.
5. The experiments indicate a multifactorial (polygenic) system of inheritance.

REFERENCES

1. Thompson, J.S. 1969. Atheromata in an inbred strain of mice. J. Atheroscler. Res. 10:113-122.

ACKNOWLEDGEMENTS

This work has been supported by grants-in-aid from the Ontario (Canada) Heart Foundation and the Physicians Services Incorporated Foundation (Ontario, Canada).

The assistance of Mrs. L. Eljas and Mrs. L.A. Wheeler is gratefully acknowledged.

DIET-INDUCED HYPERCHOLESTEROLEMIA IN THE

DIABETIC AND NON-DIABETIC CHINESE HAMSTER

M.G. Soret, M.C. Blanks, G.C. Gerritsen, C.E. Day, and
E.M. Block

The Upjohn Company
Kalamazoo, Michigan 49001

INTRODUCTION

The association of human diabetes and the development of vascular disease has been established (1-4). Since the spontaneous
diabetes in the Chinese hamster *(Cricetulus griseus)* (5) has been
considered a good experimental model of the human disease (6) it
was considered of interest to find if this animal was also suited
for the study of vascular diseases, whether induced or naturally
occurring. The present study was designed to investigate some
morphologic and metabolic effects of diet induced hypercholesterolemia in the Chinese hamster.

MATERIALS AND METHODS

Forty-two Chinese hamsters were selected for this study.
Fourteen mild diabetics and 14 non-diabetics were fed Purina Mouse
Chow containing 1.5% cholesterol while 7 mild diabetics and 7 non-
diabetics were fed a regular Purina Mouse Chow diet and served as
controls for a period of 8 months. By accident, the cholesterol-
fed group received the control diet during the 5th and 6th months
of the test. All animals were fed *ad libitum*.

The animals were killed by exsanguination from the eye orbital
plexus (7), and the blood was processed for subsequent tests.

Blood glucose levels were estimated by a Technicon Autoanalyzer
using a modification of the ferricyanide reduction method as described by Hoffman (8). Serum cholesterol levels were measured

following the methods of Block et al. (9). Lipoprotein determinations by electrophoresis followed the methods of Alexander and
Day (10).

Systematic gross examination of the aorta was made within
minutes of sacrifice. Samples of aorta, liver, kidney, adrenal,
pancreas, spleen, and heart were fixed in Bouin's solution; liver,
kidney and adrenal were fixed in methanol; and heart, aorta, and
liver were fixed in neutral formalin. For light microscopy, 5 μ
sections from all paraffin embedded tissues were stained with hematoxylin eosin (H&E) and allochrome. Pancreas was also stained by
the Scott-Halmi aldehyde fuchsin method. Formalin-fixed frozen
sections of liver, heart, and aorta were stained with Oil Red O
(ORO).

Small sections of the aortas taken 1-2 mm above and below the
renal arteries were fixed in 2% glutaraldehyde and postfixed in 1%
osmium tetroxide and embedded in Epon 812. Blocks were sectioned
with a diamond knife with the LKB-2 ultramicrotome. Ultrathin
sections were stained with uranyl acetate and lead citrate and were
examined with the Philips 301 electron microscope.

Total cholesterol concentration of the aorta, excluding the
segments submitted for microscopy, were determined by gas liquid
chromatography, after extraction with isopropanol (11), following
the procedure of Day et al. (12).

RESULTS

Metabolic Studies

The initial conditions of the 33 surviving animals in this
study are summarized in Table I.

Plasma cholesterol levels were normal for all animals at the
beginning of the tests. Non-diabetic and diabetic Chinese hamsters
fed the cholesterol diet experienced an increase of plasma cholesterol levels by the end of the first month (Figure 1a). This increase was sharp among the diabetics and moderate among non-
diabetics. The marked decrease in plasma cholesterol levels between
the 5th and 6th months among cholesterol-fed animals, reflects the
accidental switching of the cholesterol diet to the regular diet.
However, plasma levels of cholesterol increased sharply after the
animals were placed back on the cholesterol diet. No changes were
observed in the animals fed the control diet.

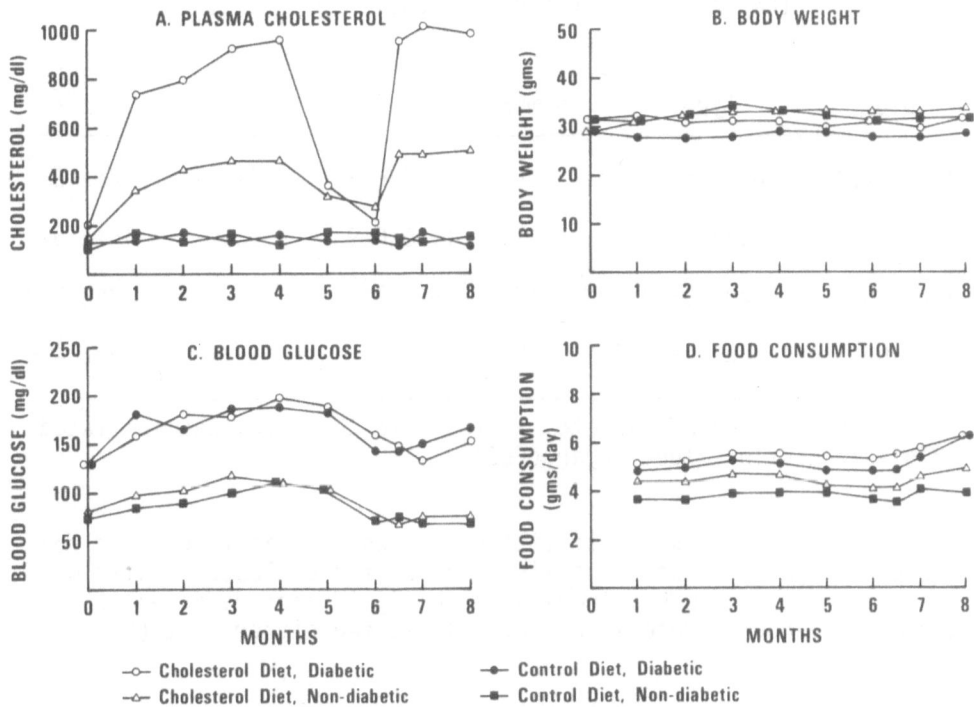

Figure 1.   a.   Comparison of plasma cholesterol levels for non-diabetic and diabetic Chinese hamsters fed the cholesterol diet or the control diet.

b.   Weight of non-diabetic and diabetic Chinese hamsters fed the cholesterol diet or the control diet.

c.   Blood glucose levels for non-diabetic and diabetic Chinese hamsters fed either the cholesterol diet or the control diet.

d.   Food consumption for non-diabetic or diabetic Chinese hamsters on the cholesterol diet or the control diet.

TABLE I

Characteristics of Chinese Hamsters at
the Beginning of the 1.5% Cholesterol Diet

Diet	Type	Number	Age(Mo)*	Duration Diabetes*	FBS mg%**
1.5% Chol.	Diabetic	9	9.2±0.8	7.7±1.1	149±12
Control	Diabetic	7	11.0±0.9	9.0±0.7	154±13
1.5% Chol.	Non-diabetic	12	9.0±1.0	--	78± 3.4
Control	Non-diabetic	5	9.5±2.5	--	83± 4.6

*Age and duration of diabetes at the time the study was initiated.
**Initial fasting blood sugar (FBS).

Figure 1b suggests that little changes in weight occurred for diabetic or non-diabetic animals, whether fed cholesterol diet or control diet. Likewise, there were no significant differences between the blood glucose levels of animals fed either diet (Figure 1c).

Since diabetics ate slightly more than non-diabetics (Figure 1d), this slight increase in dietary cholesterol intake may have contributed, in part, to the higher plasma cholesterol levels observed in the diabetics fed cholesterol-containing diet.

Terminal data are shown in Table II. Mean plasma cholesterol values of diabetics fed 1.5% cholesterol in the diet were 992 mg/dl compared with 121 mg/dl for diabetics on control diet. However, plasma cholesterol values were very variable (range 400-2000 mg/dl) as shown by the large standard error.

Figure 2 shows representative gas chromatographs of extracts of aortas after saponification, for the 4 groups of animals. The peak identified by the lower arrow has the same retention time as cholesterol. It is obvious that there were many other unidentified substances (presumably sterols) extracted from the aorta. Although considerable variation was observed, there were no obvious qualitative differences between the four groups. However, there did appear to be a general correlation in that animals with the higher plasma values tended to have the higher aortic lipid levels.

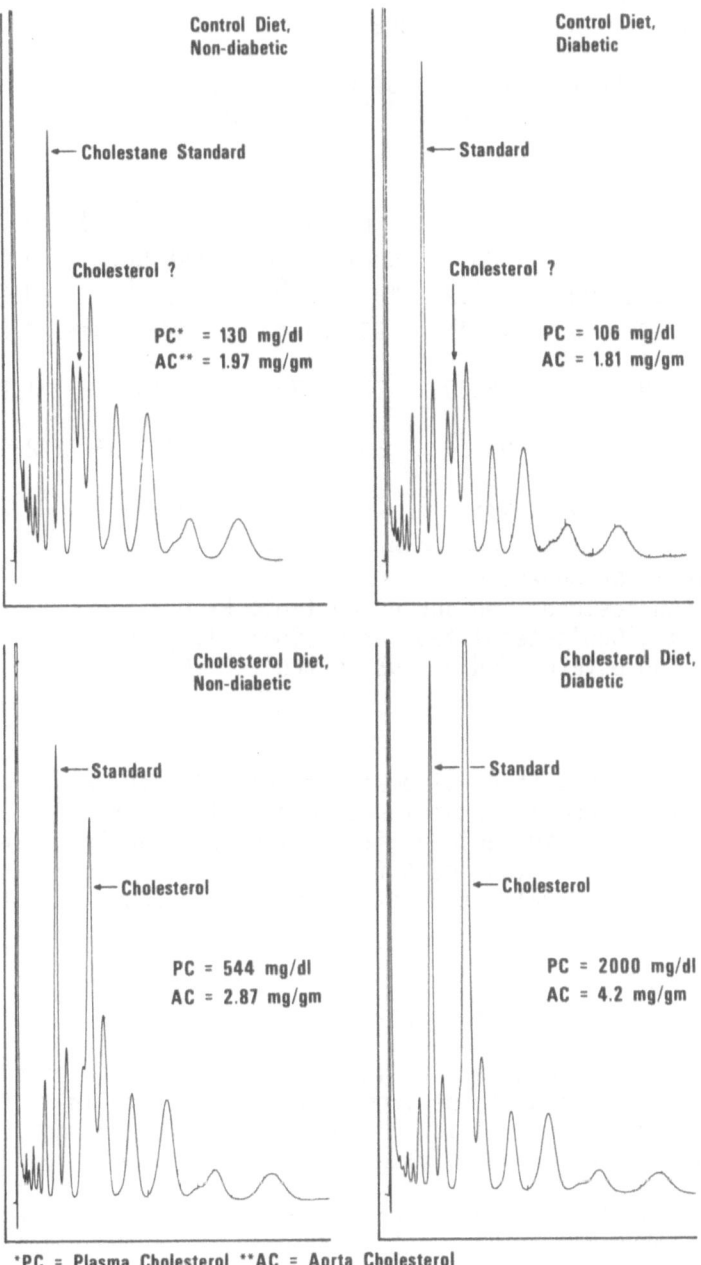

Figure 2. Representative gas chromatographs of extracts of the aortas from Chinese hamsters on the cholesterol diet or the control diet.

TABLE II

Characteristics of Chinese Hamsters
after 8 Months on a 1.5% Cholesterol Diet

Diet	Type	No.	FBS mg% ± SE	Plasma Cholesterol mg/dl ± SE	Aorta Fresh Wgt. mg ± SE	Aorta Cholesterol mg/gm ± SE
1.5% Chol.	D	9	179±14	992±219*	3.42±0.24**	3.04±0.37*
Control	D	7	162±25	121± 7	2.63±0.13	1.93±0.04
1.5% Chol.	ND	12	93± 4	507± 33*	2.89±0.33	2.99±0.35
Control	ND	5	93± 5	140± 15	3.03±0.22	2.22±0.08

D=Diabetic   ND=Non-Diabetic
*Diabetic, Cholesterol fed versus Control, P<.001.
 Non-diabetic, Cholesterol fed versus Control, P<.001.
**Diabetic, Cholesterol fed versus Control, P<.02.

Figure 3 represents densitometer tracings of the agarose gel electrophoretic serum lipoprotein pattern in the 4 groups of animals. Again, there was considerable variation from one sample to the next but in general most of the identifiable lipoprotein was in the HDL region. No obvious qualitative differences were observed between the 4 groups.

Morphologic Studies

The morphologic alterations induced after 8 months of cholesterol feeding were found to be from minor to moderate in most cases, with the exception of the liver. Some differences were noticed, however, which deserve an analysis:

A. Changes induced by the cholesterol feeding regardless of the diabetic or non-diabetic condition of the hamsters studied:

   Liver: Enlargement of hepatocytes and spongy structure of the hepatic cell (except those surrounding the central veins). (Figure 4)

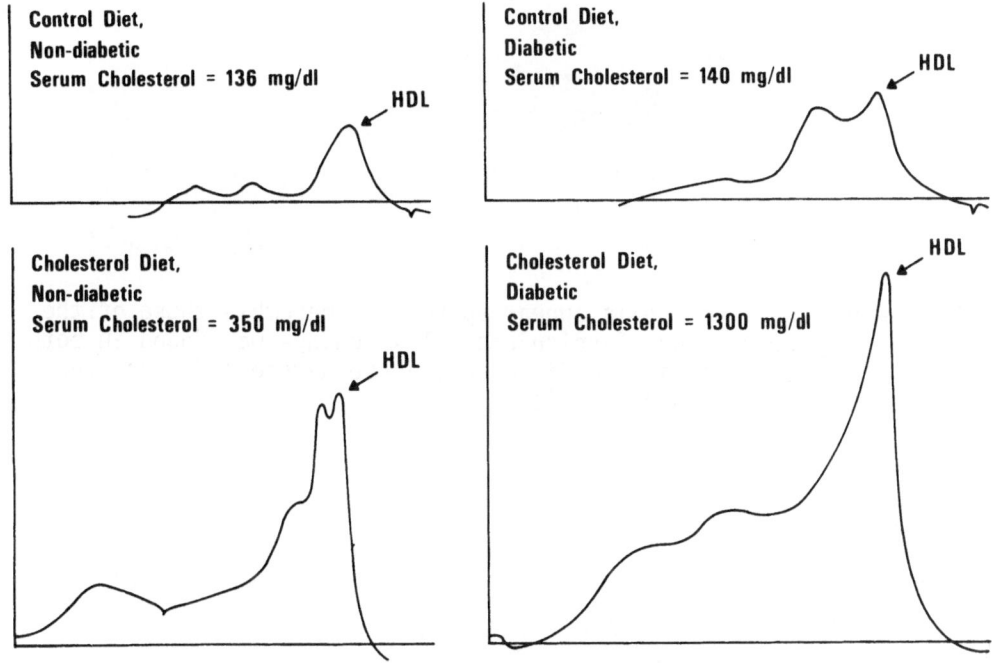

Figure 3. Densitometer tracings of the agarose gel electrophoretic
          serum lipoprotein pattern in the non-diabetic and
          diabetic Chinese hamsters fed the cholesterol diet or
          control diet.

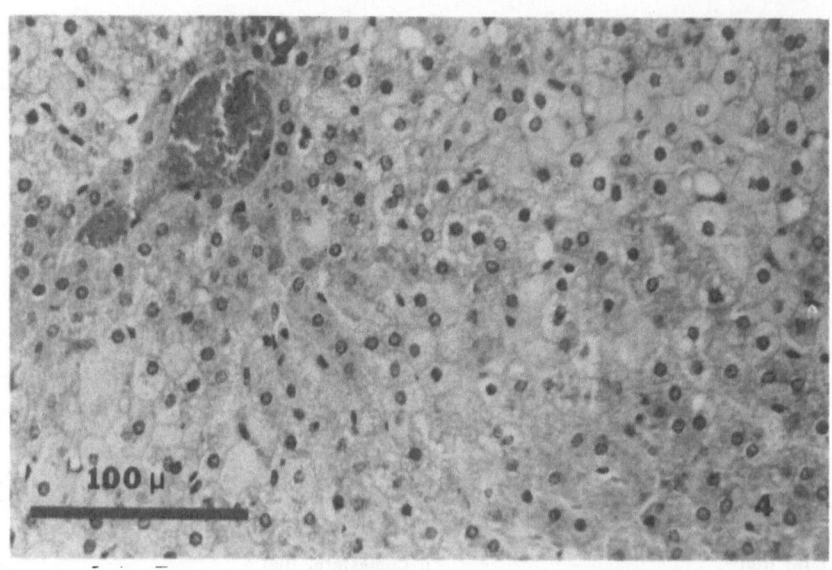

Figure 4.   The liver cells appear spongy and resemble those of the
            adrenal zona fasciculata. This change was found in both
            non-diabetic and diabetic Chinese hamsters fed the cho-
            lesterol diet. (H&E)

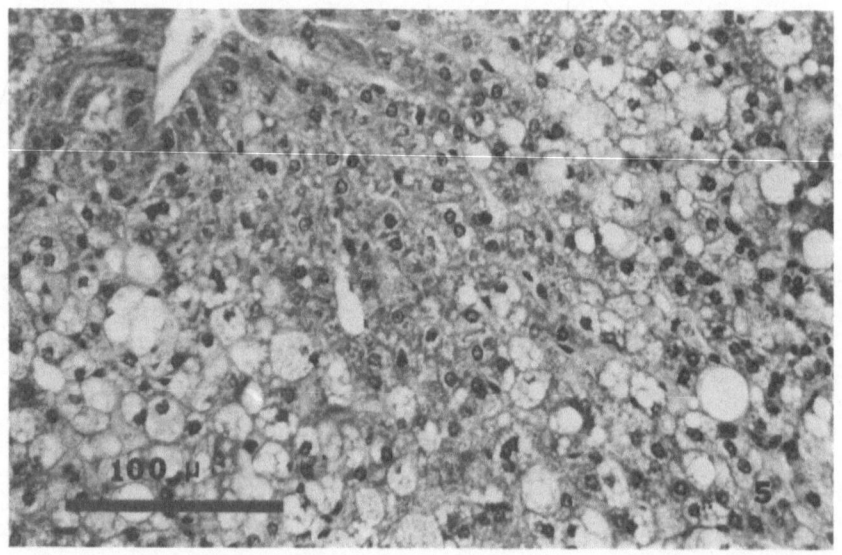

Figure 5.   Some fat infiltration was observed in the hepatocytes of
            non-diabetic and diabetic Chinese hamsters fed the
            cholesterol diet. (H&E)

Early cirrhosis

Polymorphonuclear cell infiltration

Some fat infiltration of hepatocytes (H & E method) (Figure 5)

Abundant intracytoplasmic fats (ORO method)

Kidney: Presence of hyaline casts and obsolete nephrons

Distention of the distal portion of the nephron

Spleen: Ceroid histiocytosis of the red pulp

Heart: Myocardial fat increased (ORO method)

B. Changes usually found in diabetic hamsters and not in non-diabetics, but induced by cholesterol feeding to non-diabetic hamsters:

Liver: Excessive intracytoplasmic deposit of glycogen in hepatocytes

Pancreatic Islets: Some reduction in the number and size of islets

Some degranulation of β cells

C. Changes found in diabetic hamsters induced or exaggerated by cholesterol feedings:

Liver: Passive congestion

Fatty degeneration (H & E method)

Deposit of ceroid along fibrous tracts

Kidney: Accumulation of glycogen in distal convoluted tubules

Some mesangial thickening

Aorta: Accumulation of collagen fibers beneath the endothelial basement lamina (electron microscopy)

D. Changes induced only in non-diabetic hamsters by cholesterol feeding:

Adrenal: Fatty degeneration of the zona fasciculata
           (Figure 6)

Aorta: Endothelial vacuoles containing debris (electron
           microscopy)

           Lipid droplets in endothelium (electron micro-
           scopy)

           Subendothelial macrophages containing osmiophilic
           debris (electron microscopy)

Liver: In formalin-fixed ORO-stained frozen sections:
           Large amounts of birefrigent crystals covering
           the whole section (Figure 7)

           This intracytoplasmic crystallized material,
           having the characteristics of free cholesterol,
           was minimal in sections of livers of cholesterol-
           fed diabetics.

E.   Changes commonly observed in diabetic Chinese hamsters and
     not affected by cholesterol feeding:

   Liver: Intracytoplasmic glycogen accumulation of hepa-
              tocytes

   Pancreatic Islets: Degranulation of β cells

              Reduction in size and number of islets

              β cell vacuolation (hydropic degeneration)

   Aorta: Minor vacuolation of endothelial cells (electron
              microscopy)

DISCUSSION

Because of the well-documented association between diabetes
and the development of vascular disease in humans, it was hypothe-
sized that the genetically diabetic Chinese hamster might be a
suitable model for atherosclerosis research. The diabetic syndrome
that qualifies it for a good model of human diabetes might also include atherosclerotic lesions. Or possibly the diabetic trait
could make the hamster more susceptible to the induction of experimental atherosclerosis. To test these hypotheses both diabetic and
non-diabetic Chinese hamsters were placed on an atherogenic diet
for 8 months. The monthly monitoring of serum cholesterol levels

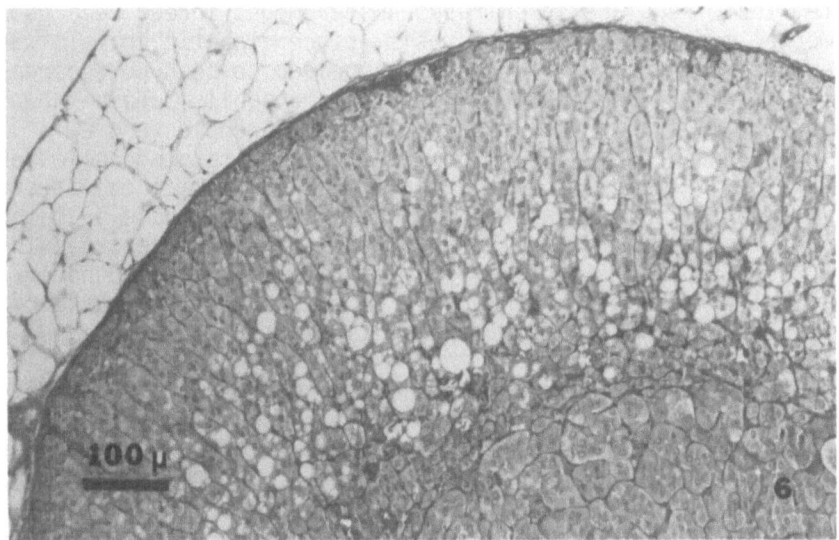

Figure 6. Fatty degeneration of the adrenal zona fasciculata
          occurred only in non-diabetic Chinese hamsters fed the
          cholesterol diet. (PAS Allochrome)

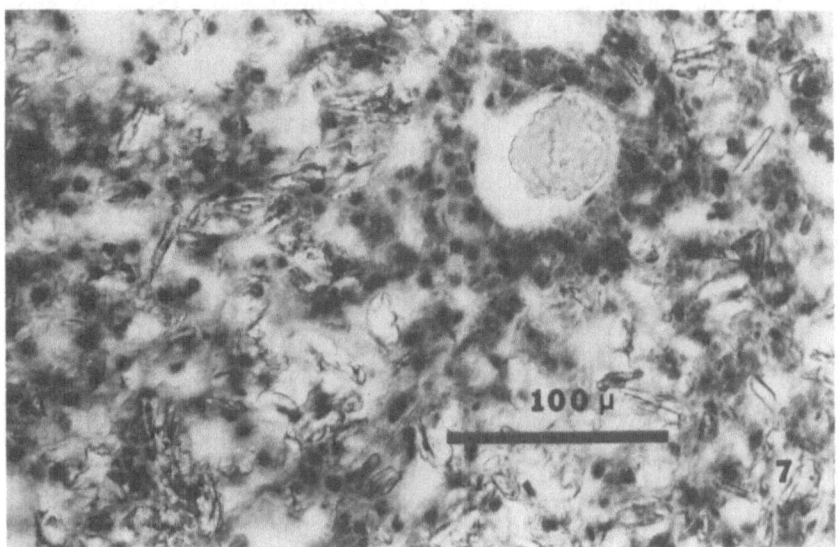

Figure 7. Birefrigent crystals (possibly, cholesterol) were ob-
          served in frozen sections of liver. These crystals
          were predominantly found in the non-diabetic Chinese
          hamster fed the cholesterol diet. (ORO)

suggested that the diabetic Chinese hamster might indeed be a good experimental model for atherosclerosis, since diabetic animals were hyperresponders whereas non-diabetics appeared to be hyporesponders. Reasons for the differences in cholesterol metabolism are unknown. Previously it was shown that spontaneously hypercholesterolemic diabetic Chinese hamsters had a reduced turnover rate of cholesterol (13). However, in the same study, diabetics with normal cholesterol levels had normal turnover rates. Therefore, since these diabetics had initial normal cholesterol levels, the difference reported in cholesterol metabolism is probably not due to decreased turnover. A more likely explanation is probably increased dietary intake of cholesterol due to hyperphagia of the diabetics.

The slight increase in aortic cholesterol was comparable to what we have observed for rats and mice in response to an athero-genic diet. An unusual feature of the hamster aorta was the numer-ous non-saponifiable lipid components (possibly sterols) that were detected on GLC analysis. These materials are not detectable in rat, mouse, quail and man, where cholesterol is virtually the only component seen under similar conditions (14).

It has been reported that cats, for example (15), fed a choles-terol-containing diet for 12 months had a marked rise in mean serum cholesterol after 1 month and declined thereafter until by the 8th month when the level was the same as in control cats. This was not the case with the Chinese hamster. Cholesterol-fed cats also showed vacuolation of the epithelial cytoplasm of proximal convoluted tubules of the kidney as well as diffuse fatty changes of the liver. Cholesterol-fed hamsters, whether diabetic or not, showed mild kidney damage and an atypical liver abnormality. This atypical swollen-spongy appearance of the liver cell was the most significant histologic alteration found in all cholesterol-fed hamsters and resembled that of the cholesterol rich cells of the adrenal zona fasciculata. ORO staining of formalin fixed-frozen sections showed that fat was more abundant in livers of cholesterol-fed hamsters. Although typical fat accumulation, when found in paraffin sections, was preferentially located in periportal areas, ORO staining demon-strated the presence of fat throughout the lobule.

Large amounts of crystallized material (probably cholesterol) were found in frozen-cut, ORO stained liver sections of cholesterol-fed non-diabetics. However, in the cholesterol-fed diabetic Chinese hamster similar liver sections had, for unknown reasons, only slight amounts of these crystals. Glycogen accumulation was found to be preferentially centrolobular. Ceroid was mostly found along fibrotic tracts in the livers of cholesterol-fed animals, though more abundant in diabetics. The hepatocyte alterations described above must have been related to the diet-induced hyper-cholesterolemia.

Neither diabetic nor non-diabetic Chinese hamsters developed gross or microscopic atherosclerotic lesions, either spontaneously or in response to cholesterol feeding. Cats, mentioned above, and rabbits fed cholesterol for 4 months (16) showed typical fatty streaks and smooth cell vacuolation which were not observed in cholesterol fed Chinese hamsters.

The human aortic intima differs from that of rodents. The endothelium of the human aorta rests on a thin basement membrane, below which is the internal elastic membrane. The subendothelium is thin and may contain a few connective tissue elements. In rabbits (17), rats (18,19) and Chinese hamsters there is a subendo- thelial space. In all Chinese hamsters examined, but more so in the cholesterol fed, there was an abundance of a subendothelial frayed or reticular material. Accumulation of collagen fibers was also found in the aortic subendothelium of cholesterol-fed diabetic hamsters. The morphologic findings discussed above indicate that the Chinese hamster, whether diabetic or not, reacts in a peculiar way to dietary-induced hypercholesterolemia.

The resistance of mice and rats to naturally occurring or induced atherosclerosis has been established (20). Such animal models have not been considered useful in the study of atherosclero- sis. This has been attributed in part to the predominance of HDL lipoproteins found in the plasma. Likewise, the resistance to the development of atherosclerosis in the Chinese hamster could possibly be attributed to the predominance of HDL over other plasma lipopro- teins. Therefore, diet induced hypercholesterolemic Chinese ham- sters, both non-diabetic and mild diabetic, do not appear to be suitable models for the study of atherosclerosis.

REFERENCES

1. Ahuja, M.M., V. Gossnian, C.K. Bhan, and V. Kumar. 1972. Vascular disease in north Indian diabetics in relation to diet and blood lipids. In Impact of Insulin on Metabolic Pathways, ed. by P. Shafrier, Academic Press, New York, p. 423.

2. Elkeles, R.J., C. Lowy, A.D.H. Wyllie, J.L. Young, and T.R. Fraser. 1971. Serum insulin, glucose, and lipid levels among mild diabetics in relation to incidence of vascular compli- cations. Lancet 1:880-883.

3. Keen, H. 1970. Minimal diabetes and arterial disease: prevalence and the effect of treatment. In Advances in Metabolic Disorders (Suppl. 1), ed. by Camerini-Davalos, R.A. and H.S. Cole, Academic Press, New York, pp. 437-440.

4. Levitas, I.M., and J.J. Kristal. 1972. Stress exercise
    testing of the young diabetic for the detection of unknown
    coronary artery disease. In Impact of Insulin on Metabolic
    Pathways, ed. by P. Shafrier, Academic Press, New York, pp.
    491-493.

5. Meier, H. and G.A. Yerganian. 1959. Spontaneous hereditary
    diabetes mellitus in Chinese hamster (*Cricetulus griseus*):
    I. Pathologic findings. Proc. Soc. Exp. Biol. 100:810-815.

6. Gerritsen, G.C. and W.E. Dulin. 1967. Characterization of
    diabetes in the Chinese hamster. Diabetologia 3:74-84.

7. Riley, V. 1960. Adaptation of orbital bleeding technique to
    rapid serial bleeding. Proc. Soc. Exp. Biol. Med. 104:754-
    760.

8. Hoffman, W.S. 1937. A rapid photoelectric method for the
    determination of glucose in blood and urine. J. Biol. Chem.
    120:51-55.

9. Block, W.D., K.J. Jarrett, Jr., and J.B. Levine. 1965. Use
    of a single color reagent to improve the automated determina-
    tion of serum total cholesterol. In Automation in Analytical
    Chemistry, ed. by L.T. Skeggs, Jr., Mediad Inc., pp. 345-347.

10. Alexander, C. and C.E. Day. 1973. Distribution of serum
    lipoproteins of selected vertebrates. Comp. Biochem. Physiol.
    46B:295-312.

11. Day, C.E. and W.W. Stafford. 1975. New animal model for
    atherosclerosis research. In Lipids, Lipoproteins, and Drugs,
    ed. by D. Kritchevsky, R. Paoletti, and W. Holmes, Plenum
    Press, New York, pp. 339-347.

12. Day, C.E., P.E. Schurr, W.E. Heyd, and D. Lednicer. 1976.
    Biological activity of a hypobetalipoproteinemic agent. In
    Atherosclerosis Drug Discovery, ed. by C.E. Day, Plenum Press,
    New York, pp. 231-249.

13. Chobanian, A.V., G.C. Gerritsen, P.I. Brecher, and M. Kessler.
    1974. Cholesterol metabolism in the diabetic Chinese hamster.
    Diabetologia 10:595-600.

14. Day, C.E. Unpublished Data.

15. Manning, P.J. and T.B. Clarkson. 1970. Diet-induced athero-
    sclerosis of the cat. Arch. Path. 89:271-278.

16. Wellmann, K.F. and B.W. Volk. 1970. Renal changes in experimental hypercholesterolemia in normal and subdiabetic rabbits. I. Short term studies. Lab. Invest. 22:36-49.

17. Bierring, F. and T. Kobayashi. 1963. Electron microscopy of the normal rabbit aorta. Acta Pathol. Microbiol. Scand. 57: 154-168.

18. Pease, D.C. and W.J. Paule. 1960. Electron microscopy of elastic arteries; the thoracic aorta of the rat. J. Ultra. Res. 3:469-483.

19. Keech, M.K. 1960. Electron microscope study of the normal rat aorta. J. Biophysic. Biochem. Cytol. 7:533-543.

20. Clarkson, T.B. 1963. Atherosclerosis - spontaneous and induced. In Advances in Lipid Research, ed. by R. Paoletti and D. Kritchevsky, Academic Press, New York, pp. 211-252.

SECTION 4

AVIAN MODELS

PRODUCED BY SELECTIVE BREEDING OF JAPANESE QUAIL

ANIMAL MODEL FOR EXPERIMENTAL ATHEROSCLEROSIS

K.P. Chapman, W.W. Stafford and C.E. Day

The Upjohn Company

Kalamazoo, Michigan 49001

ABSTRACT. The Japanese quail (Coturnix coturnix japonica) was bred selectively to produce a strain highly susceptible to experimental atherosclerosis. A population was produced where aortic atherosclerosis is contracted by 99% of the fourth generation males and 83% of the females. Forty-three percent of the males exhibited severe atherosclerosis making this line of Japanese quail a suitable model for discovering and testing anti-atherosclerosis compounds. This feature is augmented by other features such as size, disposition, and abundance which qualify them as suitable experimental subjects. A second line of Japanese quail was bred to be resistant to dietary-induced atherosclerosis. This strain may be a useful research tool for characterizing the etiology of atherosclerosis.

INTRODUCTION

The most popular animal models for screening and preliminary testing of anti-atherosclerotic drugs have been small rodents. The reasons are standard ones: ease of handling, small size, low cost, and availability. Unfortunately rats and mice have a natural resistance to atherosclerosis. A second deterrent to research on the artery itself has been the preoccupation with agents that lower serum cholesterol, the rationale being ease of measurement and the nebulous association of serum cholesterol with atherosclerosis.

A search was begun for an animal with the same attributes as the rat but with the added feature of susceptibility to dietary-induced atherosclerosis. The ideal animal model should allow high volume testing with easily measurable and meaningful parameters at the arterial level. The Japanese quail (<u>Coturnix coturnix japonica</u>) has all these features and was tested by us for their utility as an animal model for anti-atherosclerosis drug research.

When birds from the colony maintained at The Upjohn Company were first studied, the response by individual birds to experimental atherosclerosis was too varied to be useful. Clearly a population with genetic uniformity was needed in order to detect small differences between control animals and animals under treatment. In addition it was desired to develop a strain which was more susceptible to experimental atherosclerosis.

It was with this goal - to produce a strain of Japanese quail which was highly and uniformly susceptible to experimental atherosclerosis - that the following breeding program was initiated in an attempt to obtain a good animal model for detecting anti-atherosclerotic agents.

MATERIALS AND METHODS

The Japanese quail were obtained from a closed stock colony maintained at The Upjohn Company. This colony was derived from stock obtained from four separate university colonies in the U.S.A. The original mated pairs and their offspring were fed a standard chicken mash diet (1). The remaining generations were maintained on Purina Game Bird Startena® and Game Bird Layena®. Stock animals from the colony were randomly paired and placed on 2% crystalline cholesterol mixed with the ground diet. The offspring from each pair were reared concurrently. After 15 weeks, the parents were bled and sacrificed. The aorta, right brachiocephalic artery, and left brachiocephalic artery were removed, visually scored and assayed for cholesterol. These procedures have been described previously (2). Individual serum samples were assayed for cholesterol (3) and also for the following serum parameters measured by a Technicon SMA 12/60 Autoanalyzer®: calcium, inorganic phosphate, glucose, blood urea nitrogen (B.U.N.), uric acid, cholesterol, total protein, albumin, total bilirubin, alkaline phosphatase, lactate dehydrogenase (LDH) and serum glutamic-oxaloacetic transaminase (SGOT). Offspring whose parents had high artery scores and high arterial cholesterol were chosen as parents for a new line designated Susceptible to Experimental Atherosclerosis (SEA). A single pair of parent birds each having artery scores of zero produced offspring which were used exclusively to form a second line of birds named Resistant to Experimental Atherosclerosis (REA). This procedure of choosing breeding pairs for each succeeding generation based on their parents' atherosclerosis has been continued to the present. Brother-sister matings were made with the first generation, but this practice was discontinued in subsequent generations

TABLE I

Breeding Results for Various Atherosclerosis Endpoints for Male SEA Japanese Quail

GENERATION	INCIDENCE OF AORTIC ATHEROSCLEROSIS (%)	INCIDENCE OF SEVERE* AORTIC ATHEROSCLEROSIS (%)	AORTIC ATHERO-SCLEROSIS SCORE	ARTERIAL CHOLESTEROL (mg/g)	SERUM CHOLESTEROL (mg/dl)
0	48 (20/42)	17 (7/42)	29	5.87	1,205
1	68 (21/31)	29 (9/31)	41	7.37	1,195
2	76 (52/68)	10 (7/68)	26	6.19	1,073
3	88 (38/43)	21 (9/43)	37	17.66	1,482
4	99 (75/76)	43 (33/76)	76	31.62	1,894

*Atherosclerosis score ≥90.

TABLE II

Breeding Results for Various Atherosclerosis Endpoints for Female SEA Japanese Quail

GENERATION	INCIDENCE OF AORTIC ATHEROSCLEROSIS (%)	INCIDENCE OF SEVERE* AORTIC ATHEROSCLEROSIS (%)	AORTIC ATHERO-SCLEROSIS SCORE	ARTERIAL CHOLESTEROL (mg/g)	SERUM CHOLESTEROL (mg/dl)
0	40 (14/35)	0 (0/35)	12	4.05	505
1	77 (24/31)	3 (1/31)	29	4.77	375
2	67 (45/67)	4 (3/67)	30	5.65	518
3	76 (28/37)	0 (0/37)	12	8.86	678
4	83 (65/78)	0 (0/78)	14	10.63	507

*Atherosclerosis score $\geq$ 90.

of breeding based on a report of reduced fecundity after intense inbreeding of Japanese quail (4).

RESULTS AND DISCUSSION

We are now raising our fifth generation of SEA quail in our continuing attempt to selectively breed Japanese quail which respond more uniformly to dietary-induced aortic atherosclerosis. The results are summarized in Tables I and II. The SEA birds of the fourth generation are consistently susceptible to experimental atherosclerosis. The percent of male birds with severe arterial involvement (aorta scores of 90 or greater) has also increased to 43% of the population. The females show less severe involvement and are thus less suitable for experimentation. What appears to be negative selection with regard to atherosclerosis in the second generation was probably due to the change in diet at this point. The improved diet most likely ameliorated the initial apparent susceptibility of this line. However, the remainder of the effect was due to their selected genotype which was bred and improved with succeeding generations to produce a non-artifactual 99% response to an atherogenic diet in the fourth generation.

The two brachiocephalic arteries were removed from each bird along with the aorta in order to obtain sufficient tissue for cholesterol analysis and to obtain additional measurements of grossly visible atherosclerosis. Table III shows the slightly higher incidence of atherosclerosis in the right brachiocephalic artery than in the aorta; for this reason, scores for each arterial branch have been tabulated separately. It can be seen, though, that the three arteries respond similarly to cholesterol feeding.

Table III

Atherosclerotic Incidence in Three Arteries in SEA Male Quail

GENERATION	AORTA (%)	RIGHT BRACHIO-CEPHALIC (%)	LEFT BRACHIO-CEPHALIC (%)
0	48	--	--
1	68	55	58
2	77	82	82
3	88	95	91
4	99	100	99

Because development of the REA line was given secondary priority, only a few birds were mated and produced each generation. Consequently, the variation between individuals becomes more noticeable and the data less clearcut (Tables IV and V). However, there are some characteristics emerging in this line which depart from those of the original stock. One such characteristic is serum cholesterol level after cholesterol feeding which is significantly lower in the REA birds than in the original parent birds.

This result has been confirmed in a separate experiment with second generation, SEA and REA males fed chicken mash supplemented with 2% cholic acid and 3% cholesterol. After 34 days, the birds were switched to unsupplemented chicken mash. Non-fasting serum cholesterols were measured throughout the testing time, and endpoint serum chemistries were also run. Figure 1 shows the serum cholesterol levels of SEA birds reaching twice that of REA birds (1253 mg% vs 602 mg%) while on the cholesterol diet. Both lines showed a rapid drop in serum cholesterol after return to the control diet. An attempt to show a direct correlation between serum cholesterol and artery cholesterol (using data from fourth generation SEA males) was unsuccessful, but it is felt that serum cholesterol level might still serve as a partial indicator of susceptibility.

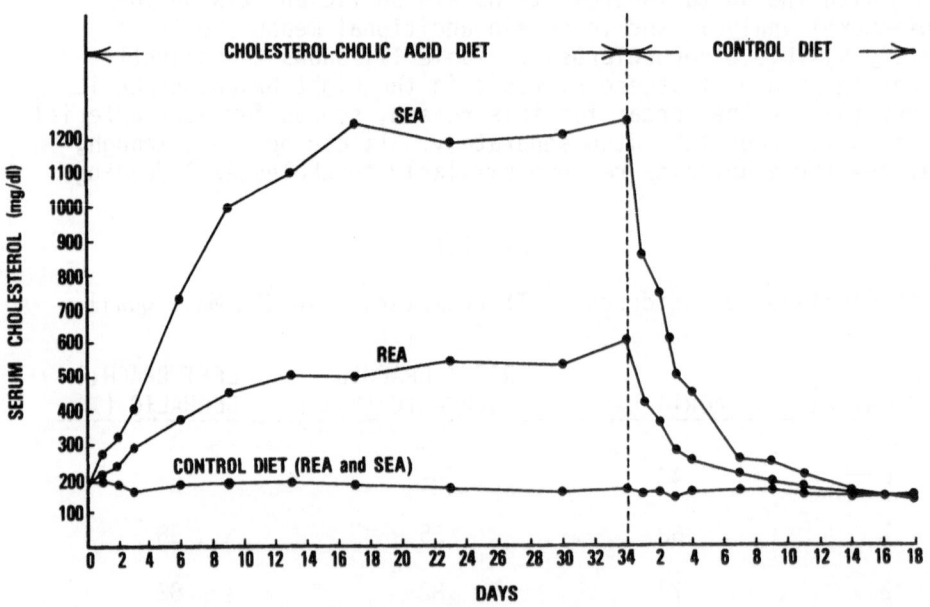

Figure 1. Serum cholesterol levels in second generation SEA and REA male Japanese quail (10 birds/group) in response to a 3% cholesterol-2% cholic acid diet followed by normal control diet.

TABLE IV

Breeding Results for Various Atherosclerosis Endpoints for Male REA Japanese Quail

GENERATION	INCIDENCE OF AORTIC ATHEROSCLEROSIS (%)	INCIDENCE OF SEVERE* AORTIC ATHEROSCLEROSIS (%)	AORTIC ATHERO-SCLEROSIS SCORE	ARTERIAL CHOLESTEROL (mg/g)	SERUM CHOLESTEROL (mg/dl)
0	48 (20/42)	17 (7/42)	29	5.87	1205
1	17 (2/12)	0 (0/12)	4	1.63	488
2	0 (0/8)	0 (0/8)	0.2	1.04	256
3	18 (2/11)	0 (0/11)	0.4	3.41	307
4	40 (4/10)	0 (0/10)	7	3.80	798

*Atherosclerosis score ≥90.

TABLE V

Breeding Results for Various Atherosclerosis Endpoints for Female REA Japanese Quail

GENERATION	INCIDENCE OF AORTIC ATHEROSCLEROSIS (%)	INCIDENCE OF SEVERE* AORTIC ATHEROSCLEROSIS (%)	AORTIC ATHERO-SCLEROSIS SCORE	ARTERIAL CHOLESTEROL (mg/g)	SERUM CHOLESTEROL (mg/dl)
0	40 (14/35)	0 (0/35)	12	4.05	505
1	8 (1/13)	0 (0/13)	1	2.19	235
2	67 (8/12)	0 (0/12)	6	1.99	228
3	60 (9/15)	0 (0/15)	2	3.44	259
4	13 (2/15)	0 (0/15)	0.3	4.20	374

*Atherosclerosis score ≥90.

TABLE VI

Serum Alkaline Phosphatase Levels in Male SEA and REA Quail

STRAIN/ GENERATION	TREATMENT	NO. OF BIRDS	ALKALINE PHOSPHATASE (IU/L)
SEA/2	Cholesterol-cholic acid diet for 34 days followed by control diet for 18 days	10	617
REA/2		9	835*
SEA/3	Normal diet	10	282
REA/3		10	417**

* Significance P<.05
** Significance P<.01

A second difference in this second generation of SEA and REA males was the serum alkaline phosphatase level. Results from the experiment just described are included in Table VI showing the serum alkaline phosphatase levels in SEA quail to be significantly lower than in REA quail. This dichotomy is evident even in third generation SEA and REA males which had never been fed cholesterol. While this particular factor may not be of any physiological importance, the finding points out the advantages of having distinct lines of REA and SEA quail. Two such lines afford the opportunity to compare various factors and thus determine possible underlying causes of atherosclerosis.

Some preliminary experiments are now being conducted to characterize more fully the rate, and nature, of experimental atherosclerosis in SEA quail as it progresses and then regresses. Our findings thus far have shown the SEA Japanese quail to be a satisfactory model for both prevention and regression studies in atherosclerosis.

REFERENCES

1. Tennent, D.M., H. Siegel, G.W. Kuron, W.H. Ott, and C.W.
    Mushett. 1957. Lipid patterns and atherogenesis in cholesterol
    fed chickens. Proc. Soc. Exptl. Biol. Med. 96:679-683.

2. Day, C.E., and W.W. Stafford. 1975. New animal model for
    atherosclerosis research. In Lipids, Lipoproteins and Drugs,
    ed. by D. Kritchevsky, R. Paoletti, and W. Holmes, Plenum
    Press, New York, pp. 339-347.

3. Block, W.D., K.J. Jarrett, and J.B. Levine. 1966. Use of a
    single color reagent to improve the automated determination of
    serum total cholesterol. In Automation in Analytical Chemistry,
    ed. by L.T. Skeggs, Mediad Inc., New York, pp. 345-347.

4. Wakasugi, N., and K. Kondo. 1973. Breeding methods for main-
    tenance of mutant genes and establishment of strains in the
    Japanese quail. Proc. ICLA Asian Pacific Meeting on Laboratory
    Animals, ed. by K. Fujiwara, ICLA Asian Pacific, Tokyo, pp. 151-
    159.

MORPHOLOGIC OBSERVATIONS ON EXPERIMENTAL

ATHEROSCLEROSIS IN SEA JAPANESE QUAIL

M.G. Soret, T. Peterson, K.P. Chapman, W.W. Stafford,
C.E. Day, and E.M. Block

The Upjohn Company, Kalamazoo, Michigan 49001

INTRODUCTION

The Japanese quail has been considered useful for the study of experimental atherosclerosis since the original reports of Ojerio et al. (1) and of Smith and Hilker (2). However, in the use of these not selectively bred animals the appearance of gross lesions was not uniform or took up to 28 months for their production. Furthermore, microscopic examination of the lesions was totally or practically neglected.

Chapman et al. (3) reported the development and evaluation of a selectively bred line of Japanese quail for the study of experimental atherosclerosis. Males in this line of quail, described as Susceptible to Experimental Atherosclerosis (SEA), had close to a 100% incidence rate of fatty streak lesions in the brachiocephalic arteries and aorta within 3 months while on a defined cholesterol supplemented diet. Cholesterol induced lesions in the SEA quail were more prominent and appeared earlier in the brachiocephalic arteries than in the aorta (3). Therefore, the structure and the development of lesions in the brachiocephalic arteries were preferentially studied by light and electron microscopy.

MATERIALS AND METHODS

Fourteen, SEA, male, Japanese quails were placed on a defined cholesterol-rich diet (3) and six on a control diet for a period of up to three months. At weekly intervals, during the first six weeks of the cholesterol feeding, two quails were sacrificed, and the last

two were sacrificed at the end of three months. The control
animals, fed Purina Wild Game Bird Layena Chow, were sacrificed
on the first and sixth week of the experiment as well as at the end
of the three months duration of the experiment. Immediately after
sacrifice gross examination was used to evaluate the progression of
the lesions (3). The thoracic and abdominal areas of the quails
were opened and the arteries were perfused with 2% glutaraldehyde
fixative. The left and right brachiocephalic arteries were removed
and placed in 2% glutaraldehyde. In addition, a segment of the
thoracic aorta ($\sim$4 mm long) and a segment of the aorta just above
and below the coeliac artery ($\sim$4mm long) were also placed in glutaraldehyde. Small cross sections of each of the 4 areas were postfixed in 1% osmium tetroxide and embedded in Epon 812. Blocks were
sectioned with a diamond knife using the LKB-2 ultramicrotome.
Thick sections, about 1 μ, were stained with toluidine blue 0 for
light microscopy. Ultrathin sections, about 80 mμ, were stained
with uranyl acetate and lead citrate and examined with the Philips
301 electron microscope.

RESULTS

Brachiocephalic Arteries of Control-fed SEA Japanese Quail

The brachiocephalic arteries of the 16 week old Japanese quail
measured about 6 mm in length and had an average diameter of $\sim$1.3 mm
(Figure 1). The intima of these arteries was quite irregular in
thickness and structure. There was no clearly outlined membrana
elastica interna, and there were multiple small masses of smooth
muscle cells within what appeared to be the subendothelium.

The continuous endothelium, made of roughly cuboidal cells,
rested on a subendothelium of variable thickness (Figure 2). The
ground substance of the subendothelium contained undifferentiated
cells and others which resembled smooth muscle cells and fibrocytes.
All of these cells were generally arranged perpendicularly to the
lumen of the artery. In some areas the endothelium was found to
rest on heavily fenestrated, thin, elastic laminae (Figure 3).
Cross sectioned, longitudinally arranged, elastic fibers were
numerous in the subendothelium.

The endothelial and subendothelial cells of the brachiocephalic arteries of the SEA Japanese quail fed a regular diet often
contained multiple vacuoles (Figure 2) which may have represented
lipid material extracted during tissue processing.

The media of the brachiocephalic arteries was composed of
12 or 13 discontinuous circular units which were better shown in
cross sections (Figure 1). Each media unit had two distinct layers.

One layer was made of closely and spirally arranged smooth muscle cells which stain deeply with toluidine blue O. These muscle layers were bordered by frequently interrupted elastic laminae. The other layer of the medial unit was slightly wider, stained poorly with toluidine blue O and was made of connective tissue. This connective tissue or interlaminar layer contained fibroblasts and undifferentiated cells, either mesenchymal or primitive smooth muscle cells. Variable amounts of collagen fibers in bundles and fine elastic fibers were also present in the interlaminar layer. Fibrocytes and smooth muscle cells of the media have also been found to contain, though infrequently, lipid inclusions in the cytoplasm (Figure 4).

Brachiocephalic Arteries of Cholesterol-fed SEA Japanese Quail

Some animals displayed cholesterol induced lesions as early as 1-2 weeks. From 2-6 weeks on the cholesterol-rich diet the number of intimal cells with fatty inclusions and the amount of fat per cell increased noticeably. After 5-6 weeks, fat was frequently found in luminal, surface, hemispheric elevations, almost 0.15 mm in diameter, containing tightly packed round foam cells in which the nuclei were still centrally located (Figure 5). Some swelling of the subendothelium, also found at this stage, caused the endothelium to protrude into the lumen of the artery (Figure 6). Other lipid laden cells of the intima and of the interlaminar layers of the media were always arranged in palisades, as if they were migrating toward the lumen.

After three months of the cholesterol diet, the lesions had further developed causing partial obliteration of the lumen (Figure 7). As it is shown in Figure 8, these lesions consisted of an expanded subendothelium and the inner layers of the media. There were three distinct areas in the lesions, two of which were in the subendothelium and the third in the media (Figure 8 a, b, c, respectively). The first area (Figure 9) was composed of a mass of tightly packed foam cells located beneath an extremely thin endothelium. The second area of the lesion was composed of undifferentiated cells (Figure 10) arranged in palisades perpendicular to the lumen. Two cell types could be found in this area, one which resembled a foam cell and another which contained multiple osmiophilic inclusions. Cells in this area were separated from each other by some ground substance and appeared to be migrating toward the lumen.

The third area of the lesion (Figure 11) comprised the outer intima and the inner layers of the media. No foam cells were found in the media. All cells of the media, whether fibrocytes, smooth muscle cells, or undifferentiated cells, contained only dense, osmiophilic inclusions.

KEY TO ABBREVIATIONS IN FIGURES

bm: basement membrane

ed: edema

el: elastic lamina

en: endothelium

foc: foam cell

gs: ground substance

in: intima

li: lipid

lu: lumen

m: media

msc: mesenchymal cell

pv: pinocytotic vesicle

rbc: red blood cell

TB: toluidine blue 0

UL: uranyl acetate-lead citrate

Figure 1.   Cross section of a brachiocephalic artery from a
            control diet fed SEA male quail. Arrow points to area
            enlarged in Figure 2. TB, Marker=0.1 mm.

Figure 2.   The intima and innermost smooth muscle cell layer of
            the media. Smooth muscle cells appear free of lipid
            inclusions. Undifferentiated subendothelial cells and
            endothelial cells may have noticeable lipid vacuoles.
            Subendothelial cells appear in palisades perpendicular
            to the endothelium. TB, Marker=10 u.

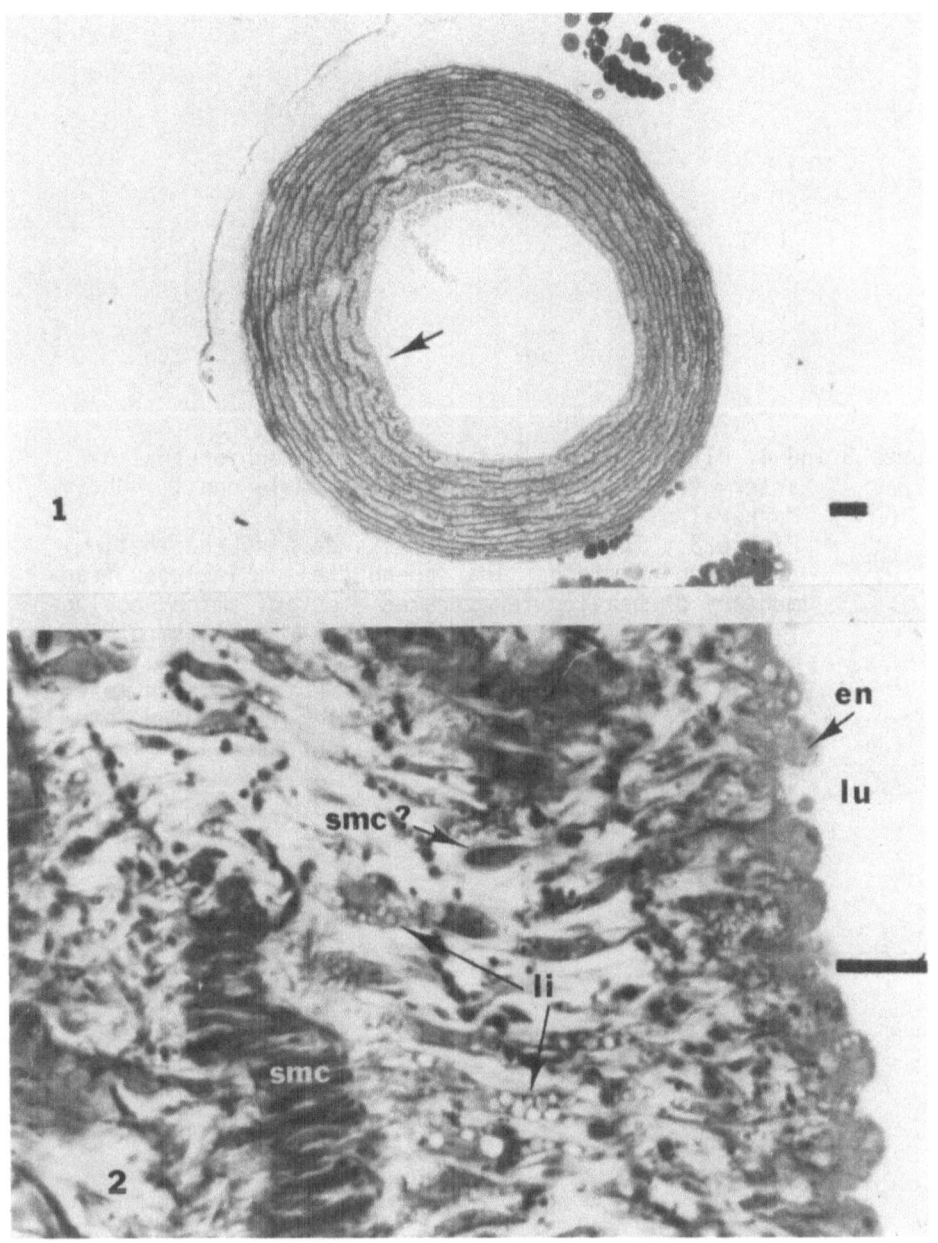

Figures 3 and 4. Ultrastructural features of a brachiocephalic
            artery from a regular diet fed SEA male quail. UL,
            Marker=1 u.
            Figure 3. The endothelium rests on a subendothelium
            of irregular width. The subendothelium includes frag-
            mentary or heavily fenestrated elastic lamina, collagen
            fibers, fibrocytes, and cells that resemble smooth
            muscle cells.
            Figure 4. Innermost area of the media. Smooth muscle
            cells usually border the elastic lamellae. The inter-
            laminar space contains a ground substance and fibro-
            cytes. Fibrocytes and undifferentiated smooth muscle
            cells contain lipid inclusions. Large arrow points
            toward the lumen.

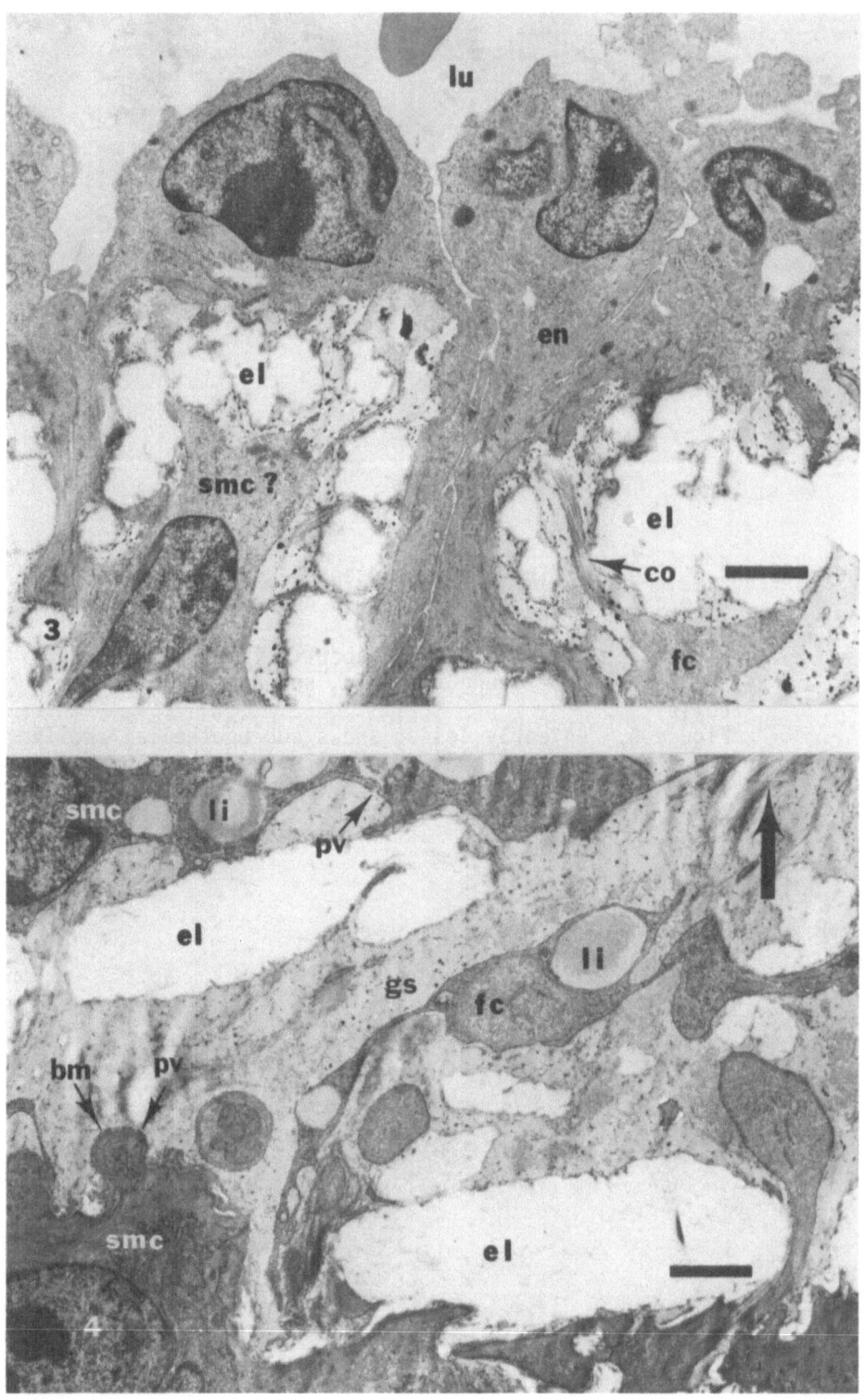

Figures 5 and 6. Lesions in the brachiocephalic arteries of a SEA
            male quail after 5-6 weeks on a cholesterol supplemented
            diet. TB, Marker=10 u.
            Figure 5. Elevated lesions about 0.15 mm in diameter
            are composed of young, spheric, subendothelial, foam
            cells.
            Figure 6. An early lesion shows subendothelial swelling
            and migration of lipid laden cells into the subendothe-
            lium.

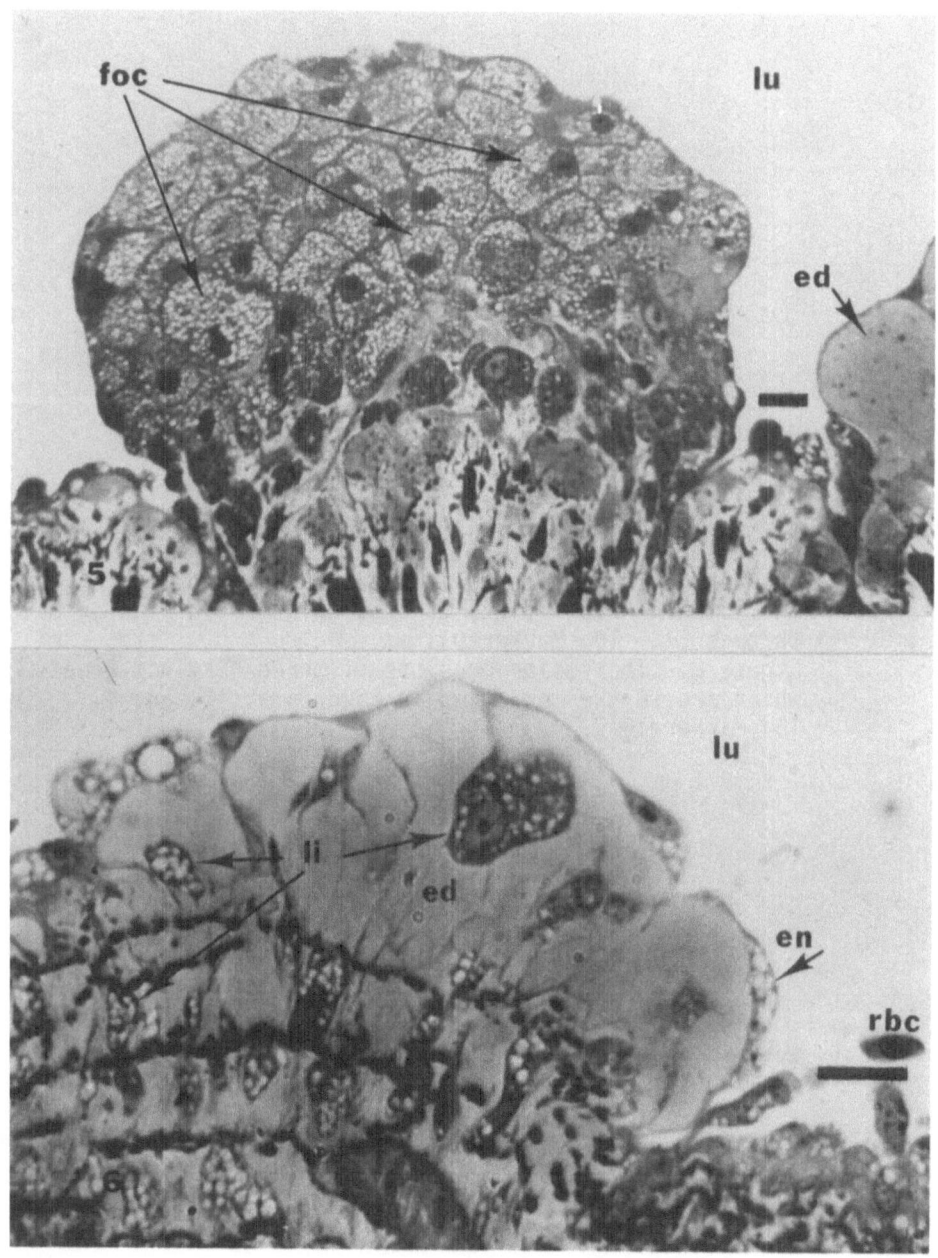

Figures 7 and 8. Cross section of a brachiocephalic artery from a
          cholesterol diet fed SEA male quail.
          Figure 7. The lesion obliterates a great portion of
          the lumen. Arrow points to area enlarged in Figures 8
          through 11. TB, Marker=0.1 mm.
          Figure 8. The lesion consists of three distinct areas
          which are further enlarged in Figures 9, 10, and 11.
          TB, Marker=10 u.

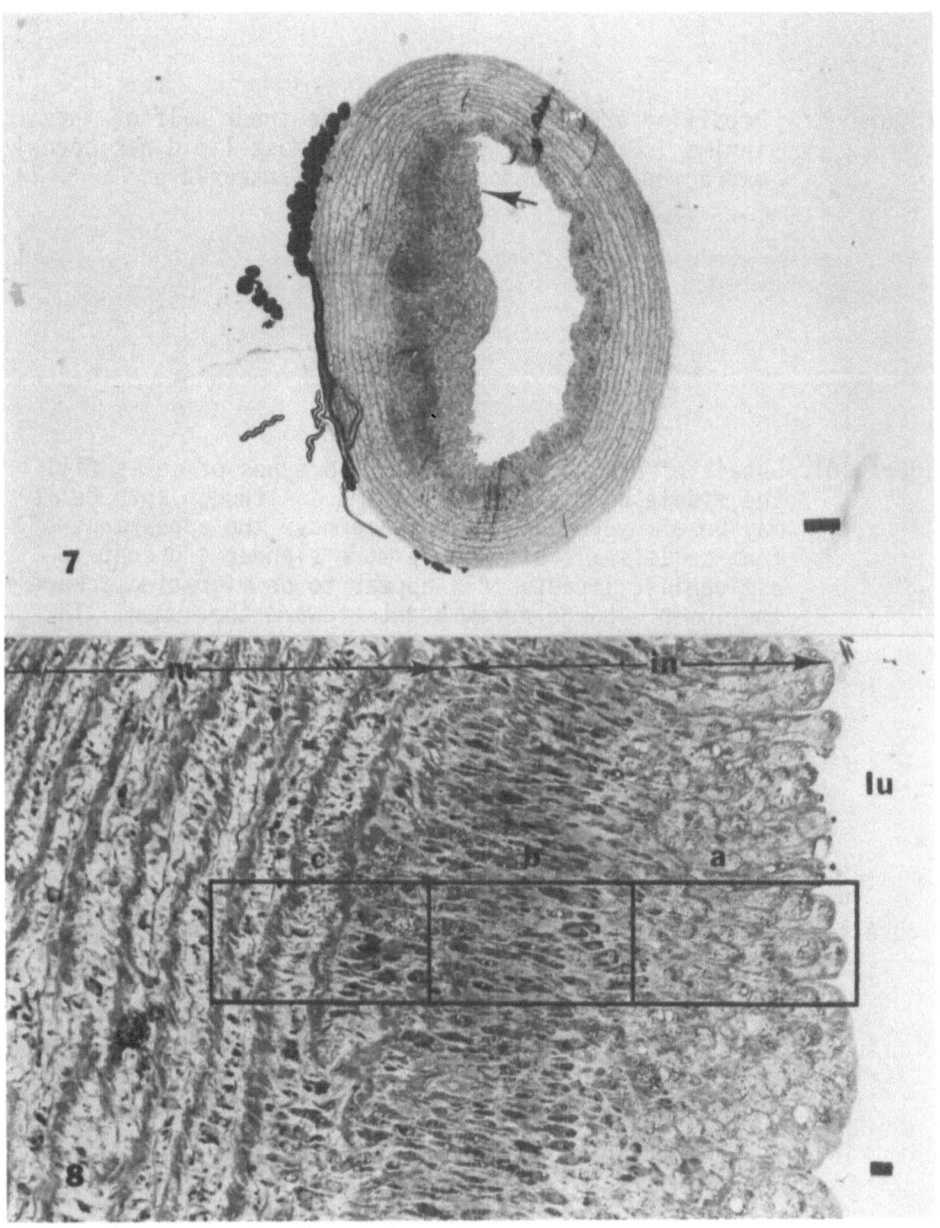

Figure 9.   Detail of area in Figure 8a. The inner half of the
             intima is a mass of foam cells. Most lipid has been
             extracted from these cells. TB, Marker=10 u.

Figure 10.   Detail of area in Figure 8b. Two types of cells fill
             the middle portion of the intima. Although both cells
             may be of myogenic origin, some have the appearance of
             foam cells while others are more slender and contain
             osmiophilic lipids. All appear to be migrating toward
             the lumen. Large arrow points toward the lumen. TB,
             Marker=10 u.

Figure 11.   Detail of area in Figure 8c. Foam cells were found
             very deep in the intima and did not appear to trans-
             cend the first muscle cell layer of the media. Cells
             of the media, whether interlaminar fibrocytes, primitive
             mesenchymal cells, or smooth muscle cells, contained
             only dense osmiophilic lipid inclusions. Large arrow
             points in direction of the lumen. TB, Marker=10 u.

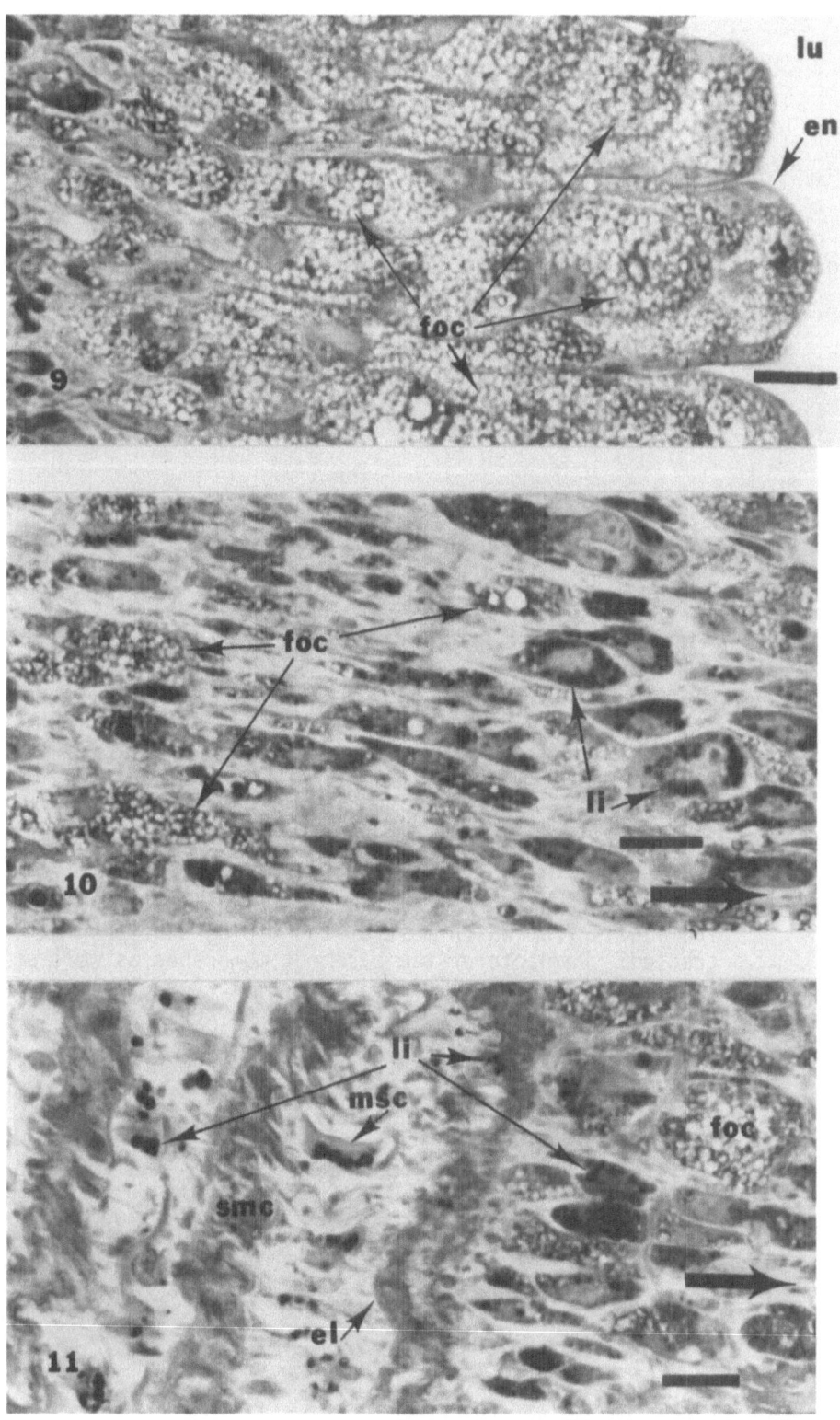

Figure 12. Ultrastructural details of the inner intima. The
            vacuoles of the endothelium and foam cells show a rim
            of osmiophilic material. This suggests the lipid
            nature of the material extracted from these vacuoles.
            UL, Marker=1 u.

Figure 13. Ultrastructural detail of the middle intima. Myogenic
            foam cells from which most of the lipids have been ex-
            tracted. Remnants of the basement membranes as well as
            junctions between cells and pinocytotic vesicles suggest
            the muscular character of the cells at center and left.
            The cell right of center is probably a fibrocyte.
            Large arrow points in direction of the lumen. UL,
            Marker=1 u.

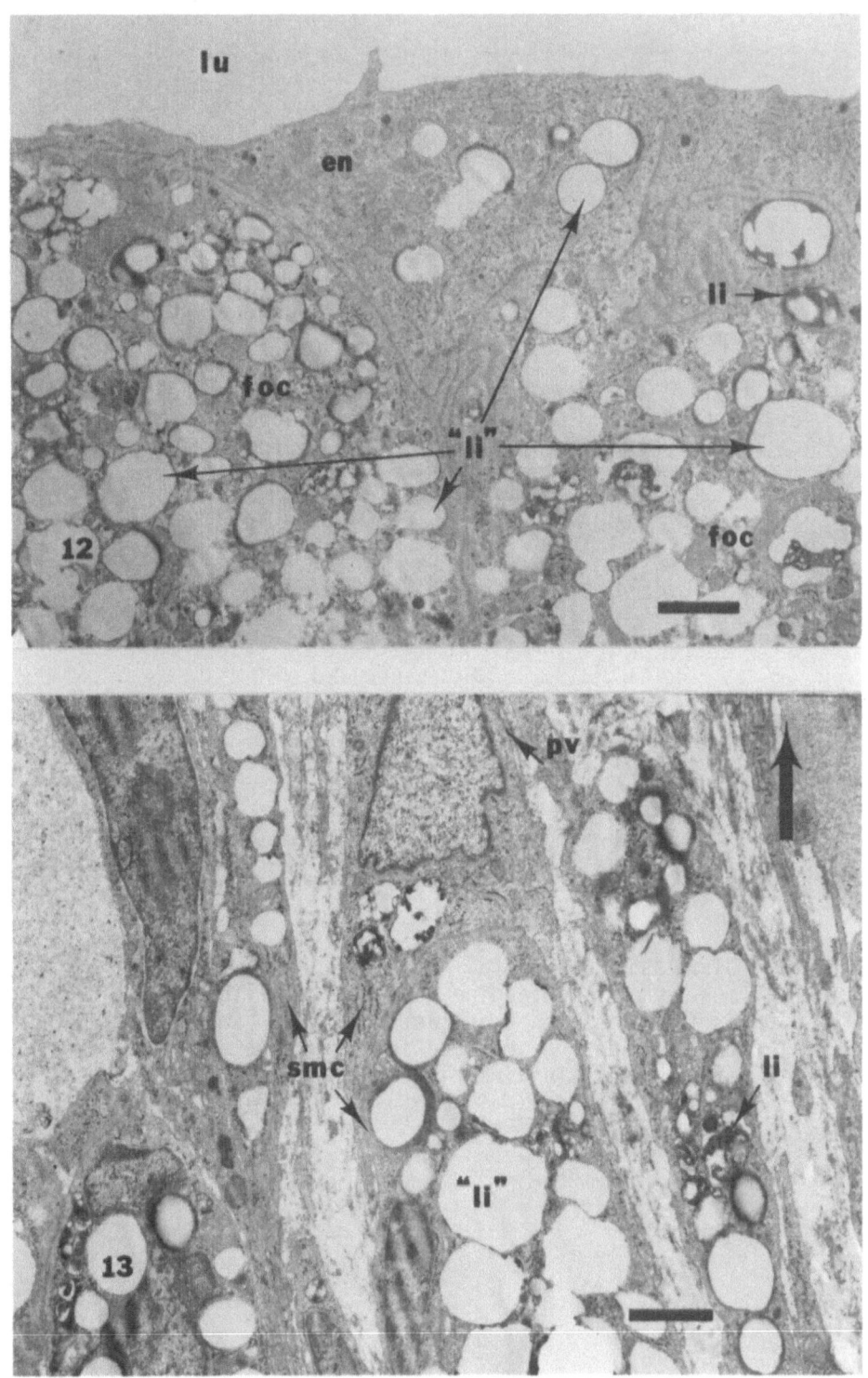

Figure 14. Ultrastructural detail of the outer intima. A smooth
            muscle cell (left), a mesenchymal cell of primitive
            smooth muscle cell (center), and a fibrocyte (right of
            center) all contain osmiophilic lipid inclusions.
            Notice the absence of collagen fibers in the ground
            substance. Fragments of elastica appear on the right.
            Large arrow points in direction of the lumen. UL,
            Marker=1 u.

Figure 15. Ultrastructural detail of inner media. A smooth
            muscle cell containing dense osmiophilic lipid inclusions
            is found between two elastic laminae. Moderate amounts
            of collagen are observed in the ground substance. Large
            arrow points in direction of the lumen. UL, Marker=1 u.

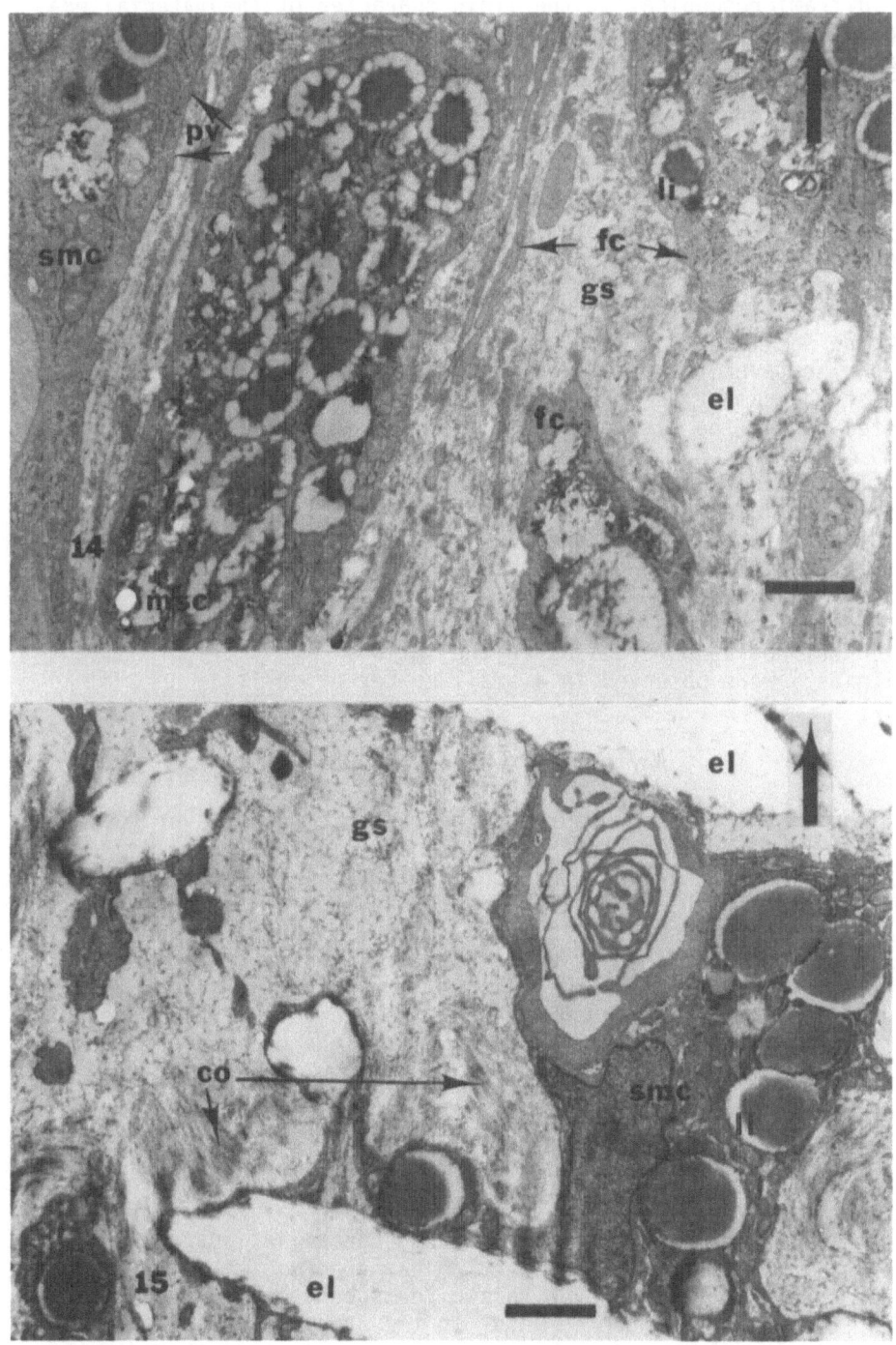

Ultramicroscopically, the lipid character of the material extracted from the vacuoles of the endothelial and foam cells was suggested by the osmiophilic rims observed in most vacuoles (Figure 12). The foam cells, although greatly enlarged by their content, appeared intact and viable.

Unlike cells of the inner intima, cells of the middle and outer intima were separated from each other by an intercellular space. Many of the cells in the middle intima (Figure 13) were probably myogenic, since they had basement membrane and pinocytotic vesicles and formed junctions with neighboring cells. However, myofilaments were difficult to find. Other slender cells, devoid of basement membrane and junctions with other cells, were identified as fibrocytes. Whatever the origin of these cells, the lipid inclusions were of the same type as those of the foam cells and also were extracted during the tissue processing.

The cells found in the outer intima (Figure 14) either resembled smooth muscle cells, fibrocytes, or undifferentiated cells. All cells in the lesions appeared intact. The absence of collagen in the intracellular ground substance was noteworthy.

Lipid inclusions of the medial cells (Figure 15) were osmiophilic but not as numerous as in the intima. Myelin figures (phospholipids?) were observed in a small number of cells.

Aorta of SEA Japanese Quail

The microscopic structure of the thoracic segments of the SEA quail aorta was similar to that of the brachiocephalic artery described above. However, at the coeliac level, there was no interlaminar layer in the media. The media was made of alternating layers of smooth muscle cells and elastic laminae. The endothelium rested on a well defined membrana elastica interna.

Lesions of the aorta, whether at the thoracic level or near the coeliac arteries, were well defined only at the end of three months on the cholesterol diet.

The membrana elastica interna of avian aortas is more noticeable and continuous the farther from the heart. After three months on the cholesterol diet, the SEA quail developed moderate fatty streaks in the aorta. Fatty streaks of the thoracic aorta were made of a few foam cells filling the subendothelial space and lipid laden cells scattered in the interlaminar spaces of the inner media. At the coeliac level, however, a swollen subendothelium containing a few foam cells was more common. In the avian lower aorta, there is no interlamellar space. Muscle cells in this area showed negligible involvement in the formation of the fatty streaks.

DISCUSSION

The predisposition of the SEA Japanese quail to the development of atheromatous lesions was clearly indicated by the presence of numerous lipid laden cells in the intima of the aorta and brachiocephalic arteries of animals fed the control diet. The response of this line of quails to an atherogenic diet was fast and reproducible (3).

The macroscopic characteristic of the lesions have features which resemble those found in early fatty streaks of humans (4), monkeys (5), rabbits (6), and White Carneau pigeons (7).

However, there are a few features peculiar to the SEA quail. The arterial lesions in pigeons are preferentially located in the lower aorta. In SEA quail and in quail studied by Smith and Hilker (2), the preferential location was found to be in the brachiocephalic arteries, although some involvement of the thoracic and abdominal aorta was observed. Aortic fatty streaks in SEA quail showed minimal involvement of the media. The relatively minor but definite involvement of the SEA quail aorta in the development of fatty streaks suggests that this artery may also become atherosclerotic but at a much slower rate than in the brachiocephalic arteries.

The initial lesion was apparently massive lipid uptake by the endothelium which was followed by a marked and widely spread swelling of the superficial subendothelium. The material causing the subendothelial swelling, which failed to stain with PAS using epon sectioned material, apparently exerted a positive attraction for subendothelial and medial cells. The resulting fatty streak of the SEA quail, within three months of cholesterol feeding, was made up of only intact lipid laden cells. Some of the lipid inclusions of cells in the outer intima vaguely resembled the filamentous type described by McGill and Geer (4).

Neither extracellular lipids nor macrophages were found even in raised lesions. In the absence of extracellular lipids and the resulting fat necrosis, no inflammatory reaction nor collagen deposition was observed. Whether the cells found in the SEA quail fatty streak were derived from smooth muscle cells (8) or from interlaminar cells (9) or from multifunctional mesenchymal cells (10) still is a matter of speculation.

REFERENCES

1. Ojerio, A.D., G.J. Pucak, T.B. Clarkson and B.C. Bullock. 1972. Diet-induced atherosclerosis and myocardial infarction in Japanese quail. Lab. Animal Sci. 22:33-39.

2. Smith, R.L. and D.M. Hilker. 1973. Experimental dietary production of aortic atherosclerosis in Japanese quail. Atherosclerosis 17:63-70.

3. Chapman, K.P., W.W. Stafford and C.E. Day. 1976. Animal model for experimental atherosclerosis produced by selective breeding of Japanese quail. In: Atherosclerosis Drug Discovery, ed. by C.E. Day, Plenum Press, New York. pp. 347-356.

4. McGill, H.C., Jr. and J.C. Geer. 1963. The human lesion, fine structure. In: Evolution of the Atherosclerotic Plaque, ed. by R.J. Jones, University of Chicago Press, Chicago, pp. 65-76.

5. Stary, H.C. 1974. Proliferation of arterial cells in atherosclerosis. Adv. Exp. Med. Biol. 43:59-81.

6. Still, W.J.S. 1963. An electron microscope study of cholesterol atherosclerosis in the rabbit. Exp. Molec. Path. 2:491-502.

7. Cooke, P.H. and S.C. Smith. 1968. Smooth muscle cells: The source of foam cells in atherosclerotic White Carneau pigeons Exp. Molec. Path. 8:171-189.

8. Geer, J.C. and M.D. Haust. 1972. Smooth Muscle Cells in Atherosclerosis. S. Karger, Basel.

9. Moss, N.S. and E.P. Benditt. 1970. The ultrastructure of spontaneous and experimentally-induced arterial lesions II. The spontaneous plaque in the chicken. Lab. Invest. 23:231-245.

10. Wissler, R.W. 1967. The arterial muscle cell, smooth muscle or multifunctional mesenchyme? Circulation 36:1-4.

A MECHANISM FOR LIPID ACCUMULATION AND CENTRAL NECROSIS

IN FIBROUS PLAQUES

L. Clarke Stout, M.D.

Dept. of Pathology

University of Texas Medical Branch
Galveston, Texas 77550

ABSTRACT   This is a step section study of 3 fibrous plaques from
the abdominal aorta of an ostrich. The distribution of gelatinous
like lesions in these plaques suggested that the gelatinous lesions
were formed by the influx of plasma at the plaque shoulders. Two
gelatinous lesions extended like tunnels into the center of one of
the plaques. The presence of focal necrosis and large cholesterol
crystals in one of these gelatinous tunnels deep within the plaque
suggested that gelatinous lesions might represent one mechanism by
which fibrous plaques are converted to atheromatous plaques.

INTRODUCTION

We do not really know why some fibrous plaques develop necrotic
lipid rich centers. It is thought that excessive lipid accumulates
in smooth muscle cells leading to cell death with release of the
lipid into the extracellular space. This extracellular lipid then
stimulates the proliferation of additional smooth muscle cells which
eventually form a "fibrous cap" over the pool of extracellular lipid.
Although this theory may be correct, it will not be totally accept-
able to those who feel that fatty streaks are not the precursors of
fibrous plaques. In this paper, I will present morphologic observations which suggest a different mechanism for lipid accumulation
and central necrosis in fibrous plaques.

MATERIALS AND METHODS

This study is part of an autopsy survey of vascular disease in

405 mammals and birds dying in The Oklahoma City Zoo between 1964
and 1969. Details of the methodology and results have been previously
published (1). The present report is based on the study of 3 fibrous
plaques from the abdominal aorta of a young male ostrich (Struthio
camelus). This bird died with sepsis following surgical correction
of a prolapsed rectum. Each plaque was step-sectioned completely on
a cyrostat at approximately 200 micron intervals. The sections were
stained with Oil Red O and hematoxylin. Other stains were employed
as needed including H and E, Weigert's elastic stain, and the Schultz
modification of the Liebermann-Burchardt reaction for cholesterol.

RESULTS

     The 3 plaques in question were composed primarily of orderly rows
of smooth muscle cells and elastic fibers. The largest plaque was
up to 4 times as thick as the underlying media. The media and adventitia adjacent to all of the plaques were unremarkable. The remarkable feature about these plaques was the distribution of the multiple
gelatinous like lesions which were present, particularly in the largest plaque. This plaque had a very complex surface contour, apparently because it had arisen around two branch orifices (Figure 1). The
gelatinous like lesions were located at the shoulders of the plaque,
particularly those shoulders created by the exit of branch arteries.
Two of the gelatinous like lesions extended into the plaque like tunnels, each staying within the same tissue plane regardless of the
depth of penetration (Figure 1, sections 5,6 and sections 8,9). Areas of focal necrosis and accumulations of large cholesterol crystals
(Figure 2) were found in one of these gelatinous like lesions, being
located at a depth of 1 to 3 millimeters from the apparent point of
entry at the plaque surface (Figure 1, sections 8,9). Because the
tissue planes in fibrous plaques tend to lie parallel to the internal
elastic membrane, a gelatinous like lesion may start at the intimal
surface at the plaque shoulder and end in the outermost layer of the
intima (the layer adjacent to the media) deep within the center of
the plaque.

     The 2 remaining plaques contained gelatinous like lesions which
were smaller than those in the largest plaque, and which were confined
to the subendothelial portions of the plaque shoulders. This finding,
plus the fact that all deep gelatinous like lesions in the largest
plaque could be traced to the surface, suggested that the gelatinous
like lesions developed at the plaque surfaces and extended from there
toward the plaque centers.

     Morphologically, the gelatinous like lesions appeared to be focal
collections of edema with disruption of elastic lamellae within the
lesions and compression of adjacent elastic lamellae. The smooth
muscle cells within the gelatinous like lesions were randomly oriented

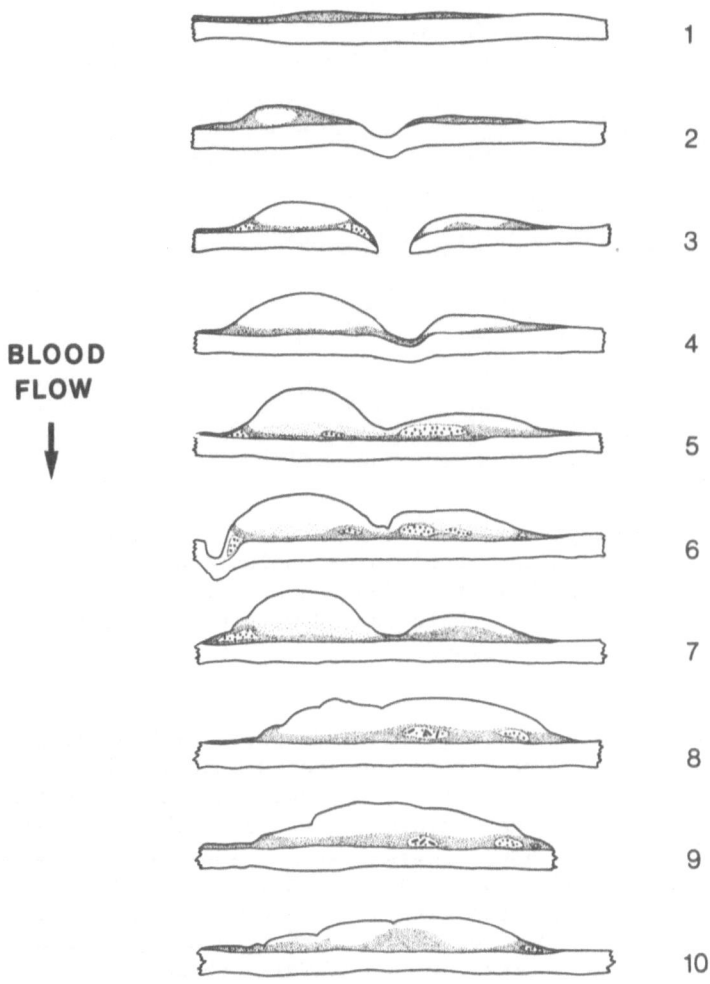

Figure 1.   Free hand drawing of the largest plaque.   The sections
are at approximately 2 millimeter intervals.   Finely stippled areas
represent perifibrous lipid.   Coarsely stippled areas represent gelatinous lesions.   Black lines within gelatinous lesions in sections 8
and 9 represent large cholesterol crystals.

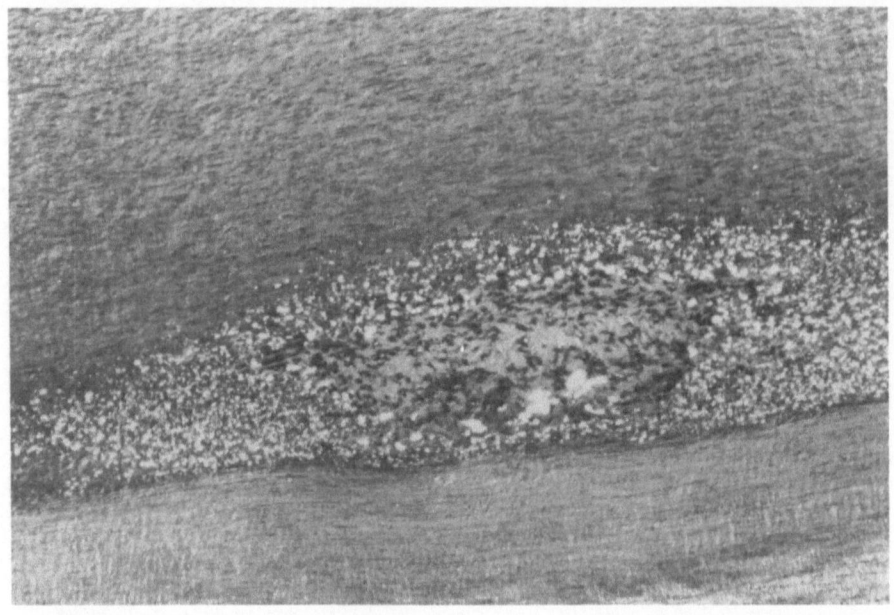

Figure 2.   Histologic section of gelatinous lesion (Figure 1, section 8) showing accumulation of large cholesterol crystals.   The
smaller crystals are cholesterol esters in perifibrous lipid.   Oil
Red O - hematoxylin X 80, photographed with polarized light.
(Reduced 10% for reproduction.)

and frequently contained large lipid droplets within their sarcoplasm.   This was in contrast to the smooth muscle cells in the adjacent plaque which were uniformly oriented and had only fine droplets of lipid in their sarcoplasm (Figure 3).   This suggested that
the metabolism of the smooth muscle cells within the gelatinous like
lesions was disturbed.   The areas of necrosis seen in one gelatinous
like lesion deep within the largest plaque were small acellular areas
which occasionally contained granules of blue and pink staining material presumed to be nuclear or cytoplasmic debris.

DISCUSSION

I interpret these morphologic changes as follows: Gelatinous
like lesions developed in preexisting fibrous plaques, probably as
a result of endothelial damage due to hemodynamic stresses and toxins
from the septicemia.   Although we did not have ultrastructural studies
of the endothelium overlying the gelatinous like lesions, the finding
of a small hyalin mural thrombus adjacent to one gelatinous like lesion was good indirect evidence of endothelial damage.   In the larg-

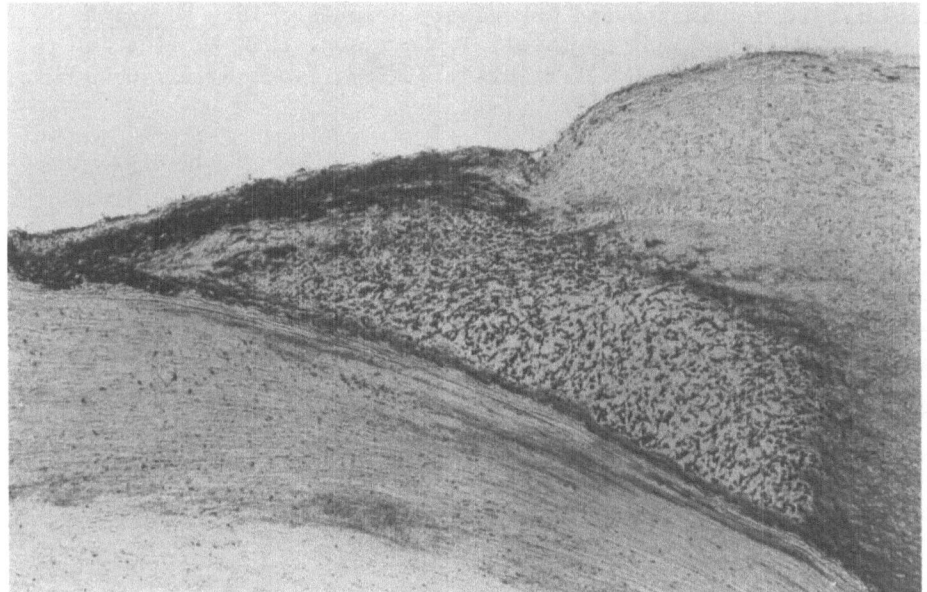

Figure 3.   Histologic section of gelatinous lesion (Figure 1, section 7) showing compression of adjacent elastic fibers which are
coated with perifibrous lipid, random orientation of smooth muscle
cells and large lipid droplets within smooth muscle cells. Lipids
appear black. Oil Red O X 80. (Reduced 10% for reproduction.)

est plaque, the influx of plasma components created gelatinous like
tunnels into the plaque. These gelatinous tunnels appeared to stay
within existing tissue planes, and, therefore, were able to extend
deeply into the central portion of the plaque remaining in the zone
immediately adjacent to the media. The development of small areas
of focal necrosis and the accumulation of large cholesterol crystals
in one of these gelatinous tunnels were probably due to alterations
in cell nutrition as well as the increased influx of lipoprotein.
Although the areas of necrosis and cholesterol accumulation seen in
this ostrich plaque were not as large as those seen in the usual
human atherosclerotic plaque, the qualitative resemblance between
the two is clear. I suggest that the above described pathogenic
sequence could well be one mechanism for the conversion of a fibrous
plaque into an atheromatous plaque.

REFERENCES

1. Stout, C. and F. Bohorquez. 1973. Arteriosclerosis and other

vascular diseases in zoo and laboratory animals. In: <u>Research Animals in Medicine</u>, Ed. by Lowell T. Harmison, DHEW Publication No. (NIH) 72-333, U.S. Gov't Printing Office, Stock No. 1740-0338, Washington, D.C. pp 841-859.

ACKNOWLEDGMENTS

    This project was initiated by Dr. Marshall E. Groover and was facilitated by Dr. Philip Ogilvie and The Oklahoma Zoological Society. My colleague, Federico Bohorquez, helped with much of the work. Histological sections were prepared by Zelma Proctor and Rosemarie Winkler. The project was supported in part by Grants HE 08725 and HE 11044 from The National Heart and Lung Institute, USPHS.

THE INFLUENCE OF SOME DIETARY FACTORS AND/OR TREADMILL EXERCISE

ON RAT AND CHICKEN TISSUE LIPIDS AND SERUM LIPOPROTEINS

K. Ananth Narayan and William K. Calhoun

Nutrition Group, Food Sciences Laboratory
U.S. Army Natick Development Center
Natick, Massachusetts 01760

ABSTRACT

Four different experiments, one with cockerels and three with rats, are described which relate to the effect of dietary factors and/or exercise on serum and liver lipids as well as on serum lipoproteins. Several classes of lipoproteins were isolated by preparative ultracentrifugation, and their purity assessed by gel electrophoresis. The lipid composition and protein content of serum lipoproteins and tissue were also determined. Dietary cholesterol produced an enormous increase (200 fold) in serum very low density lipoproteins in cockerels. This lipoprotein was apparently of very large particle size because it failed to penetrate the spacer gel during disc electrophoresis. In rats fed a cholesterol-supplemented diet, the increase in very low and low density lipoproteins was relatively insignificant in comparison with the cockerels. However, in both species, the liver was overloaded with cholesterol. Further, the serum high density lipoproteins, HDL_2 were greatly diminished in both species as a result of cholesterol ingestion for 7 weeks. As a possible explanation for these related observations, it was proposed that HDL_2 was utilized in the formation of cellular membranes by cholesterol-burdened, hyperplastic livers. A very high level of dietary corn oil (40% by weight) caused drastic changes in rat liver lipid levels and in serum lipoprotein profiles. Specifically, liver cholesterol and triglycerides were increased about 200% over normal. In another experiment, tissue lipids and serum lipoprotein levels were determined in treadmill-exercised rats and in sedentary controls. Two levels (4 and 40%) of a fat mixture (1:1, hydrogenated coconut oil: corn oil) were used in this study. The serum cholesterol was

unchanged in the 4 groups, while the serum triglycerides were reduced in exercised rats given 4% but not 40% fat as compared to
respective controls. Rats fed 40% fat and exercised had near normal levels of liver lipids which was in sharp contrast to their
sedentary controls. The low density lipoproteins were surprisingly
higher in exercised rats given high fat than in sedentary controls.
It was suggested that the direct synthesis of these lipoproteins by
the liver may be necessitated under unusual conditions. In conclusion, considering the central role of liver in lipid and lipoprotein metabolism, greater attention should be focused on this
organ in future experiments on the control of hyperlipoproteinemia.

INTRODUCTION

There are many approaches for the possible prevention and
treatment of atherosclerotic disease in man, for example, dietary
adjustments, physical exercise, drug therapy and surgical interven-
tion. In almost all treatments, the invariant happens to be close
control of diet (1) with respect to total energy, fat calories,
cholesterol content and polyunsaturated to saturated fat ratio.
In most species (primates, dogs, rabbits and chickens) dietary
cholesterol enhances the concentration of serum cholesterol as well
as serum total low density lipoproteins. The accumulation of
cholesterol in liver and arterial walls as a result of greatly
increased exogenous supply is well documented in rabbits, chickens,
nonhuman primates, swine and dogs. In the human diet, this sterol
is plentiful in egg and egg products; appreciable amounts are contributed by meat and dairy products. Furthermore, high levels of
dietary fat stimulate cholesterogenesis. The nature and type of
fat has a considerable effect on this complex transformation, involving as it does approximately 43 steps from acetate to cholesterol. In several species including human, the dietary saturated
fatty acids, myristic and palmitic acids but not stearic acid,
increase while linoleic acid decreases the level of serum
cholesterol. Due to cholesterol biosynthesis _in vivo_ and its
stimulation by low cholesterol foods through regulatory control
mechanisms, it is not possible to control hyperlipoproteinemia
by dietary restrictions alone. Epidemiological studies have
identified serum cholesterol level as a major risk factor in human
coronary heart disease. Further, there is overwhelming evidence
that cholesterol is an abundant lipid species in human atheromatous
depositions. On the other hand, in certain resistent species,
either high fat diet, high cholesterol diet or both have failed
to influence serum cholesterol levels. Therefore, we undertook a
comparative study of dietary factors on serum lipids and blood
lipoproteins in two species which react differently to cholesterol
supplementation. In addition, in order to critically assess the

consequences of physical exercise, the influence on these parameters in sedentary and treadmill-exercised rats fed two widely divergent levels of fat has been investigated.

EXPERIMENTAL

Animals and Diet

Chickens. In experiment I, one day old chickens (New Hampshire - Columbian cross) were placed on control diet A (10% corn oil and 90% poultry ration) or diet B (1% cholesterol, 10% corn oil and 90% poultry ration). Water and feed were given ad libitum. After 3 and 7 weeks on the diets, blood was obtained by heart puncture from several animals in each group per each time period. The liver was quickly excised and frozen until used for analysis.

Rats. With this species, three separate experiments (II, III and IV) were completed. In all cases, a semipurified diet consisting of glucose, casein, fat, minerals and vitamin mixture were used. In experiment II, 30 male, Holtzman rats (200g) were divided into two equal groups (C and D) and were fed a semipurified diet containing 10% corn oil by weight without and with 1% cholesterol, respectively (2). Blood and liver samples were obtained from both groups after 2 and 7 weeks on the diets.

In experiment III, 90 male Holtzman rats (300g) were divided into three equal groups (E, F and G) and were fed a semipurified diet containing 0%, 10% and 40% corn oil by weight, respectively (3). At selected time periods (1, 2, 4 and 10 weeks), several rats from each group were withdrawn for the collection of blood and tissues.

In experiment IV, 20 selected rats and 20 other rats (male, Holtzman, 350g) were further subdivided into two equal groups each (H, I, J and K), respectively (4). The animals were fed either a low fat (4%) or a high fat (40%) diet. Concurrently, the selected rats (groups J and K) were treadmill-exercised with increasing intensity 5 days/week for a period of 6 weeks. In the final weeks of training, the exercised rats ran 80-85 minute/day on a belt moving at 23 m/minute at an inclination of 8.5°. At the end of 6 weeks, blood and tissues were obtained in the resting state from the 4 groups of rats. In all experiments, feed and water were available ad libitum.

Chemical analysis. The procedures followed for lipid extraction of tissues and serum lipoproteins, assay for protein, total

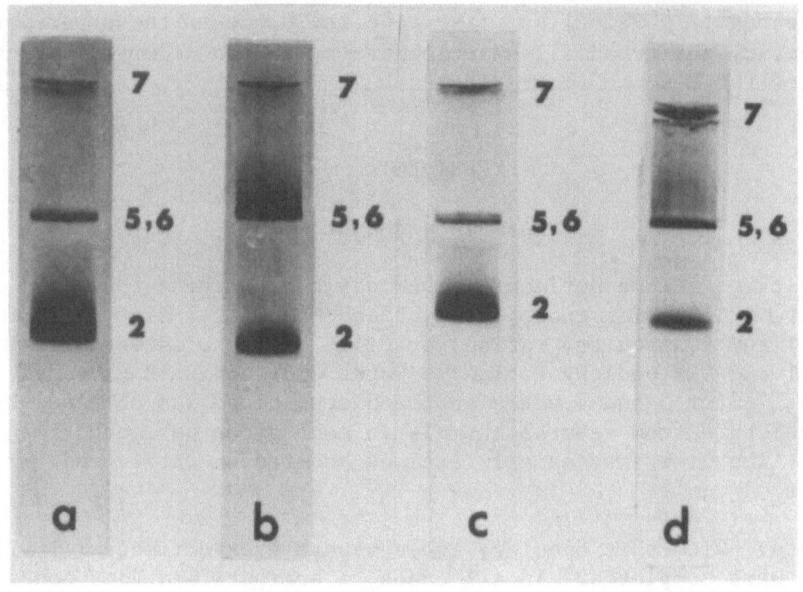

FIGURE 1

Electrophoresis of chicken serum lipoproteins. 3.75% polyacrylamide gel using Sudan black B-prestain. a, b, and c, d, weeks 3 and
7 on diets. a, c, and b, d, control and cholesterol groups.

lipids, cholesterol and phospholipids were the same as indicated
earlier (2). Triglycerides were determined by the procedure of
Van Handel and Zilversmit (5).

   Polyacrylamide gel electrophoresis. The method has been
described in detail elsewhere (6). In general, a 3.75% separating
gel and either Sudan black B prestain or an Amido black 10B stain
was used.

   Preparative ultracentrifugation. The isolated sera samples
were sequentially ultracentrifuged at several densities (2). In
general, the following density fractions were obtained after prolonged centrifugation (20-24 hr) at 114,480 x g at 10°C: very
low density lipoproteins, VLDL (d < 1.006); low density lipoproteins,
LDL (1.006 < d < 1.050); high density lipoproteins, HDL_1 (1.050 < d <
1.063); HDL_2 (1.063 < d < 1.125) and HDL_3 (1.125 < d < 1.21).

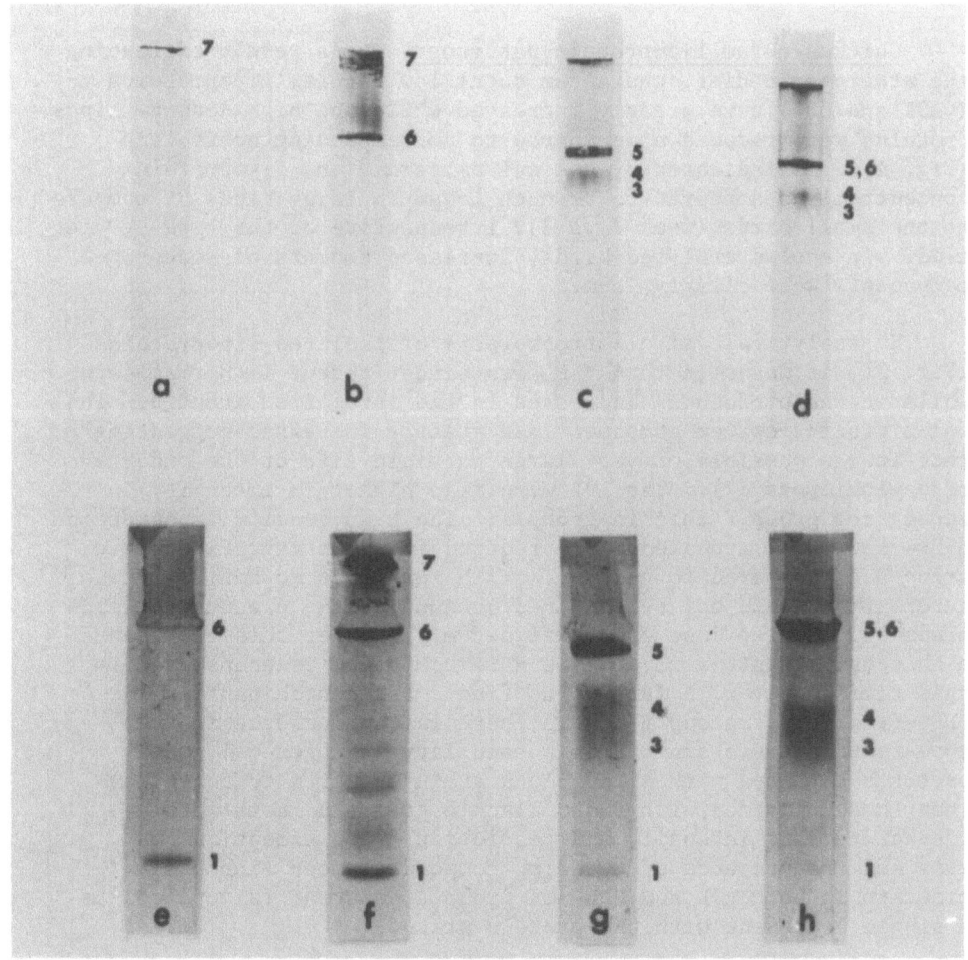

FIGURE 2

Electrophoresis of isolated chicken serum lipoproteins. 3.75%
polyacrylamide gel using Sudan black B-prestain (top panel) and
Amido black 10B stain (bottom panel). a,b, e,f are VLDL and c, d,
g, h are LDL. The first pattern in each set is control, and the
second is from cholesterol group. Band 7 is the very high particle
size component of VLDL present in cholesterol group which does
not penetrate the spacer gel.

RESULTS

Experiment I

Chicken serum lipoprotein patterns.   As a result of feeding
the atherogenic diet, the serum total low density lipoproteins
(VLDL and LDL) were greatly increased while the high density lipoproteins were reduced as compared to corresponding controls
(Fig. 1). As indicated by the gel patterns, the lipoprotein
concentrations appeared to be much lower in large birds as compared
to the small birds (week 7 vs 3), irrespective of the type of diet
used. In cholesterol-fed birds, increased amounts of spacer gel
components were clearly seen.

By analytical gel electrophoresis of isolated lipoproteins
(Fig. 2), it was seen that VLDL was almost absent in normal serum
while it was profoundly increased in the serum from group B. The
non-migrating spacer component was greatly increased suggesting
that it was possibly of very large particle size of the order
of chylomicrons (7). The LDL were also higher in intensity in
serum from group B than in group A. The high density lipoproteins
(HDL_2 and HDL_3) appeared to be reduced in intensity (Fig. 3) in
group B as compared to group A. With reference to HDL_1, precise
information could not be obtained because of the presence of slow
bands only in the case of normal serum. Whether this represents
a LDL contaminant or is truly a HDL_1 component is unanswered at
this time. However, a failure to find a LDL contaminant in the
HDL_1 fraction of group B, where there was an increase in LDL,
appears to argue against this possibility. In general, the
patterns obtained with Amido black stain appeared to be better
than those obtained with Sudan black B prestain, both with
respect to band intensity and resolution. One exception to
this was the presence of two slow components seen with the
prestain in both LDL and HDL_1 of group A, whereas it appeared as
a single component with the protein stain.

Chicken serum lipids and lipoproteins. The enormous increase
in total serum lipids (about 3-fold), in phospholipids (about
1-fold) and particularly in cholesterol (about 5-fold) in cholesterol-fed birds as compared to controls is clearly seen in Table I.
Ultracentrifugal fractionation of these sera indicated that the
greatest change was in the concentration of VLDL. These lipoproteins were present to an insignificant extent in normal chicken
serum but were increased 200-fold in serum from group B. The
LDL were also increased about 2-fold in group B, whereas HDL_1
appeared to be somewhat decreased in group B as compared to group
A. Among the major high density lipoproteins, only HDL_2 appeared
to be impressively lower in group B than in group A. The cholesterol percent of the total lipids was predictably higher in all
lipoproteins, especially VLDL and LDL, from group B as compared
to group A.

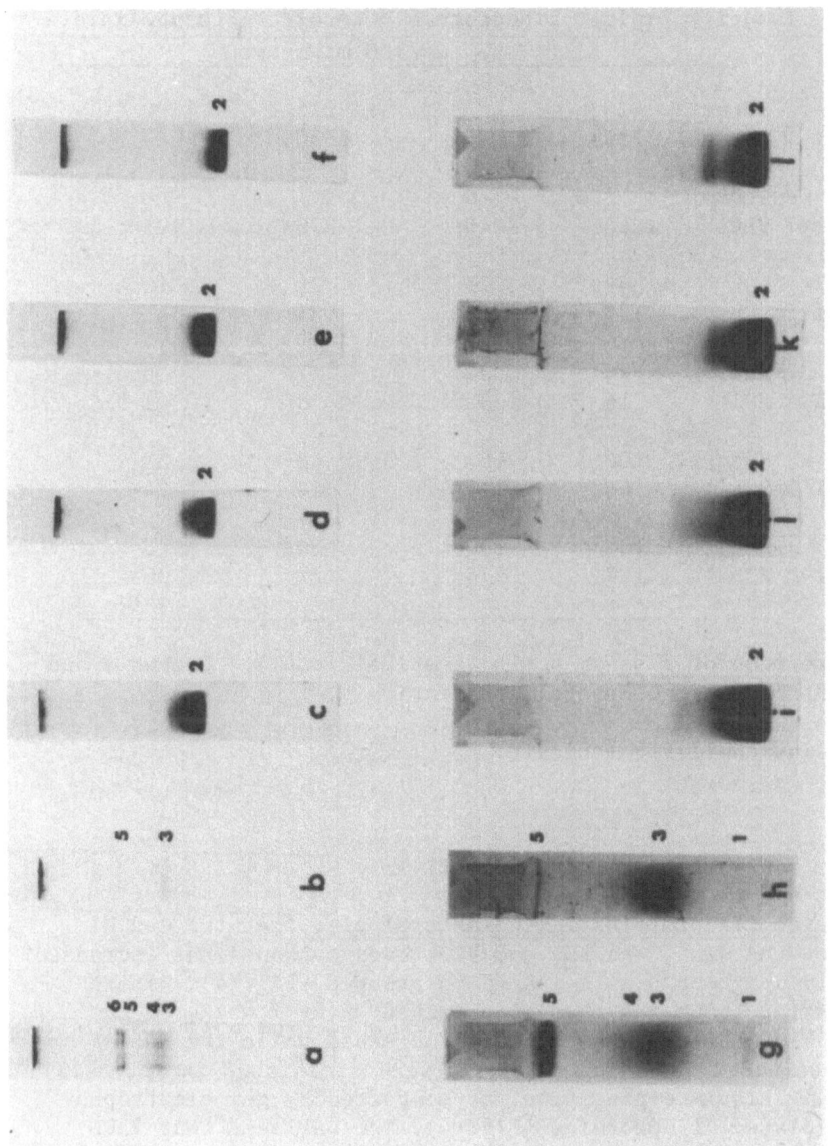

FIGURE 3.   Electrophoresis of isolated chicken serum lipoproteins. 3.75% polyacrylamide gel with Sudan black B prestain (top panel) and Amido black 10B stain (bottom panel). a, b, g, h are HDL1; c, d, i, j, are HDL2; and e, f, k, l are HDL3. The first and second pattern in each set is from control and cholesterol group, respectively.

TABLE I

Effect of Dietary Cholesterol on Chicken Serum Lipoproteins[a]

Group	Sample Identity	Total Lipid	Lipoprotein	Choles- terol[b]	Phospholipid
		mg/100 ml serum			
Control	Serum	420		215	190
Cholesterol	Serum	1730		1350	320
Control	VLDL	2.6	6		
Cholesterol	VLDL	1060	1240	830	135
Control	LDL	49	71	29	16
Cholesterol	LDL	175	223	135	41
Control	HDL_1	24	39	12	8
Cholesterol	HDL_1	16	32	8	4.5
Control	HDL_2	106	187	48	53
Cholesterol	HDL_2	66	125	44	24
Control	HDL_3	132	260	66	70
Cholesterol	HDL_3	127	256	77	36

[a] Values are mean of 2 serum pools (4 animals/pool). Groups A and
   B are control and cholesterol, respectively.

[b] Expressed as cholesterol oleate.

Experiment II

Rat serum lipoproteins and cholesterol diet. At the end of
two weeks on the diet, the LDL and VLDL band was somewhat increased
in intensity in group D as compared to group C (Fig. 4). There
was no question about the changes observed after 7 weeks on the
diet. The VLDL-LDL band was greatly increased while the HDL_1
(intermediate bands) and HDL_2 (band 2) were diminished in intensity
in group D. This interpretation was supported by gel electrophoresis of isolated lipoproteins (Fig. 4). It was seen that VLDL
and LDL, particularly the latter, were present in much greater
concentration in group D than in group C. On the other hand, HDL_1
and HDL_2, but not HDL_3, were lower in cholesterol-fed rats than in
controls. Further, the LDL in group D were apparently of greater
particle size than the LDL from group C.

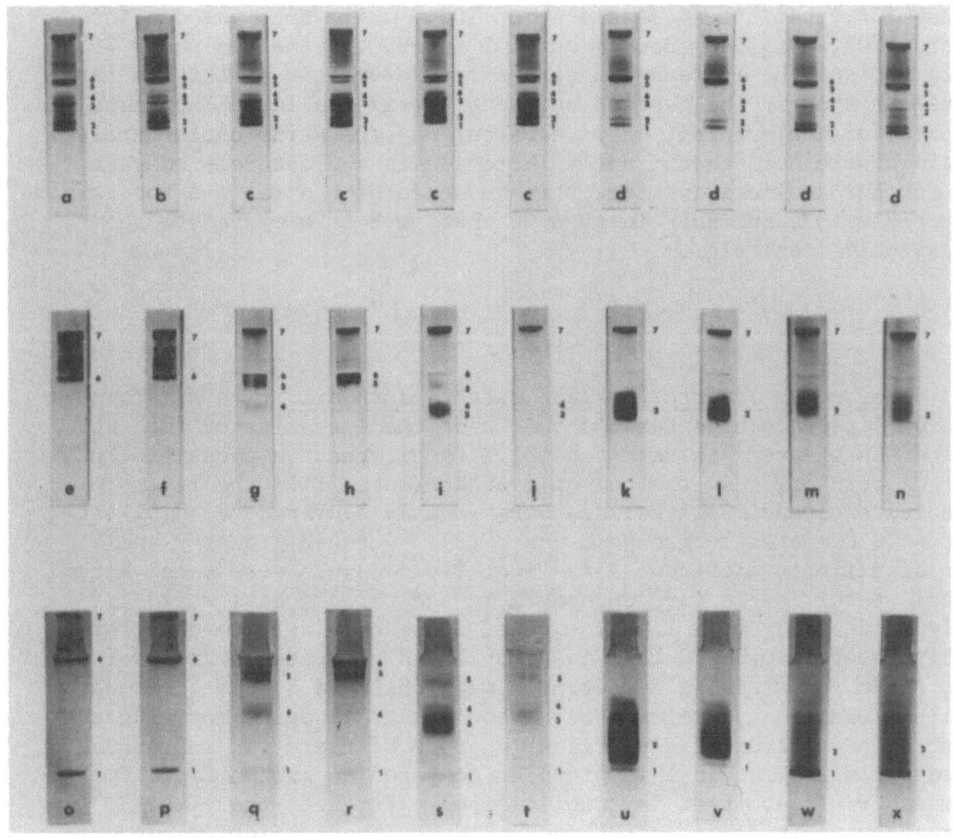

FIGURE 4

Electrophoresis of rat serum lipoproteins in 3.75% gel. Top panel,
Sudan black B-prestained serum patterns a, b and c, d weeks 2 and
7 on diets. a, c, and b, d, are from groups C and D. Middle panel
(Sudan black B prestain) and bottom panel (Amido black stain).
e, f, o, p are VLDL; g, h, q, r are LDL; i, j, s, t, HDL₁; k, l, u,
v are HDL₂; m, n, w, x are HDL₃. The first in each set is control
and the second is from cholesterol group.

That the rat behaves differently from the chicken with respect
to dietary cholesterol is indicated by the lack of any major changes
in rat serum lipids in group D as compared to group C (Table II),
which may be contrasted with the large changes seen in Table I
with chickens. It is further seen that VLDL was increased less
than 20%, that LDL increased about 100%, while HDL_1 was decreased
about 70%, HDL_2 decreased about 50% and HDL_3 decreased about 20%
(2). Since the increase in either rat serum VLDL or LDL was far
smaller than in the case of chickens provided a large exogenous
source of cholesterol, it is apparent why the serum cholesterol
levels were not exhorbitantly increased in cholesterol-fed rats.
A further ameliorative factor in the case of the rat was the larger
decrease in serum HDL_2 in group D than in B as compared to their
respective controls.

Experiment III

Rat serum lipoproteins and dietary corn oil. The prestained
serum lipoprotein patterns showed that the intensity of the LDL
band was greater in rats fed 40% corn oil than in those fed 10%
or 0% corn oil. At the end of 4 weeks (Table III) the liver
cholesterol and triglycerides were grossly elevated (P < 0.01) in
group G compared to groups E and F (3). Between groups E and F,
no significant differences in liver lipid levels were seen. Serum
cholesterol levels were unchanged in the three groups while triglycerides and, to a lesser extent, phospholipids were considerably lower in group G than in group E and F. Between groups E and
F, again, no striking differences were observed. Subsequent work
with isolated lipoproteins have shown that, in agreement with the
decrease in serum triglycerides in group G, there was a pronounced
reduction in VLDL in this group as compared to groups E and F
(manuscript submitted for publication). Further, there was a
progressive increase in LDL and its constituent moieties, especially cholesterol, as the level of dietary corn oil was increased
from 0 to 40%. The phospholipid and protein components of HDL_2
were reduced significantly in group G as compared with group F
and/or group E. However, the decrease was not as profound as
that observed in experiment II.

Experiment IV

Treadmill exercise and serum and liver lipids. The serum
cholesterol and total lipids were relatively unchanged (Table IV)
as a result of either diet or exercise (4). Both high fat (group
I) and exercised low fat (group J) groups had lower serum
triglycerides than the low fat group (group H). In exercised high
fat (group K), serum triglycerides were not lower than in controls
(group I) but tended to be higher. In group I, most liver lipids

TABLE II

Effect of Dietary Cholesterol on Rat Serum Lipoproteins[a]

Group	Sample Identity	Total Lipid	Lipoprotein	Choles- terol[b]	Phospholipid
			mg/100 ml serum or g liver		
Control	Serum	243		80	77
Cholesterol	Serum	213		89	61
Control	Liver	56		6	
Cholesterol	Liver	185		77	
Control	VLDL	62	84	7.1	9.9
Cholesterol	VLDL	77	99	23	12
Control	LDL	20	33	6.8	3.7
Cholesterol	LDL	42	62	24	7.2
Control	HDL_1	21			
Cholesterol	HDL_1	6.4			
Control	HDL_2	93	164	45	33
Cholesterol	HDL_2	46	87	23	14
Control	HDL_3	22	83		5.8
Cholesterol	HDL_3	17	67		2.2

[a] Values are mean of 6, 2, 2 serum pools, respectively, for serum, liver and lipoproteins. Groups C and D are control and cholesterol, respectively.

[b] Expressed as cholesterol oleate.

were considerably higher than in group H. A beneficial effect of exercise was noted in the drop to near normal liver lipid levels in group K.

Heart and muscle lipids. These tissues have also been examined and the results have indicated no striking changes in the case of heart lipids. The muscle concentration of cholesterol, but not phospholipids, was significantly greater in group K than in all other groups. This observation, considered together with the decrease in liver cholesterol of the same group, may suggest a transfer of cholesterol from the liver to other sites as a

TABLE III

Effect of Dietary Corn Oil on Rat Liver and Serum Lipids[a]

Group % Corn Oil	Sample Identity	Total Lipid	Cholesterol[b]	Phospho- lipid	Triglyceride
			mg/g liver or 100 ml serum		
0	Liver	37	1.9	24	7.5
10	Liver	43	2.2	24	10
40	Liver	68	5.6	25	23
0	Serum	320	58	110	57
10	Serum	310	57	120	54
40	Serum	260	55	99	39

[a] Values are mean of 4 livers and 8 serum pools, respectively, at the end of 4 weeks on the diets. Groups E, F and G correspond to 0, 10 and 40% corn oil, respectively.

[b] Expressed as unesterified cholesterol.

result of dietary high fat level and exercise.

Serum lipoproteins. The high fat diet reduced serum VLDL level (Table IV) as compared to low fat diet but the differences were not statistically significant. Exercised rats on the low fat diet had significantly less serum VLDL than corresponding controls. Exercised rats fed high fat had much lower levels of serum VLDL than their sedentary controls but the differences were not significant (P >0.05)

The LDL were greatly elevated (Table IV) in group I as compared to group H. In both exercised groups J and K, the LDL values were considerably higher than in their controls. However, only the differences between groups K and I were significant (P <0.01). There were only minor differences in the three density classes of HDL among the 4 groups.

DISCUSSION

Dietary cholesterol and serum lipoproteins. While the formation of atheromatous lesions was not investigated here, it is known that lipid deposits form easily in the arterial walls of several species such as rabbits and chickens given a cholesterol-

TABLE IV

Effect of Exercise on Rat Serum Lipoproteins[a]

Group and Fat Level	Sample Identity	Total Lipid	Lipo-protein	Choles-terol[b]	Trigly-ceride
		mg/100 ml serum or g liver			
Control 4%	Serum	310		64	97
Control 40%	Serum	310		68	66
Exercise 4%	Serum	300		65	71
Exercise 40%	Serum	320		72	84
Control 4%	Liver	42		2.1	9.3
Control 40%	Liver	76		3.8	18
Exercise 4%	Liver	48		2.1	17
Exercise 40%	Liver	46		2.0	8.7
Control 4%	VLDL	47	49	2.4	30
Control 40%	VLDL	35	37	2.0	17
Exercise 4%	VLDL	23	24	1.2	16
Exercise 40%	VLDL	18	19	1.1	9.2
Control 4%	LDL	21	25	3.8	8.1
Control 40%	LDL	40	50	11	10
Exercise 4%	LDL	29	36	7.6	7.9
Exercise 40%	LDL	54	67	15	13

[a] Values are mean of 8, 4 and 4 serum pools, respectively, for serum, liver and lipoproteins. Groups H, I, J, K correspond to control 4%, control 40%, exercise 4% and exercise 40%, respectively.

[b] Expressed as unesterified cholesterol.

supplemented diet. Based on blood chemistry, the rat appears to be almost immune to dietary cholesterol unless other agents such as bile acids or thiouracil are also provided. The data obtained suggest that the deposition of cholesterol in tissues in the chicken may be related to the enormous concentration of VLDL in this species given a cholesterol-supplemented diet. In rats given a cholesterol diet, the increase in both VLDL and LDL was very small by comparison and may, therefore, protect it from unusual accumulations. In what manner is the rat able to prevent the accumulation of VLDL and LDL in blood is not clear at this time. Whether this is in any way related to the differential response of the adipose tissue of the two species in relation to total fatty acid synthesis in vivo (8) remains to be determined. Even in the human (9), the adipose tissue appears to be largely a site for deposition of fat as in the case of chickens rather than for fat synthesis as in the rat.

In terms of chemical composition, the VLDL species in the serum of cholesterol-fed birds have a remarkably low level (6%) of triglycerides (10). The increased accumulation seen here is perhaps related to decreased catabolism of these cholesterol-rich VLDL remnants (11). In the rat, special atherogenic and thrombogenic diets have also led to the accumulation of VLDL in serum. Therefore, the manner in which the rat is able to prevent excessive hyperlipoproteinemia under conditions of cholesterol-supplementation alone merits further study.

The drastic reduction in serum HDL_2 in both chicken and rats given a cholesterol diet may be due to transfer of small molecular peptides (12) which are common to HDL and VLDL. However, the recent report concerning the decreased synthesis of apoHDL in cholesterol-fed rats by Frnka and Reiser (13) lends some support to a previous hypothesis (2) that HDL_2 secretion into circulation may be curtailed because of its utilization in the biogenesis of cellular membranes. In order to accomodate excessive amounts of a slowly degradable compound such as cholesterol, compensatory hyperplasia of the liver may be encountered (2). During liver regeneration, a similar reduction in serum HDL_2 concentration as well as a large decrease in radioactive leucine incorporation into HDL_2 was observed (14). A reduction in HDL, in addition to the well known increase in LDL,is generally observed in humans with atherosclerotic disease. Further, an Air Force longitudinal survey has documented a progressive decrease in the serum HDL of 400 West Point graduates (15). Thus, the role of serum HDL may be more important than hitherto recognized. A recent report by Langdon (16), which has provided additional immunological and chemical evidence for the presence of apolipoproteins in human erythrocyte membrane proteins, is in consonance with the previous postulate (2, 14, 17) concerning serum HDL and membrane biosynthesis.

Dietary corn oil and serum lipoproteins. Because of recent emphasis upon the beneficial aspects of polyunsaturated fat, we have examined the effect of a very high level of corn oil in rats. In this species this level (40% by weight) caused the accumulation of cholesterol and triglycerides in the liver, reduced serum VLDL, greatly augmented LDL and slightly reduced HDL_2 as compared to controls. In comparison with experiment II, the increase in LDL was almost as large in experiment III (group G) whereas the decrease in HDL_2 was only nominal. It is possible that this is related to the differing accumulations of cholesterol in the two experiments (experiment II, 45 mg/g liver, and experiment III, 6 mg/g liver).

The manner in which polyunsaturated fat decreases serum cholesterol in humans is not known. Several investigators (18, 19) have suggested that there is increased oxidation and excretion of cholesterol,while others (20) have concluded that there is re-distribution of cholesterol between serum and tissues including the liver. Since high levels of cholesterol have been reported in apparently healthy subjects (21, 22), there is need for great caution in the selection of suitable foods in the human diet. Although an extremely high level of corn oil was used in experiment III, such levels have by no means been excluded from clinical studies (23, 24). On the basis of available information, levels of linoleate exceeding 10% by weight do not seem to be justified.

Dietary fat level, physical exercise and serum lipoproteins. The beneficial effect of exercise on general well-being and morale does not require documentation. The reduction in serum lipids, more often triglycerides and less often cholesterol, as a result of physical exercise is well known (25, 26). In experiment IV, we chose a moderate degree of exercise which generally reflects the norm and have evaluated its effect on tissue lipids and serum lipoproteins in rats given two levels of fat. Under these condi-tions, the serum cholesterol level was not altered significantly in any of the 4 groups. Furthermore, the serum triglycerides, which were reduced in exercised rats given a low fat diet, failed to do so in exercised rats given a high fat diet.

Possibly the most interesting observation of this study was the significant elevation in serum LDL in exercised rats given high fat as compared to their sedentary controls. At the same time, the liver cholesterol in these exercised rats were near normal. Based on the observations of Wong et al. (27) with cockerels, it is possible that further increase in the intensity of exercise may have considerably decreased serum cholesterol and LDL in exercised rats fed the high fat diet. But as indicated earlier, the moderate exercise program used in the present experiment represents the norm and, therefore, may have some implications concerning the development of atherosclerosis in humans consuming a high fat diet.

In both exercised groups in the resting state, the trigly-ceride-rich VLDL were diminished as compared to controls. Askew et al. (28) have observed no significant differences in the lipo-protein lipase activity in the muscle and heart as a result of a rigorous exercise program. This suggests that there was no increased utilization of triglycerides in exercised-rested rats.

The reduced level of serum VLDL (Table IV) may perhaps be due to certain adaptive changes in these animals resulting in diminished synthesis of VLDL.

Although it is presently recognized (29) that LDL arises to a significant extent from VLDL, the reduced level of VLDL and the unaltered activity of the enzyme lipoprotein lipase in exercised-rested rats make it unlikely that increased LDL arises from accel-erated transformation of VLDL to LDL. It appears likely that there is increased direct synthesis of LDL under certain conditions, such as a high fat diet. Enhanced synthesis of cholesterol has been reported in exercised rats. It may be postulated that the increase in LDL in either sedentary or exercised rats fed high fat diet may be due to increased synthesis of LDL, which may be necessary to accelerate the rate of removal of cholesterol from the liver.

Concluding remarks. The liver plays a dominant role in lipid and lipoprotein metabolism and a multitude of factors influence the function of the liver. These include those that are provided by exogenous sources, those that are synthesized in vivo, hormonal or humoral factors, those that evoke or produce physical or emo-tional stress on the organism. An everchanging interplay of this vast array of variables acting in harmony or in opposition in an unpredictable manner provokes responses that cannot be described or mimicked in laboratory experiments with simple animal models. Nevertheless, animal experiments may provide us with guidance of a general nature. Furthermore, they will hopefully provoke further search in other areas and may ultimately provide us with an integrated concept.

The data furnished here suggest that the rat is uniquely different from other species in its handling of high levels of dietary fat and cholesterol, that high levels of corn oil produce drastic alterations in rat liver lipids and serum lipoproteins and that the interaction of a high fat diet and moderate treadmill-exercise results in unexpected alterations in rat serum lipo-protein profiles. In our experience, with these and other experi-ments, the lipids of the liver reflect, to a large extent, the dietary and nutritional status of the animal. It is therefore suggested that, in studies on atherosclerosis using animal models, the important contribution of the liver in causing specific alter-ations in lipoprotein profile be given due consideration.

ACKNOWLEDGEMENTS

A part of this work represents earlier work completed by
K. A. Narayan at the University of Illinois where it was supported

by a grant from the Chicago and Illinois Heart Association and a grant CA-01932 from U.S.P.H.S.

REFERENCES

1. Levy, R.I. and N. Ernst. 1973. Diet, Hyperlipidemia and Atherosclerosis. In: Modern Nutrition in Health and Disease. Ed. by R.S. Goodhart and M.E. Shils, Lea and Febiger, Philadelphia, pp. 895-916.

2. Narayan, K.A. 1971. Lowered serum concentration of high density lipoproteins in cholesterol-fed rats. Atherosclerosis 13: 205-215.

3. Narayan, K.A., J.J. McMullen, D.P. Butler, T. Wakefield, and W.K. Calhoun. 1974. The influence of a high level of dietary corn oil on rat serum and liver lipids. Nutr. Rep. Int. 10: 25-33.

4. Narayan, K.A., J.J. McMullen, D.P. Butler, T. Wakefield, and W.K. Calhoun. 1975. Effect of exercise on tissue lipids and serum lipoproteins of rats fed two levels of fat. J. Nutr. 105: 581-587.

5. Van Handel, E. and D.B. Zilversmit. 1957. Micromethod for direct determination of serum triglycerides. J. Lab. Clin. Med. 50: 152-157.

6. Narayan, K.A., H.L. Creinin, and F.A. Kummerow. 1966. Disc electrophoresis of rat plasma lipoproteins. J. Lipid Res. 7: 150-157.

7. Narayan, K.A., W.E. Dudacek, and F.A. Kummerow. 1966. Disc electrophoresis of isolated chylomicrons. Clin. Chim. Acta 14: 797-801.

8. O'Hea, E.K. and G.A. Leveille. 1969. Influence of feeding frequency on lipogenesis and enzymatic activity of adipose tissue and the performance of pigs. J. Animal Sci. 28: 336-341.

9. Patel, M.S., O.E. Owen, L.I. Goldman, and R.W. Hanson. 1975. Fatty acid synthesis by human adipose tissue. Metabolism 24: 161-173.

10. Kruski, A.W. and K.A. Narayan. 1972. The effect of dietary supplementation of cholesterol and its subsequent withdrawal on the liver lipids and serum lipoproteins of chickens.

Lipids $\underline{7}$: 742–749.

11. Kruski, A.W. and K.A. Narayan. 1972. Lipoprotein synthesis in chickens fed cholesterol. Atherosclerosis $\underline{15}$: 141–145.

12. Bersot, T.P., W.V. Brown, R.I. Levy, H.G. Windmueller, D.S. Fredrickson, and V.S. Lequire. 1970. Further characterization of the apolipoproteins of rat plasma lipoproteins. Biochemistry $\underline{9}$: 3427–3433.

13. Frnka, J. and R. Reiser. 1974. The effects of diet cholesterol on the synthesis of rat serum apolipoproteins. Biochim. Biophys. Acta $\underline{360}$: 322–338.

14. Narayan, K.A. 1970. Incorporation of U–^{14}C-leucine into serum lipoproteins and proteins of partially hepatectomized rats. Lipids $\underline{5}$: 156–158.

15. Clark, D.A., M.F. Allen, and F.H. Wilson. 1967. Longitudinal study of serum lipids. 12 year report. Am. J. Clin. Nutr. $\underline{20}$: 743–752.

16. Langdon, R.G. 1974. Serum lipoprotein apoproteins as major protein constituents of the human erythrocyte membrane. Biochim. Biophys. Acta $\underline{342}$: 213–228.

17. Narayan, K.A. 1971. Rat serum lipoproteins during carcinogenesis of the liver in the preneoplastic and the neoplastic state. Int. J. Cancer $\underline{8}$: 61–70.

18. Connor, W.E., D.T. Witiak, D.B. Stone, and M.L. Armstrong. 1969. Cholesterol balance and fecal neutral steroid and bile acid excretion in normal men fed dietary fats of different fatty acid composition. J. Clin. Invest. $\underline{48}$: 1363–1375.

19. Nestel, P.J., N. Havenstein, M.H. Whyte, T.J. Scott, and L.J. Cook. 1973. Lower plasma cholesterol after eating polyunsaturated ruminant fats. New Eng. J. Med. $\underline{288}$: 379–382.

20. Grundy, S.N. and E.H. Ahrens, Jr. 1970. The effects of unsaturated dietary fats on absorption, excretion and synthesis and distribution of cholesterol in man. J. Clin. Invest. $\underline{49}$: 1135–1152.

21. Frantz, I.D., Jr. and J.B. Carey, Jr. 1961. Cholesterol content of human liver after feeding of corn oil and hydrogenated coconut oil. Proc. Soc. Exp. Biol. Med. $\underline{106}$: 800–801.

22. Maruhama, U., A. Yanbe, H. Tadaki, M. Ohtsuki, A. Ohneda, R. Abe, and S. Yamagata. 1974. Liver lipids in patients with endogenous hypertriglyceridemia. Tohuku J. Exp. Med. 114: 247-252.

23. Kasper, H., H. Thiel, and M. Ehl. 1973. Response of body weight to a low carbohydrate, high fat diet in normal and obese subjects. Am. J. Clin. Nutr. 26: 197-204.

24. Little, J.A., B.L. Birchwood, D.A. Simmons, M.A. Antar, A. Kallos, G.C. Buckley, and A. Csima. 1970. Interrelationship between the kinds of dietary carbohydrate and fat in hyper-lipoproteinemic patients. Part I. Sucrose and starch with polyunsaturated fat. Atherosclerosis 11: 173-181.

25. Oscai, L.B., J.A. Patterson, D.L. Bogard, R.J. Beck, and B.L. Rothermel. 1972. Normalization of serum triglycerides and lipoprotein electrophoretic patterns by exercise. Am. J. Cardiol. 30: 775-780.

26. Campbell, D.E. 1965. Influence of several physical activities on serum cholesterol concentrations in young men. J. Lipid Res. 6: 478-480.

27. Wong, H.Y.C., S. David, and S.O. Orimilikwe. 1973. Reversal of induced experimental atherosclerosis of cholesterol fed cockerels by exercise. Fed. Proc. 32: 238.

28. Askew, E.W., G.L. Dohm, R.L. Huston, T.W. Sneed, and R.P. Dowdy. 1972. Response of rat tissue lipases to physical training and exercise. Proc. Soc. Exp. Biol. Med. 141: 123-129.

29. Eisenberg, S., D.W. Bilheimer, R.I. Levy, and F.T. Lindgren. 1973. On the metabolic conversion of human plasma very low density lipoprotein to low density lipoprotein. Biochim. Biophys. Acta 326: 361-377.

SECTION 5

TISSUE CULTURE

EFFECTS OF CHOLESTEROL DERIVATIVES ON STEROL BIOSYNTHESIS

Harry W. Chen and Andrew A. Kandutsch

The Jackson Laboratory

Bar Harbor, Maine   04609

Atherosclerosis is a condition marked by the formation of plaques in the endothelium of the arterial system which in the earliest stage are composed largely of cholesterol. The etiology of the disease is not known,although it appears that an elevated serum cholesterol level may contribute to the development and the progression of atherosclerosis in animals and in man. The production of atherosclerotic lesions in experimental animals on a cholesterol-supplemented diet suggested a connection between cholesterol and atherosclerosis.

Cholesterol in animals is derived from two sources, first the intake and absorption of dietary cholesterol and second the biosynthesis of cholesterol from acetate by various organs or cells of the body, e.g., liver, intestine, and skin. While the control of cholesterogenesis in vivo has been extensively studied, the exact biochemical mechanism by which sterol synthesis is regulated is not understood. During the last few years we have been employing tissue culture techniques in studies of the factors which affect the rate of sterol synthesis and the activity of the rate-limiting enzyme in the sterol synthetic pathway 3-hydroxy-3-methylglutaryl Coenzyme A (HMG-CoA) reductase. The results of these studies indicate that a number of oxygenated derivatives of cholesterol are potent and specific inhibitors of HMG-CoA reductase and thus of sterol synthesis (1-5). These compounds do not affect the general metabolism of a cell culture during short term incubation, whereas exposure to the inhibitors for prolonged

---

Abbreviations used are: HMG-CoA, 3-hydroxy-3-methylglutaryl Coenzyme A; MVA, mevalonic acid.

periods of time results in retarded cell growth. Presumably the
effect of the inhibition upon cell growth is due to the unavailability of sterols for the formation of new membranes.

PROCEDURE FOR TESTING THE INHIBITION OF STEROL SYNTHESIS

To study the regulation of sterol synthesis in cell cultures
it is desirable to have cells grown in chemically defined medium.
Serum contains large quantities of cholesterol and small amounts of
other steroids and their presence in the medium resulted in
suppression of cholesterol synthesis. To induce sterol synthesis
in cells which depend on serum for growth delipidized serum can be
used (6,7). Alternatively, the serum can be removed from half
confluent cultures for investigations that can be carried out
during the one or two days that the cells are able to maintain
nearly normal metabolism in its absence. However, the ability of
cells to synthesize cholesterol after serum removal is very variable in different cell cultures. Mouse lymphocytes and some
embryonic cell cultures can be induced to synthesize cholesterol
by this manipulation (5) while other types of cells cannot.

In testing a compound for its effect upon sterol synthesis it
is important to investigate whether or not it acts specifically at
a single site in the sterol synthetic pathway and whether or not it
affects other pathways of metabolism. The flow chart shown in
Figure 1 illustrates procedure for the complete testing of the effect
of a sterol on sterol synthesis. First we measure the effect of
the compound on the incorporation of $(1-^{14}C)$acetate into fraction of
digitonin precipitable sterols, of fatty acids, and of CO_2. The
steroid is added to the medium over a range of at least four concentrations. If it inhibits the conversion of acetate into the
sterol fraction and at the same time has no depressing effect on
the synthesis of fatty acids or production of CO_2, then the compound
is regarded as a potentially specific inhibitor of sterol synthesis.
Decreased CO_2 evolution in a treated culture within a period of a
few hours may be due to general toxic effects of a sterol; and
reduced synthesis of fatty acids as well as of sterol can be the result of interference with the formation of acetyl-CoA or the
transport of acetate into the cells. Since HMG-CoA reductase is the
rate-limiting enzyme for the synthesis of sterol (9,10), the assay
of its activity offers further evidence regarding the specificity
of the effect of a chemical on sterolgenesis. The half life of the
enzyme is relatively short (about 2 hours, see ref. 4,10) so that
repression of its synthesis can diminish the enzyme to bring about
a rapid decline in enzyme activity. Frequently the effect of a
chemical upon the incorporation of (^{14}C)mevalonic acid (MVA) into
sterol is also examined. This study in conjunction with data

FIGURE 1

Scheme for Assaying the Effect of Sterols on Sterol Synthesis in Cell Culture

Monolayer cells grown to half confluent in plastic flask fed 20 ml fresh medium overnight (75 cm²).

Discard medium, add test sterol suspended in 5 ml fresh medium, incubated at 37°C for 4 hrs. with constant shaking at 60 gyration per min.

Labeled with 0.1 ml of $(1-^{14}C)$acetate (20 μCi, 29 μmole) in medium; stoppered the flask with septum stoppers fitted with plastic cup; incubated & shaken for additional 2 hrs.

End the incubation with the acidification of 0.3 ml of 12 NH_2SO_4.

Add 0.3 ml hyamine to the plastic cup with a syringe and shake the flask at room temperature for 15 min. to collect CO_2.

Add 1 ml of 90% KOH, stand overnight at room temperature.

Saponification (8)

*Duplicate flasks for assaying the effect of sterol on DNA, RNA, and protein synthesis and cellular content of cyclic AMP.

*Assay of $(2-^{14}C)$MVA incorporation to sterol (1).

Duplicate flask for assay of HMG-CoA reductase.

Count 0.1 ml of hyamine solution to determine the production of $^{14}CO_2$.

1 ml for analysis of DNA content.

Saponifiable fraction

Solvent extraction
Count aliquote for (^{14}C)fatty acids.

Nonsaponifiable fraction

Count aliquote for (^{14}C) nonsaponifiable fraction

Digitonin precipitation, solvent extraction
Count aliquote for ^{14}C-sterol

*These analyses were not routinely carried out.

obtained from acetate incorporation can ascertain the specific
effect of a compound on HMG-CoA reductase. If the chemical,
without general toxic effect nor diminishing fatty acid or CO_2
production, decreases the incorporation of acetate as well as
MVA into sterol, then it may inhibit steps beyond HMG-CoA reductase.
As a final test of the effect of a compound upon the general
metabolism of cells we also determine its effect upon the cellular
content of cyclic AMP, the incorporation of thymidine into DNA, of
uridine into RNA, and of amino acids into proteins.

When a highly purified preparation of cholesterol was tested
under the conditions shown in Figure 1, we were surprised to find
that it had little or no effect upon sterol synthesis although a
considerable amount of cholesterol was taken up by cells (1, 4).
On the other hand the addition of a commercial cholesterol preparation to the medium inhibited sterol synthesis. The inhibitory
contaminants present in the commercial preparation were precipitated
by digitonin indicating that they were sterols. They were slightly
more polar than cholesterol and were concentrated in the mother
liquid obtained by crystalizing the cholesterol, but we have not yet
purified enough of the contaminants to characterize them more
extensively. Larger quantities of inhibitory sterols were found
to be present in a mixture of sterols isolated from a mouse prepu-
tial gland tumor, and the most potent of these were identified as
7α-hydroxycholesterol, 7β-hydroxycholesterol, and 7-ketocholesterol
(1). Further studies indicated that 20α-hydroxycholesterol,
25-hydroxycholesterol, and several other oxygenated derivatives of
cholesterol were more potent inhibitors of sterol synthesis than
any of the 7-oxygenated sterols (2). For example, 25-hydroxy-
cholesterol at the concentration of 0.05 to 0.07 μM will inhibit
the rate of sterol synthesis by 50% in 6 hours. At a higher concentration (2.5μM) 25-hydroxycholesterol depressed the activity of
HMG-CoA reductase almost totally within 2 hours (2).

Some of these sterol inhibitors have been tested on various
cell types. Table 1 demonstrates the effects of various concentrations of 25-hydroxycholesterol and 7-ketocholesterol on sterol
synthesis in several different kinds of cultured cells, and
in one kind of rat hepatoma cells. In all of these cell cultures
sterol synthesis was depressed by both inhibitors, although the
sensitivity of the various cell types to the inhibitions varied.
L cells and lymphocytes were more sensitive to inhibition than
were two types of liver cell cultures and leukemic cells.

STRUCTURAL FEATURES OF STEROLS REQUIRED FOR
INHIBITORY ACTIVITY

In the last few years we have tested more than 70 different
steroids in a search for effective inhibitors of sterol synthesis.

TABLE 1
Inhibition of Sterol Synthesis by Oxygenated Derivatives of
Cholesterol in Various Cell Types

	% of controls					
	25-hydroxy cholesterol			7-keto cholesterol		
	1µg/ml	2µg/ml	5µg/ml	2µg/ml	5µg/ml	10µg/ml
L cells	5	2		20	7	
Liver cells (primary cultures)	22	17	8		47	30
FL83, liver cells		45	25		40	20
Embryonic cells in tissue culture SWR/J		17	6		10	5
SFHMT cells (Rat hepatoma cells adapted to grow in serum-free medium				21	8	6
Lymphocytes (PHA stimulated)	5	5	4			
AKR/J leukemic cells	39	24		49	17	4
AKR/J leukemic cells (PHA stimulated)	29	13		77		2

The procedure for assay of sterol synthesis has been described
in the text, in Figure 1 and extensively in reference (1,2). Cells
were incubated with or without inhibitors for 6 hours, the last 2
hours with (1-^{14})acetate. SWR/J embryonic cells in culture were
grown in EMEM medium (Microbiological Associate, Bethesda, Maryland)
plus 10% fetal calf serum. Serum was removed 12 hours before
experiment. Data for lymphocytes has been previously reported(5).

Table 2 shows the results obtained in a representative test of a
series of structurally related sterols. The numbers in Table
2 represent the concentration of sterol required to achieve a 50%
inhibition of sterol synthesis and HMG-CoA reductase activity in
L cells and primary liver cell cultures. The former parameter was
calculated from the ratio of (^{14}C) sterol to (^{14}C) fatty acids to
compensate for differences in general metabolic activities of groups
of cultures used in the numerous tests. The table illustrates a
number of important points. Inhibitory potency varies with seeming-
ly minor changes in structure such as the displacement of a hydroxyl
function from one position in the side chain to an adjacent carbon
atom. The best inhibitors are highly potent, 25-hydroxycholesterol
being effective in L cells at 0.05 μM. Sensitivity to the
inhibitors, as mentioned before, varies with cell types. In general,
cells grown in chemically defined medium are more sensitive to
inhibition than are cells grown in serum containing medium, and
established cell lines are more susceptible than primary cell
cultures. From Table 2 it can be seen that while 22-ketocholesterol
is a potent inhibitor in L cells it is not very effective in the
primary cultures of liver cells.

    The structures of inhibitory sterols identified so far are
shown in Figure 2. All of the compounds are derived from cholestane
by the introduction of one functional group, either a ketone or
hydroxyl function, at position 3 and a second functional group
(ketone or hydroxyl) in the 6,7,15,20,22,24, or 25 positions.
A nuclear double bond in the 4 or 5 position is not required. The
complete 8-carbon side chain is necessary for full activity. The
loss of one of the terminal methyl groups of the side chain results
in the loss of 70% of activity, whereas elimination of the three
terminal carbon atoms results in the loss of all activity. According to structural features mentioned above the number of compounds
which are inhibitory seems to be large, however, the inhibitory
potencies of many of them are relatively weak. Some of the better
inhibitors are listed in the order of decreasing activity on the
basis of tests with L cells: 25-hydroxycholesterol, 14α-methyl-
cholest-7-en-3β,15α-diol, 24(α,β)-hydroxycholesterol, 25-ketochol-
esterol, 20α-hydroxycholesterol, 22β-hydroxycholesterol, 7-keto-
cholestanol, 22-ketocholesterol, 6-ketocholestanol, 7-ketocholesterol,
7β-hydroxycholesterol, cholest-4-en-3,6-dione, 5α-cholestan-3,6-dione,
and 22α-hydroxycholesterol.

EFFECTS OF DIETARY STEROLS ON HEPATIC
CHOLESTEROGENESIS AND PLASMA CHOLESTEROL

    It has been long recognized that certain dietary sterols
including cholesterol, bile acids and other related sterols depress

TABLE 2

EFFECTS OF MODIFICATIONS OF THE STEROL SIDE CHAIN ON INHIBITORY ACTIVITY

| Steroid | Concentration required for 50% inhibition | | | |
| | Cell Cultures | | Primary Cultures of liver cells | |
	Sterol Synthesis*	HMG-CoA Reductase	Sterol Synthesis*	HMG-CoA Reductase
		(μM)		
20α-Hydroxycholesterol	1.2	1.5	5.7	3.2
22-Ketocholesterol	1.7	3.2	37.0	62.0
22α-Hydroxycholesterol	3.7	3.5	6.0	5.8
22β-Hydroxycholesterol	1.0	3.5	6.0	7.5
24(α,β)-Hydroxycholesterol	0.5	0.3	9.0	6
24-Ketocholesterol	0.7	1.3	2.5	16
25-Hydroxycholesterol	0.07	0.05	1.0	3.0
Cholest-5-en-3β, 17α, 20α-triol	>15.0			
β-Sitosterol	>15.0			
Stigmasterol	>15.0			
Ecdysterone	>15.0			
Kryptogenin	1.2	2.5	7.4	6.1
Tigogenin	12.0	>20.0	>75.0	>75.0
Diosgenin	11.0	>20.0	20.0	49.0

*Calculated as the ratio, ^{14}C-sterols to ^{14}C-fatty acids.

The preparation of sterol suspensions, conditions for incubating cultures with steroid-containing media, procedures for measuring the metabolism of acetate to digitonin-precipitable sterols, fatty acids, and CO_2 and methods for assaying HMG-CoA reductase, protein and DNA have been described (1,2). The sources of some of the sterols and values for their inhibitory activities have been reported previously (2). 24-ketocholesterol was purchased from Analabs. 24(α,β)-hydroxycholesterol was prepared by NaBH$_4$ reduction of 24-ketone. The mixture of epimeric diols was purified by preparative thin layer chromatography on silicic acid (solvents:ethylacetate-benzene; 30-60)-under conditions which did not result in their separation (11).

cholesterol synthesis in liver (9,10,12). The mechanism by which
the dietary sterols inhibit cholesterol synthesis is not well understood. Some regulatory fluctuations in the rate of sterol synthesis,
such as a diurnal cycle in the rate of sterol synthesis and
increases in sterol synthesis resulting from injecting Triton
WR1339 or by feeding the bile acid sequestering agent cholestyramine, are brought about by changes in the rate at which HMG–CoA
reductase is synthesized (8,11). Data presented by Higgins and
Rudney (13) indicate that dietary cholesterol affects sterol
synthesis by repressing the synthesis of HMG-CoA reductase, but in
addition inactivation of the enzyme seems to occur.

FIGURE 2
Sterols that Inhibit Sterol Synthesis and Depress HMG-CoA
Reductase Activity.

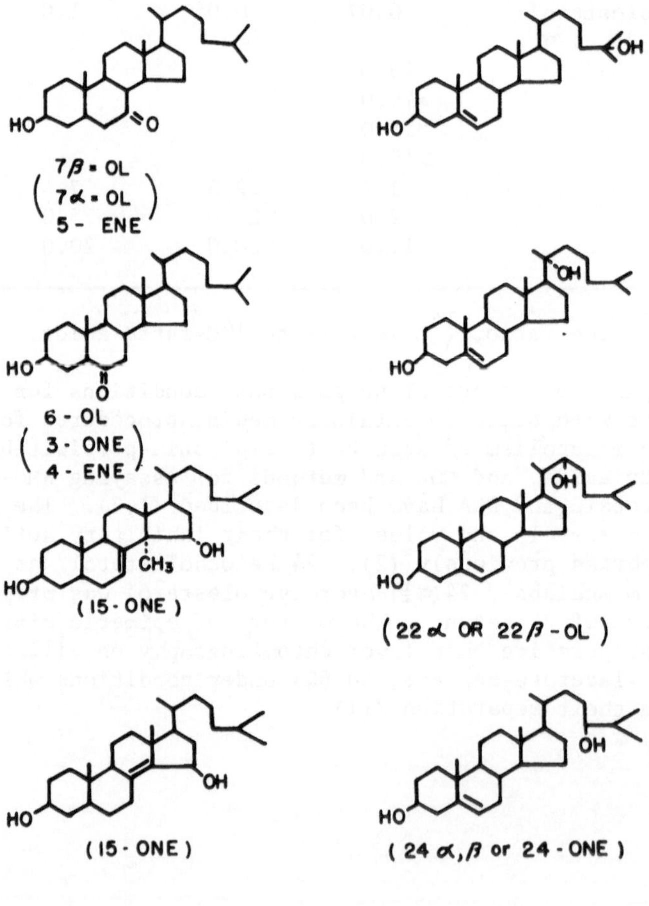

TABLE 3

EFFECTS OF DIETARY STEROLS ON HEPATIC CHOLESTEROGENESIS

Steroid*	0.25% of the Diet	0.1% of the Diet
	(% of the Control)	
Cholesterol	20 ± 5[a],[b]	61 ± 19[c]
Impure cholesterol	31 ± 10[a]	
7-Ketocholesterol	52 ± 20	
7(α,β)-Hydroxycholesterol	40 ± 8[a]	155 ± 23[a]
7-Ketocholestanol	98 ± 45	
6-Ketocholestanol	27 ± 6[a]	73 ± 16
5α-Cholestan-3,6-dione	54 ± 15[a]	138 ± 60
5α-Cholestan-3,6-diol	35 ± 11	42 ± 11[a]
Cholest-4-en-3,6-dione	20 ± 8[a]	48 ± 10[a]
5α-cholestan-3β,5α,6β-triol	93 ± 27	
20α-Hydroxycholesterol	105 ± 58	
20-Butyl-5-Pregnen-3β, 20α-diol	245 ± 35[a]	
20-Pentyl-5-Pregnen-3β, 20α-diol	90 ± 12	
22-Ketocholesterol	69 ± 1	
25-Hydroxycholesterol	24 ± 5[a]	75 ± 9
27-Nor-25-ketocholesterol	58 ± 15	
Kryptogenin	200 ± 39[a]	

[a]   Significant at the level of 0.029 or lower.

[b]   Average mean and standard error for 6 experiments.

[c]   Average mean and standard error for 2 experiments.

Pure cholesterol was obtained by passing Sigma CH-S grade cholesterol through the dibromide derivative followed by crystallization from methanol. The impure cholesterol preparation was the second crop of sterols obtained by crystallizing from methanol a standard cholesterol preparation from Schwartz/Mann. 7(α,β)-Hydroxycholesterol was purchased from Schwartz/Mann. 7-Ketocholesterol, 5α-cholestan-3,6dione, and 5α-cholestan-3β,5α,6β-triol were obtained from Steraloids and cholest-4-en-3,6-dione was from British Drug House (BDH). 5α-cholestan-3,6-diol was produced from 6-keto-cholestanol by NaBH$_4$ reduction followed by crystallization from

methanol: m.p. 192° (corrected) (ɑ)ᴅ + 12.8° ± 1.7 in chloroform
(ȼ= 2.5 g/100 ml). Sources of other sterols were as described
previously (1,2). Steroids were added to unpelleted Old Guilford
(Guilford, Conn.) chow containing 19% protein, 6% fat and other
nutrients and fed overnight (18 hours) to groups of 4 male C57BL/6J
mice 3 to 4 months of age as described previously (12). Rates of
acetate metabolism to sterols, fatty acids and CO_2 in liver slices
incubated in vitro were determined as described previously (1,8).

     Since certain derivatives of cholesterol which repress sterol
synthesis in cultured cells (1,2) are metabolites of cholesterol in
vivo   it is possible that one or more of these regulate sterol
synthesis in vivo and that the effect of dietary cholesterol upon
hepatic cholesterogenesis is due to its role as a precursor of an
inhibitory sterol. Whether or not inhibitors identified in studies
with cultured cells have a regulatory role in vivo it was of interest·
We determined their ability to inhibit hepatic cholesterogenesis when
they are fed with the diet.

     As is demonstrated in Table 3, when fed at a concentration of
0.25% of the diet 25-hydroxycholesterol, 6-ketocholestanol, and
cholest-4-en-3,6-dione and cholesterol inhibited the incorporation
of acetate into sterol by as much as 70 to 80%. Other sterols
including 7(ɑ,β)-hydroxycholesterol, 5ɑ-cholestan-3,6-diol, 7-keto-
cholesterol, 5ɑ-cholestan-3,6-dione, and 27-nor-25-ketocholesterol
appeared to be somewhat less effective so that sterol synthesis was
depressed to about one half of the control value. Two compounds,
20ɑ-hydroxycholesterol and 7-ketocholesterol, are effective in the
cell culture system but did not inhibit sterol synthesis to any
appreciable extent in vivo. It is possible that these sterols are
rapidly metabolized to other noninhibitory sterols upon feeding.
The interpretation of the data from experiments involving dietary
sterols is complex. The inhibitory activities, in vivo, of the
sterols measured under our conditions may be affected by the
extent to which they are absorbed, transported, and metabolized
within the animals. So far we have not studied these parameters.

     The effects of long term feeding of inhibitory sterols have not
yet been investigated thoroughly,in part, because of the cost of
sterols. Table 4 shows the effect upon plasma cholesterol levels of
feeding one of the more readily available sterols, 6-ketocholestanol,
to strains of mice for as long as 12 days. 6-Ketocholestanol is a
relatively good inhibitor of sterol synthesis in cell cultures and
also in liver after overnight feeding as shown in Table 4. However,
the compound did not significantly lower the plasma cholesterol level
after up to 12 days of feeding to AKR/J mice or to a partially inbred
line of mice which was selected for high plasma cholesterol. The
control of the plasma cholesterol level in animals is complex,and

it is quite stable in mice. Factors which regulate the synthesis of cholesterol, the uptake of dietary sterol, elimination of choles- terol either unchanged or as bile acids, and sizes of the pools of free and esterified cholesterol can all contribute to the level of cholesterol in blood. Thus, inhibition of hepatic cholesterogenesis may not produce an appreciable effect upon the overall level of cholesterol in blood during a short period of time.

TABLE 4

THE EFFECT OF FEEDING 6-KETOCHOLESTANOL ON PLASMA
CHOLESTEROL LEVELS IN MICE

Mice	Day 0	Day 3	Day 5	Day 7	Day 12
AKR/J	157 ± 6	-	115 ± 11	-	145 ± 5
High cholesterol line	338 ± 11	330 ± 14	-	333 ± 0.07	-

Values are expressed as mean $\pm$ S.E. of mg cholesterol per 100 ml of plasma. 6-Ketocholestanol was fed to groups of 6 mice, 3-5 months of age. Cholesterol was assayed in 20 μl of plasma using a Hycel reagent (Hycel, Inc., Houston, Texas) for AKR/J mice and perchloric acid-phosphoric acid-ferric chloride reagent (14) for the high plasma cholesterol line of mice. The latter line of mice was originally selected for high plasma cholesterol (15) then maintained by brother-sister mating for 16 generations.

Hopefully, our studies of steroid inhibitors of sterol synthesis will provide a basis for the identification or preparation of other compounds which can be used to control sterol synthesis in vivo. Ideally such an inhibitory compound should be absorbed and transported effectively to sterol synthesizing cells and should be metabolized at a low rate.

ACKNOWLEDGEMENTS

This study was supported by a research grant CA02758 from the National Cancer Institute. The Jackson Laboratory is fully accredited by the American Association for Accreditation of Laboratory Animal Care.

REFERENCES

1. Kandutsch, A. A. and H. W. Chen. 1973. Inhibition of sterol
synthesis in cultured mouse cells by 7α-hydroxycholesterol,
7β-hydroxycholesterol, and 7-ketocholesterol. J. Biol. Chem.
248:8408-8417.

2. Kandutsch, A. A. and H. W. Chen. 1974. Inhibition of sterol
synthesis in cultured mouse cells by cholesterol derivatives
oxygenated in the side chain. J. Biol Chem. 249:6057-6061.

3. Chen, H. W., A. A. Kandutsch, and C. Waymouth. 1974. Inhibition
of cell growth by oxygenated derivatives of cholesterol. Nature
251:419-421.

4. Kandutsch, A. A. and H. W. Chen. 1975. Regulation of sterol
synthesis in cultured cells by oxygenated derivatives of
cholesterol. J. Cell. Physiol. 85:415-424.

5. Chen, H. W., H.-J. Heiniger, and A. A. Kandutsch. 1975.
Relationship between sterol synthesis and DNA synthesis in
phytohemagglutinin-stimulated mouse lymphocytes. Proc. Nat.
Acad. Sci. U.S.A. 72:1950-1954.

6. Rothblatt, G. 1969. The effect of serum components on sterol
synthesis in L cells. J. Cell. Physiol. 74:163-170.

7. Rothblatt , G. H., C. H. Burns, R. L. Connor and J. R. Landrey.
1970. Desmosterol as the major sterol in L-cell mouse fibroblasts
grown in sterol-free culture medium. Science 169:880-882.

8. Kandutsch, A. A. and S. E. Saucier, 1969. Prevention of cyclic
and Triton-induced increases in hydroxymethylglutaryl coenzyme A
reductase and sterol synthesis by puromycin. J. Biol. Chem.
244:2299-2305.

9. Siperstein, M. D. 1970. Regulation of cholesterol biosynthesis
in normal and malignant tissues. Curr. Top. Cell. Regul. 2:65-100.

10. Rodwell , V. W., D. J. McNamara and D. J. Shapiro. 1973.
Regulation of hepatic 3-hydroxy-3-methylglutaryl coenzyme A
reductase. Adv. Enzymol. 38:373-412.

11. Van Tier, J. E. and L. L. Smith. 1970. Sterol metabolism XIII.
Chromatographic resolution of the epimeric 24-hydroxycholesterols.
J. Chromatog. 49:555-575.

12. Kandutsch, A. A. and R. M. Packie. 1970. Comparison of the
effects of some C_{27}-, C_{21}-, and C_{19}- steroids upon sterol

synthesis and hydroxymethylglutaryl-CoA reductase activity. Arch, Biochem. Biophys. 140:122-130.

13. Higgins, M., and H. Rudney. 1973. Regulation of rat liver β-hydroxy-β-methylglutaryl-CoA reductase activity by cholesterol. Nature 246:60-61.

14. Momose, T., Ueda, Y., Yamamoto, K., Masumura, T. and Ohta, K. 1963. Determination of total cholesterol in blood serum with perchloric acid-phosphoric acid-ferric chloride reagent. Anal. Chem. 35:1751-1753.

15. Weibust, R. S. 1973. Inheritance of plasma cholesterol levels in mice. Genetics 73:303-312.

MECHANISM OF INHIBITION OF CHOLESTEROL UPTAKE BY THE ARTERIAL WALL

R.J. Bing, J.S.M. Sarma, R. Fischer, S. Ikeda

Huntington Memorial Hospital, Pasadena, and University
of Southern California, Los Angeles, California
100 Congress Street, Pasadena, California 91105

Our early studies on in vitro perfused aortas and coronary
arteries have dealt with lipid synthesis and cholesterol (cholest-
5-en-3β-ol) uptake by the arterial wall. In the course of these
studies, we noticed that the addition of 7-ketocholesterol (3β-
hydroxycholest-5-en-7one) to the perfusion fluid resulted in a
significant inhibition of cholesterol uptake by the arterial wall
of different species, without interfering with lipid synthesis.
Because of this finding, this report will be primarily concerned
with this inhibition and its mechanisms. However earlier studies
on lipid synthesis and cholesterol uptake by isolated perfused
arteries will also be discussed since the technique and the results
have a bearing on inhibitory effects of 7-ketocholesterol.

MATERIALS AND METHODS

Our methods have been described in detail in a number of
publications (1,2,3,4,5). Briefly for the studies in vitro, coronary arteries from human cadavers and rabbit aortas were
perfused in vitro. The human material was obtained from autopsy
material up to five hours after death using sterile techniques.
The length of the vessels used in the perfusion experiments ranged
from 2 to 3 cm. After dissection, the vessels were perfused for a
period of 4 hours at 37° C with a perfusion pressure of 130/100 mm
Hg at a pulsatile rate of 80. A modified Carrel-Lindbergh pump
was employed in all experiments (6).

The basic perfusion fluid consisted of sterile autologous
plasma. [3H]1,2-cholesterol (250μCi) in benzene solution was placed

in a test tube and evaporated under a stream of nitrogen. After
addition of 5 ml of human plasma, the mixture was sonicated in an
ice-water bath three times for 1 minute each at intervals of about
1 minute, using a Biosonik III with a microtip. The sonicated
mixture was then made up to a volume of about 125 ml with plasma
and shaken for two hours at room temperature. The tritium radioactivity was located mainly in the β and pre β lipoprotein fractions
and to a smaller extent in chylomicrons. When lipid synthesis was
studied, the incubated mixture was combined with a basic perfusion
fluid to which 250 μCi of $[^{14}C]$ acetate had been previously added.
The total perfusion mixture was made up to 250 ml. After extraction according to the method of Folch, analyses were carried out
on the vascular wall with the exception of the adventitia. The
tissues were weighed and frozen in liquid nitrogen and crushed
in a mortar.

     Separation of lipids was accomplished by thin-layer chroma-
tography on silica gel according to the method of Freeman and West
(7). The separate fractions were eluted from thin-layer plates
with elution solvents appropriate for the corresponding fraction.
7-ketocholesterol gave a distinct spot, detectable by ultraviolet
light, which could be quantitated as the trimethyl-silyl ether
derivative by gas chromatography column at 280o C (8). Radioactivity was counted in a Tri-Carb liquid scintillation spectrometer. The method of Zak was used for determination of
cholesterol in plasma extract and in the eluate (9).

     When 7-ketocholesterol was added to the perfusion fluid, a
100 mg sample of 7-ketocholesterol was dissolved in 5 ml of
chloroform/methanol (2:1) mixture and the solution was equally
divided into 10 different test tubes. Each tube was then quickly
evaporated in order to obtain a fine coating of 7-ketocholesterol.
About 5 ml of plasma was then placed in each test tube and
sonicated as described above. After sonication the contents of
the test tubes were pooled and brought to a volume of 125 ml with
fresh plasma and incubated in a shaker bath for two hours at 37o
C (4). In experiments in vivo rabbits were intravenously injected
with ketocholesterol using a bile salt (sodium glycocholate) as
the solubilizing agent (5). Control animals received only the
bile salt. It could be shown that bile salts alone do not interfere with the uptake of 7-ketocholesterol by the vascular wall
(Fig. 1). Sonication of cholesterol was carried out in a manner
similar to that described earlier: about 5 ml of the animal's
own plasma were sonicated with 250 μCi of $[^{3}H]$ 1,-2cholesterol,
which was injected into the rabbit through an ear vein (5). The
rabbit was sacrificed 1 1/2 hours later and the aorta was dissected,
cleaned and washed. A blood sample was collected just prior
to killing the animal.

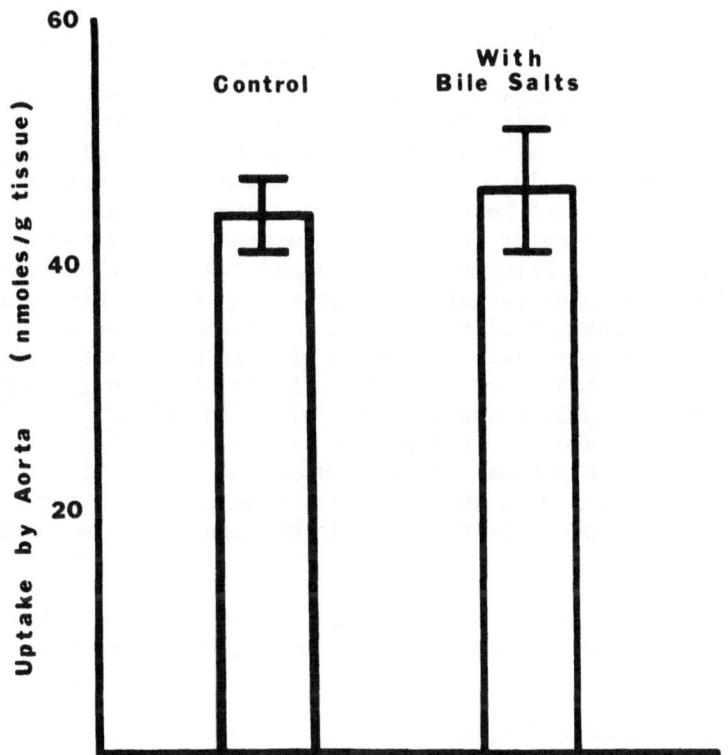

Figure 1. The effect of i.v. injection of six boli (50 mg bile salts each) at 15 minute intervals.

The aorta and plasma were analyzed as described previously.
A water soluble complex of sodium glycocholate and 7-ketocholesterol
(molecular ratios 2:1), which remained clear for about 3 minutes,
was prepared as follows: 25 mg of 7-ketocholesterol and 50 mg of
bile salt were dissolved in about 1.5 ml of 2:1 chloroform/methanol
mixture. The solution was then evaporated at a fast rate. Five
ml of sterile saline were then added. The mixture dissolved in
saline, forming a clear solution which was immediately injected
into the animal (5). If the saline solution was left standing,
7-ketocholesterol began to separate after 3 minutes. If this
solution was injected into the rabbits after separation, the
animal died within a few minutes. The animals received 4 to 6
injections in equal intervals during a 1 1/2 hour period. When
7-ketocholesterol was administered by stomach tube, 200-400 mg of
7-ketocholesterol along with an equal amount of sodium glycocholate
were dissolved in about 15 ml Folch mixture and the solvent was
evaporated in vacuo. The resultant solid mixture was suspended
in 20 ml of saline by means of a glass homogenizer and fed to the
rabbit through a No. 7 Foley catheter introduced into the stomach.
The balloon of the Foley catheter was partially filled with gastro-
graphin to verify its position below the diaphragm under a fluoro-
scope. For feeding purposes, the ratio of bile salt to steroid
was reduced to 1:1 because of laxative effects of the bile salt.
About 5 ml of fresh plasma was labelled with 250 μCi of [3H]-choles-
terol, as described above. This plasma was then injected into the
rabbit from which the plasma had been obtained. Extraction of the
lipids of the arterial wall was carried out as described above,
and separation of lipids was carried out by means of thin-layer
chromatography.

Analysis and countings were carried out as described above.
The cholesterol uptake by the aorta was calculated using the
formula:

cholesterol uptake (nmoles/gm) =

$$\frac{[3H] \text{ DPM/gm aorta} \times \text{free cholesterol content (nmoles/ml) plasma}}{[3H] \text{ DPM/ml plasma}},$$

where DPM represents the "disintegrations per minute"

RESULTS

It is apparent from the in vitro perfusion experiments, that
under these experimental conditions, neither cholesterol nor cholesteryl esters are synthesized by human coronary arteries (2,3).
Synthesis of other lipid fractions from [14C] acetate was observed
in all species perfused. In rabbit and pig arteries there was some

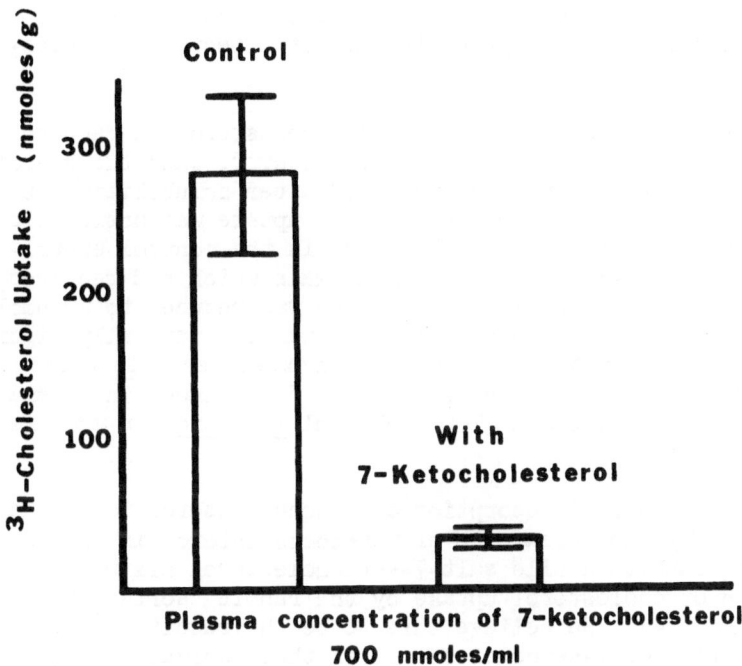

Figure 2.   Competitive inhibition of cholesterol uptake by
7-ketocholesterol in vitro.

synthesis of cholesterol; however it did not exceed 5% of the total [^{14}C] radioactivity.

The main thrust of our investigation was based on our finding that the addition of 7-ketocholesterol to the perfusion fluid significantly diminished cholesterol uptake by coronary arteries and aortas of man, rabbit, and pig (4,5). These results are summarized in Fig. 2 which shows a significant reduction of cholesterol uptake from 280 to 50 nmoles/g tissue, using concentrations of 7-ketocholesterol of approximately 700 nmoles/ml plasma in the perfusion fluid. This difference was highly significant (p < .001). The inhibition was reduced at 7-ketocholesterol concentrations below 50 nmoles/ml. Lipid synthesis was not affected by 7-ketocholesterol (4).

Inhibitory effects in vivo of 7-ketocholesterol in rabbits were more difficult to demonstrate (5). However, when the steroid was administered by intravenous injection after solubilizing it in bile salts, some inhibition of cholesterol uptake was noticeable (Fig. 3). The mean uptake of cholesterol in the control experiments was 30 nmoles (± 8).   In animals which had received the inhibitory steroid, cholesterol uptake was reduced to 20 nmoles (± 5) (Fig. 3). Although this difference was statistically significant (p < .05), it was less than that in experiments in vitro (Fig. 2). This is probably the result of differences in plasma concentration of the steroid (700 nmoles/ml in vitro, as compared to 13 nmoles/ml in vivo).

Although intestinal absorption of ketocholesterol takes place as illustrated by the appearance of 7-ketocholesterol in plasma after feeding rabbits a bile salt-7-ketocholesterol mixture (10), no inhibition of cholesterol uptake by the rabbit aortas was noticeable (Fig. 4). We believe this to be the result of relatively low concentration of 7-ketocholesterol in these animals. Figure 4 illustrates that the plasma concentration of 7-ketocholesterol achieved was only 2.2 ± 0.4 nmoles/ml plasma.

DISCUSSION

The experiments described deal with lipid synthesis and cholesterol uptake in isolated perfused coronary arteries and aortas of a variety of species (man, rabbit and pig), and with the inhibitory effect of 7-ketocholesterol in both in vitro and in vivo animal preparations. The advantages of the in vitro technique employed here are maintenance of sterility and flexibility of experimental design. Thus, in previously published reports from this laboratory, human saphenous veins could be perfused with a variety of pressures and human coronary arteries were exposed to a wide

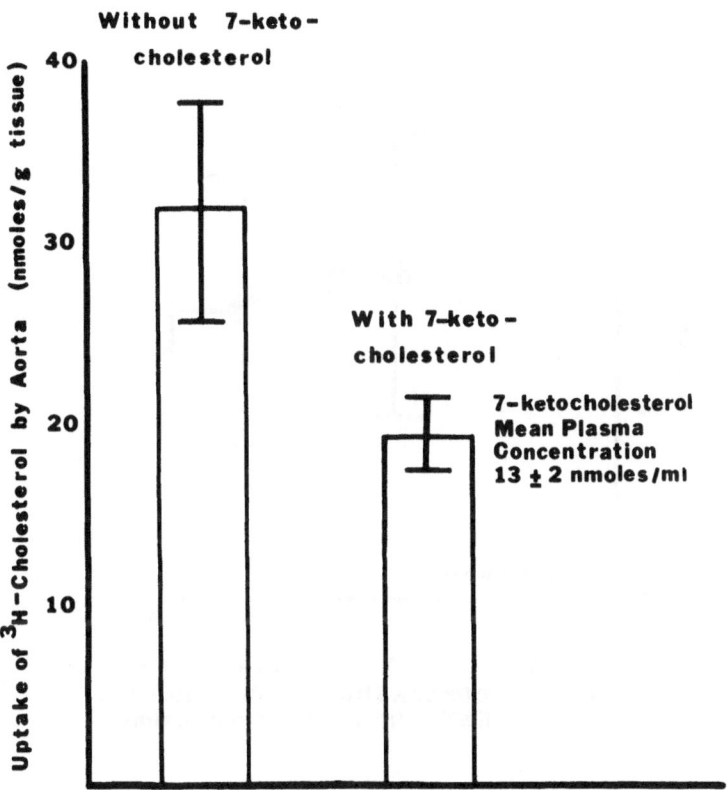

Figure 3. The effect of i.v. injection of four and six boli (25 mg 7-ketocholesterol and 50 mg bile salts each) at 20 minute intervals.

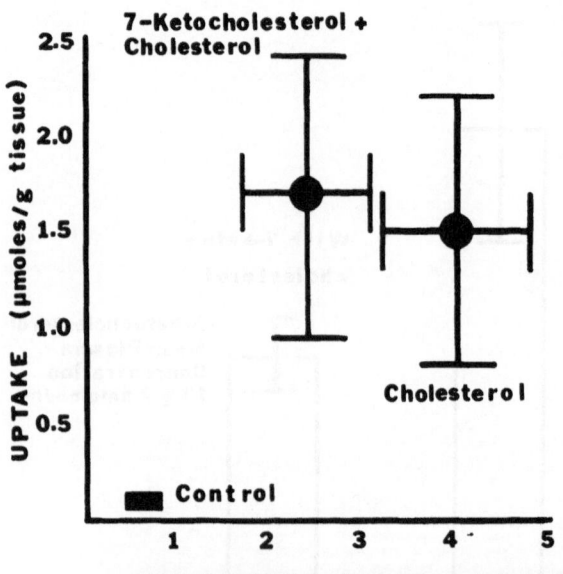

Figure 4. ^{3}H-cholesterol uptake versus plasma free cholesterol
after three weeks of gastric feeding.

range in carboxyhemoglobin concentrations of the perfusion fluid
(2,3). Other advantages of perfusion in vitro are a relatively
steady concentration of both carrier lipids and of labelled cholesterol in the perfusion fluid. Zilversmit has stressed that after
a single i.v. injection of the label into animals, the specific
activity of plasma cholesterol continuously decreases, while the
specific activity of cholesterol in the artery increases (11). In
our experiments in vitro, the specific activity of plasma cholesterol remained constant. Solubilizing the labelled cholesterol
in plasma represented a major difficulty. We chose to sonicate
the [3H] cholesterol in the animals own plasma, rather than using
a detergent or alcohol. Nilsson and Zilversmit have demonstrated
that after injection of an alcoholic solution, the steroid is
taken up by the Kupfer cells in the liver or by macrophages (12).
When sonicating the labelled cholesterol with plasma, we found
that the tritium radioactivity was located mainly in the β and pre
β lipoprotein fractions and to a smaller extent in the chylomicrons.
When 7-ketocholesterol was fed to rabbits, it was solubilized with
the salt of a bile acid (Na glycocholate). Under these conditions
radioactivity appeared in the plasma within 2 hours, reaching a
peak after 10 hours (10).

Failure of the human and pigs artery to form cholesterol from
[14C]-acetate is in line with the reports of some workers (13,14).
However others concluded that arterial cholesterol was subject to
turnover (15,16). It is likely that differences in species and
experimental conditions play a role in the differences observed.
In the studies of Zilversmit (13) and of Dayton and Hashimoto
(17), Jensen (18) and of Day et al (19), uptake of labelled cholesterol by the arterial wall in vivo appeared to be similar to
that observed in vitro. Inactivation of enzymes by metabolic
inhibitors, or by boiling strips of aorta prior to incubation with
labelled cholesterol, had no effect on cholesterol uptake (20,21).
From experiments published in this and other laboratories on the
effect of carbon monoxide or collagenase it is clear however that
a barrier exists, which when removed leads to an augmented influx
of cholesterol into the vascular wall (3,22). These findings are
also supported by the conclusions of Somer and Schwartz (23) and
of Bondjers and Björkernd (24). We also determined that cholesterol
uptake in perfused human saphenous veins increases with the perfusion pressure (2).

Two questions raised by these results concern the nature and
fate of 7-ketocholesterol in the body, and the mechanism of inhibition of cholesterol uptake.

Mitton and coworkers have found that certain conditions summarized as autoxidation, or non-enzymic degradation of cholesterol,
are responsible for the formation of cholesterol oxidation products

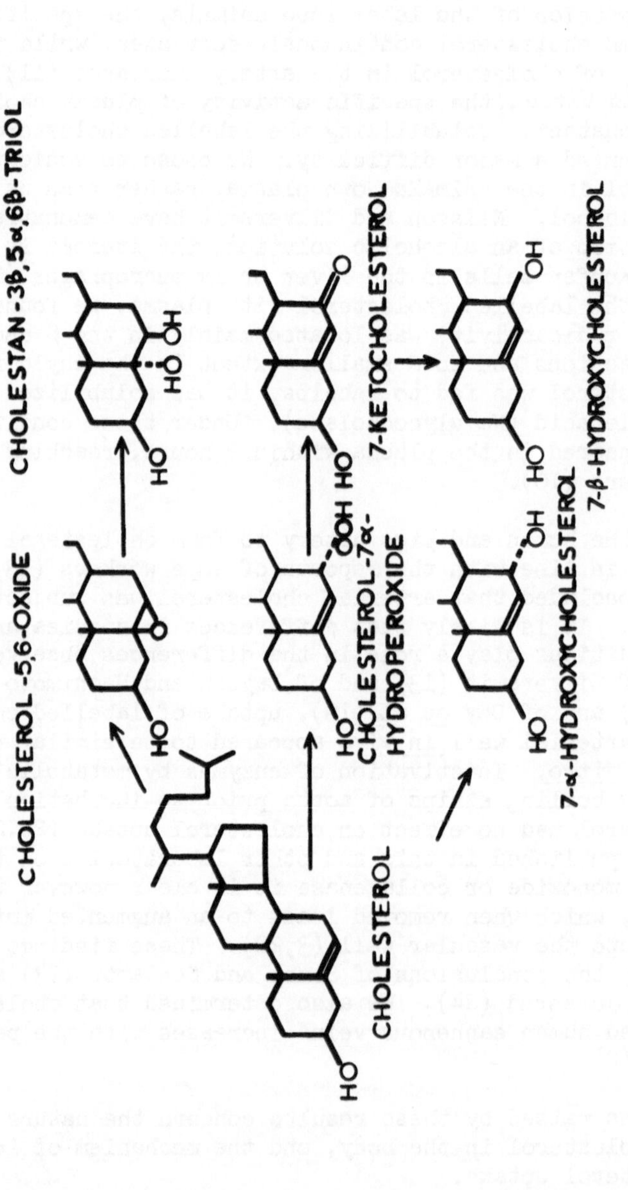

Figure 5

such as 7-ketocholesterol, 7β-hydroxycholesterol and cholestan-
3β, 5α, 6β-triol (25) (Fig. 5). These three compounds, in contrast
to 7α-hydroxycholesterol, which is the product of 7α-hydroxylation
in liver microsomes, are not converted to bile acids (25). 7-keto-
cholesterol may be present in blood vessels in vivo. Van Lier
and Smith found this steroid, together with some other 20 odd
sterol-like components, in the polar lipid fraction of the human
aorta (26). These authors do not believe that 7-ketocholesterol
encountered in human aortal tissue was generated by their analytical
and isolation technique. 7-ketocholesterol also was isolated from
whole aortas by Hardegger and his associates (27), by Kantiengar
and Morton (28) and by Brooks and associates (29).

The isolation of 7-ketocholesterol by analytical techniques
presents considerable difficulties. Mitton and coworkers demonstrated that several 7-ketocholesterol-like sterols have similar
mobilities on thin-layer plates (25). Furthermore, they found,
in thin-layer chromatogram scans on reduction of the 7-ketocholes-
terol fraction with lithium aluminum hydride, a diversity of compounds with a mobility similar to 7-ketocholesterol (25). There
was no evidence that 7α-hydroxycholesterol is formed in significant
amounts from authentic 7-ketocholesterol or from the isolated 7-
ketocholesterol fraction (25). However, when 7-ketocholesterol is
incubated with liver fractions, 7β-hydroxycholesterol is formed in
the organism as well as by autoxidation in vitro. However, the
formation of 7-ketocholesterol and 7β-hydroxycholesterol represents
a metabolic cul de sac: neither 7-ketocholesterol nor 7β-hydroxy-
cholesterol are precursors of bile acids.

The inhibitory effects of 7-ketocholesterol on cholesterol
synthesis were first described by Kandutsch and Chen and later by
Brown and Goldstein (30,31). In order to consider the question
on the mechanism of inhibition of cholesterol uptake by 7-keto-
cholesterol, the relevance of the results of Goldstein and Brown
to our results is challenging. The pertinent features of their
work can be briefly outlined: using tissue cultures they found
that the enzyme 3-hydroxy-3-methylglutaryl coenzyme A reductase
was low in normal fibroblasts grown in standard tissue culture
medium containing whole serum. When the low density lipoprotein
(LDL) fractions of serum were removed from the culture medium,
enzyme activity was 40-fold. When the low density lipoproteins were
replaced, HMG-CoA reductase declined (31,32).

Cells from homozygotes with familial hypercholesterolemia had
a much higher level of HMG-CoA reductase activity, which did not
increase when lipoproteins were removed, nor did it decrease,
when LDL were returned to the medium (30,31). It was suggested
that the homozygote's cells possess a genetically determined resistance to feedback suppression by LDL. When cholesterol was added

to an LDL-free culture medium from both normal and homozygous cell
lines, the response was a reduction of HMG-CoA reductase activity.
This effect was 100 times greater with 7-ketocholesterol. Several
conclusions were drawn by the authors from these observations
(30,31):

A normal feedback suppression of HMG-CoA reductase by LDL
exists in cells from normal individuals. It is initiated by LDL.

Resistance to feedback suppression by LDL is present in
homozygotes with familial hypercholesterolemia.

The homozygous cell possesses all the factors to suppress HMG-
CoA reductase,   provided that cholesterol is able to reach the
intracellular space.

In the normal cell, an increase in low density lipoproteins
leads to a reduction in activity of HMG-CoA reductase, but stimulates both cholesteryl esterification and the transfer of cholesterol into the cell. Non-lipoprotein cholesterol results in
these cell lines in a reduced activity of HMG-CoA reductase, and
an increase in intracellular cholesteryl esterification and transfer of cholesterol into the cell.

The crux of their work lies in the assumption of the presence
of LDL receptors at the cell wall.

If their conclusions are applicable to our findings, inhibition
of cholesterol uptake by perfused coronary arteries could result
from inhibition of HMG-CoA reductase activity in the arterial wall.
However, since human coronary arteries do not form cholesterol, it
is unlikely this mechanism is of importance. The difficulty in
applying the conclusions of Goldstein and coworkers to our findings
lies mainly in the fact that we do not deal with cholesterol synthesis, but with cholesterol uptake. Our results may eventually
be explained by assuming that an increase in 7-ketocholesterol in
plasma or perfusion fluid leads to an increase in intracellular
7-ketocholesterol, thus inhibiting cholesterol transfer across the
cell membrane. What role, if any, binding sites at the cell surface play in this mechanism is not yet clear. There is the possibility, as yet unproven, that both cholesterol and 7-ketocholesterol
actively compete for identical and specific binding sites on the
cell surface. Incubating low concentrations of I^{125}-labelled LDL
with monolayer of fibroblasts, Goldstein and Brown found a time-
dependent binding of LDL to the normal cell (31). When the amount
of unlabelled native LDL was increased, the binding of I^{125} LDL
was markedly reduced, indicating that the isotopically marked LDL
and the native LDL competed for the same specific binding sites.
We found that both 7-ketocholesterol and cholesterol compete for

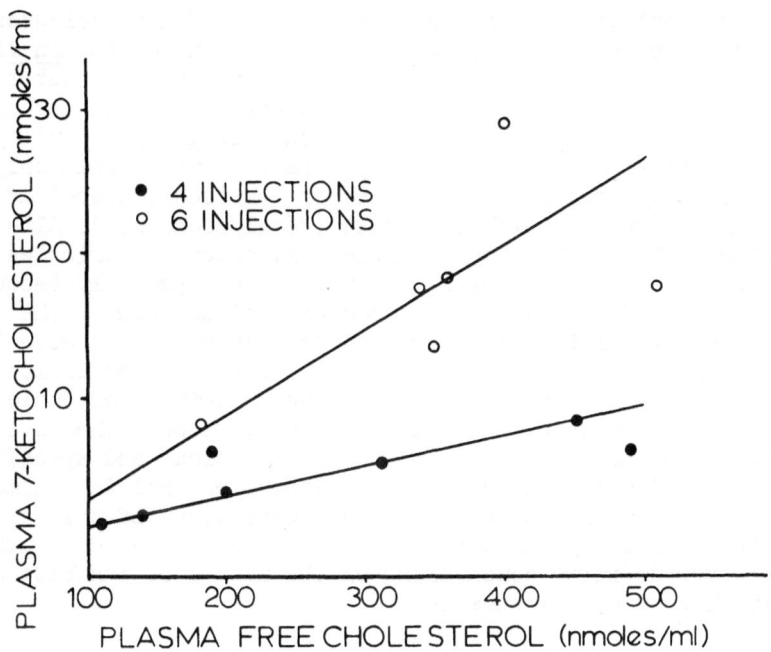

Figure 6

binding sites with plasma proteins, presumably LDL (5). This is illustrated in Fig. 6 which demonstrates a direct relationship between plasma cholesterol and plasma 7-ketocholesterol, following the intravenous infusion of 7-ketocholesterol. This suggests that the two steroids compete with the carrier proteins in plasma. A similar competition may exist at the cell surface.

SUMMARY

Experiments have been described dealing with lipid synthesis and cholesterol uptake in perfused human and pig coronary arteries, rabbit aortas, and with the inhibitory effect of 7-ketocholesterol on cholesterol uptake in these preparations and in rabbits in vivo. Human and pigs coronary arteries failed to synthesize cholesterol in vitro. 7-ketocholesterol inhibited cholesterol uptake in human coronary arteries and aortas of pigs and rabbits in vitro and by rabbit aortas in vivo. The inhibitory effect in vivo could only be shown after repeated i.v. injections of 7-ketocholesterol after solubilizing the steroid with bile salt (Na-glycocholate). Although 7-ketocholesterol was absorbed from the G.I. tract, gastric feeding of the bile salt steroid complex was ineffective, probably because of inadequate blood levels of 7-ketocholesterol achieved. The metabolic fate of 7-ketocholesterol and the nature of its effect on cholesterol are discussed. It is not likely that inhibition of HMG-CoA reductase is responsible for the inhibition of cholesterol uptake. The possibility was discussed that both cholesterol and 7-ketocholesterol actively compete for identical and specific binding sites or that an increase in 7-ketocholesterol in plasma leads to an increase in intracellular concentrations of this steroid thus inhibiting cholesterol transfer across the cell membrane. However, definite conclusions on the nature of inhibition must await further experimentation.

ACKNOWLEDGEMENT

We wish to acknowledge with thanks the Margaret W. and Herbert Hoover, Jr. Foundation, the Kenneth T. and Eileen L. Norris Foundation and the Council for Tobacco Research--U.S.A., Inc. for their support of this work.

REFERENCES

1. Morita, T. and R.J. Bing. 1972. Lipid metabolism in perfused human coronary arteries. Proc. Soc. Exp. Biol. Med. 140: 617-622.

2. Hashimoto, H., H. Tillmanns, J.S.M. Sarma, J. Mao, E. Holden, and R.J. Bing. 1974. Lipid metabolism in perfused human non-atherosclerotic coronary arteries and saphenous veins. Atherosclerosis 19:35-45.

3. Sarma, J.S.M., H. Tillmanns, S. Ikeda, A. Grenier, E. Colby, and R.J. Bing. 1975. Lipid metabolism in perfused human and dog coronary arteries. Amer. J. Cardiol. 35:579-587.

4. Bing, R.J. and J.S.M. Sarma. 1975. In vitro inhibition of cholesterol uptake in human and animal arteries by 7-ketocholesterol. Biochem. Biophys. Res. Comm. 62:711-716.

5. Sarma, J.S.M., R. Fischer, S. Ikeda, and R.J. Bing. In vivo inhibition of cholesterol uptake in rabbit aortas by 7-keto-cholesterol. In press.

6. Carrel, A., and C.A. Lindbergh. 1938. The Culture of Organs. Harper and Row, New York.

7. Freeman, C.P. and D. West. 1966. Complete separation of lipid classes on a single thin-layer plate. J. Lipid Res. 7:324-328.

8. Van Lier, J.E. and L.L. Smith. 1968. Sterol metabolism II. Gas chromatographic recognition of cholesterol metabolites and artifacts. Anal.Biochem.24:419-430.

9. Zak, B., R.C. Dickenman, E.G. White, H. Burnett, and P.J. Cherney. 1954. Rapid estimation of free and total cholesterol. Amer. J. Clin. Path. 24:1307-1315.

10. Sarma, J.S.M., R. Fischer, S. Ikeda, and R.J. Bing. The fate of labelled 7-ketocholesterol in the body (in preparation).

11. Zilversmit, D.B. 1975. Mechanisms of cholesterol accumulation in the arterial wall. Amer. J. Cardiol. 35:559-566.

12. Nilsson, A., D.B. Zilversmit. 1972. Fate of intravenously administered particulate and lipoprotein cholesterol in the rat. J. Lipid Res. 13:32-38.

13. Zilversmit, D.B. 1968. Cholesterol flux in the atherosclerotic plaque. Ann. N.Y. Acad. Sci. 149:710-724.

14. Newman, H.A.I. and D.B. Zilversmit. 1962. Quantitative aspects of

cholesterol flux in rabbit. J. Biol. Chem. 237:2078-2084.

15. Chobanian, A.V., W. Hollander. 1962. Body cholesterol meta-
    bolism in man. I. The equilibration of serum and tissue cho-
    lesterol. J. Clin. Invest. 41:1732-1737.

16. Gould, R.G., R.W. Wissler, R.J. Jones. 1963. The dynamics of
    lipid deposition in arteries. In: Evolution of the athero-
    sclerotic Plaque. Edited by R.J. Jones. University of Chicago
    Press, Chicago, pp. 205-214.

17. Dayton, S., S. Hashimoto. 1970. Recent advances in molecular
    pathology: cholesterol flux and metabolism in arterial tissue
    and in atheromata. Exp. Mol. Pathol. 13:253-268.

18. Jensen, J. 1967. The kinetics of the in vitro cholesterol up-
    take at the endothelial cell surface of the rabbit aorta.
    Biochem. Biophys. Acta 135:544-556.

19. Day, A.J., M.L. Wahlqvist, D.J. Campbell. 1970. Differential
    uptake of cholesterol and of different cholesterol esters by
    atherosclerotic intima in vivo and in vitro. Atherosclerosis
    11:301-320.

20. Newman, H.A.I., D.B. Zilversmit. 1966. Uptake and release of
    cholesterol by rabbit atheromatous lesions. Circ. Res. 18:293-
    302.

21. Dayton, S., S. Hashimoto. 1966. Movement of labeled cholesterol
    between plasma lipoprotein and normal arterial wall across the
    intimal surface. Circ. Res. 19:1041-1049.

22. Zilversmit, D.B., H.A.I. Newman. 1966. Does a metabolic barrier
    to circulating cholesterol protect the arterial wall? Circu-
    lation 33:7.

23. Somer, J.B., C.J. Schwartz. 1971. Focal ^{3}H-cholesterol uptake
    in the pig aorta. Atherosclerosis 13:293-304.

24. Bondjers, G., S. Björkerud. 1973. Cholesterol accumulation and
    content in regions with defined endothelial integrity in the
    normal rabbit aorta. Atherosclerosis 17:71-83.

25. Mitton, J.R., N.A. Scholan and G.S. Boyd. 1971. The oxidation
    of cholesterol in rat liver subcellular particles. The choles-
    terol-7α-hydroxylase enzyme system. Eur. J. Biochem. 20:569-
    579.

26. Van Lier, J.E. and L.L. Smith. 1967. Sterol metabolism. I.

26-hydroxycholesterol in the human aorta. Biochem. $\underline{6}$:3269-3278.

27. Hardegger, E.L. Ruzicka, and E. Tagmann. 1943. Untersuchungen über Organextrakte zur Kenntnis der unverseifbaren Lipoide aus arteriosklerotischen Aorten. Helv. Chim. Acta. $\underline{26}$:2205-2221.

28. Kantiengar, N.L. and R. A. Morton. 1955. Cholesta-3:5-dien-7-one in human atherosclerotic aortas. Biochem. J. $\underline{60}$:25-28.

29. Brooks, C.J. W., W. A. Harland, G. Steel. 1966. Squalene, 26-hydroxycholesterol and 7-ketocholesterol in human athero-matous plaques. Biochem. Biophys. Acta. $\underline{125}$:620-622

30. Kandutsch, A.A., H. W. Chen. 1973. Inhibition of sterol synthe-sis in cultured mouse cells by 7α-hydroxycholesterol,7β-hydroxy-cholesterol, and 7-ketocholesterol. J. Biol. Chem. $\underline{248}$:8408-8417.

31. Brown, M.S., and J.L. Goldstein. 1974. Suppression of 3-hydroxy-3-methylglutaryl coenzyme A reductase activity and inhibition of growth of human fibroblasts by 7-ketocholesterol. J. Biol. Chem. $\underline{249}$:7306-7314.

32. Brown, M.S., J.R. Faust, and J.L. Goldstein. 1975. Role of the low density lipoprotein receptor in regulating the content of free and esterified cholesterol in human fibroblasts. J. Clin. Invest. $\underline{55}$:783-793.

LIPOPROTEIN UPTAKE AND DEGRADATION BY CULTURED HUMAN ARTERIAL

SMOOTH MUSCLE CELLS

Edwin L. Bierman, M.D. and John J. Albers, Ph.D.

Departments of Medicine and Biochemistry, University of

Washington School of Medicine, Seattle, Wash. 98195

ABSTRACT: The multipotential smooth muscle cell (SMC) is the predominant cell in intima and media of large arteries, proliferating early in the development of atheroma to become the lipid-laden foam cell. Homogeneous cultures of human SMC have now been successfully grown from explants of normal pieces of artery obtained during surgery. In contrast to previous results with rat SMC, human SMC preferentially bind and take up large, lipid-rich lipoproteins (I^{125} labeled low density and very low density lipoproteins)(LDL and VLDL), in comparison to smaller, high density lipoproteins (HDL). This species selectivity appears to be related to differences both in cells and in lipoproteins. Specific binding of lipoproteins by SMC, analyzed by release of radioactive protein from the cell surfaces by trypsin, accounted for approximately half of the protein radioactivity associated with the cell layer during the first few hours of incubation. Specific binding appears to be related to the presence of apoprotein B on the lipoproteins. Lipoproteins progressively accumulate within cells as a function of incubation time. Lipoprotein degradation, assessed by appearance of TCA soluble, non-iodide radioactivity in the incubation medium, increased rapidly after an initial delay of 2 to 4 hours. Cells grown under hypoxic (5% O_2) conditions instead of the usual room air showed impaired degradation of lipoproteins. These results suggest that there are receptors on arterial SMC, highly specific for different lipoproteins (as shown for skin fibroblasts). This tissue culture system

may be useful for assessment of the effects of a variety
of hormones, metabolites, and drugs on the handling of
lipoproteins by arterial smooth muscle cells.

The arterial smooth muscle cell appears to play a fundamental
role in the pathogenesis of atherosclerosis in both man (1) and
experimental animal (2). This is the cell that proliferates early
in the development of atherosclerotic lesions in response to a
variety of stimuli or "injury" (3), and accumulates intracellular
lipids in the presence of increased concentrations of extracellular lipoprotein to become the "foam cell" that characterizes
the lesion as the process progresses. In addition, these cells
may also be involved in the deposition of lipids in the extracellular connective tissue matrix. Thus abnormalities in metabolism of these cells, particularly with regard to their ability
to bind, internalize, and degrade triglyceride-rich and cholesterol-rich lipoproteins may be crucial to the development of
atherosclerosis.

The method for growing homogeneous cultures of diploid arterial smooth muscle cells from subhuman primates was developed
by Ross (3,4) and successfully applied to growing cells from
human arteries. This method is now generally available; in addition to human and monkey cells, rat (5), guinea pig (4), rabbit
(6), and pig (7), arterial smooth muscle cells have been grown and
maintained in tissue culture. It has previously been shown that
cultured arterial smooth muscle cells proliferate in response to a
variety of stimuli, including low density lipoproteins (LDL) (3),
a potent platelet factor (8), and physiological concentrations of
insulin (9). These observations are consistent with the hypothesis that the sequence of events involved in atheroma formation
begins with "injury" to the endothelium and exposure of subendothelial tissues to plasma constituents including lipoproteins,
hormones and platelet factors.

Thus the ability to study these cells growing in culture in
response to a variety of agents provides a useful experimental
technique which may have relevance to the processes involved in
atherogenesis. Human arterial smooth muscle cell cultures have
now been successfully obtained from explants of intimal-medial
segments of tissue obtained during vascular surgery of the aorta,
iliac, femoral and renal arteries from both normals and individuals
with atherosclerosis. No obvious differences related to the site
of origin of the cells have been observed to date. These cells
share the morphological and growth characteristics of smooth muscle
cells cultured from other species, and the cultures are free of
fibroblast contamination. They differ from human fibroblasts
(both skin and adventitial) by their longer lag period before out-
growth from explants, their slower growth rate (logarithmic growth

ends at about 7 to 10 days) (Fig. 1), and their characteristic morphology (3). Smooth muscle cells contain abundant myofilaments with dense bodies, and grow in multilayers with hills and valleys rather than in a single monolayer (Figs. 2 and 3).

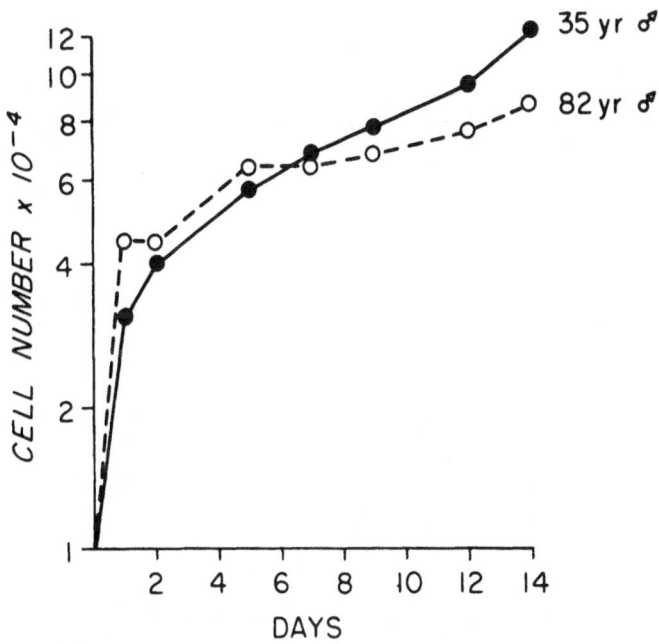

Fig. 1. Growth curves of cultures of arterial SMC obtained from explants of popliteal artery from 35 yr man and femoral artery from 82 yr man. On day 0, 10^4 cells after 3rd passage were plated in 35mm Petri dishes in 2ml Dulbecco-Vogt medium containing 10% fetal calf serum. Medium was changed 3x/wk. Data points represent mean of 4 cell counts in 2 replicate dishes.

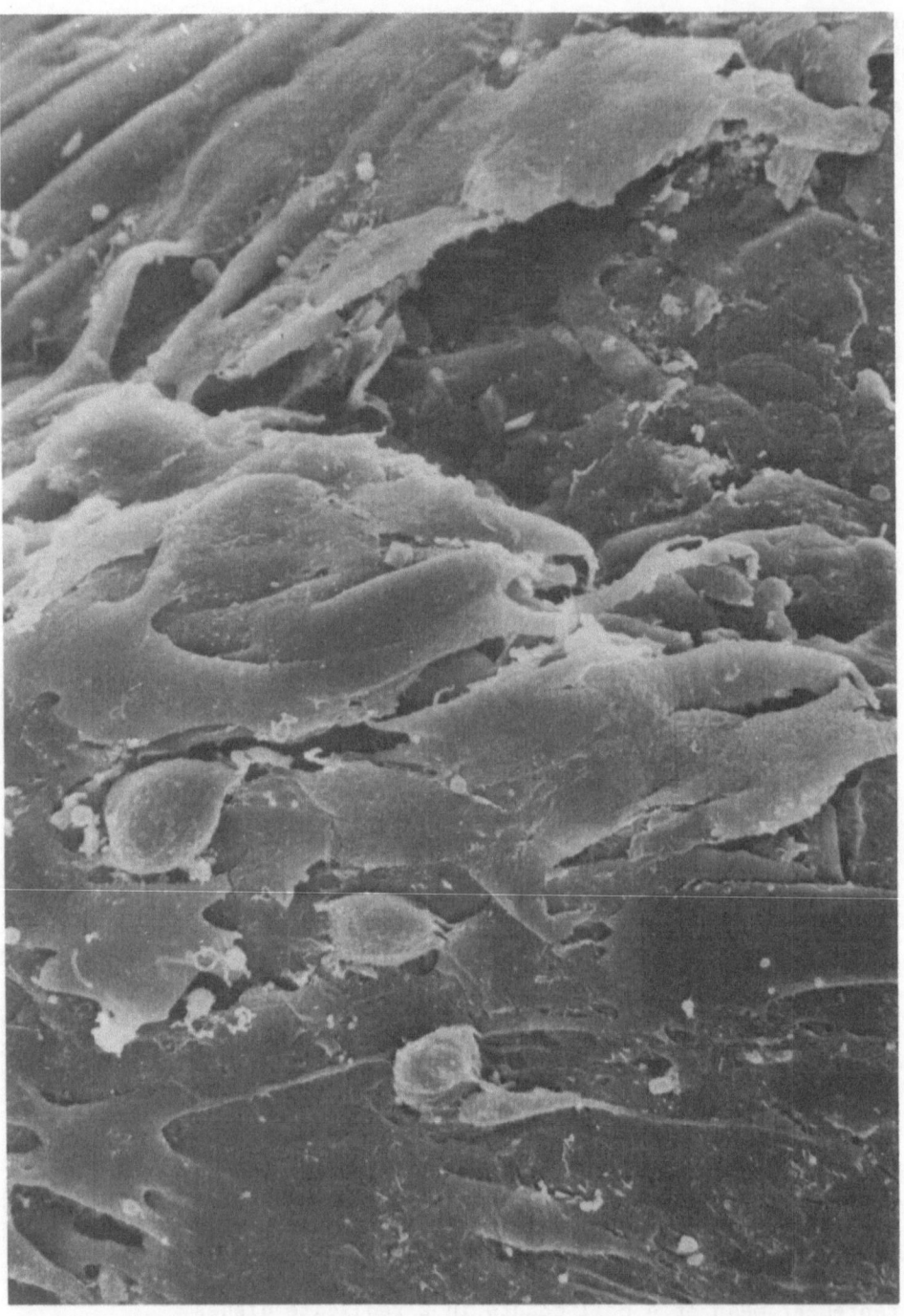

Figs. 2 and 3.   Scanning electron micrographs of human aortic
smooth muscle cells obtained from aorta of a 1 year old donor.
Cells have formed a multi-layered colony. Note uneven surface of
colony.   X 900.   (Performed by Dr. Phillip H. Smith)

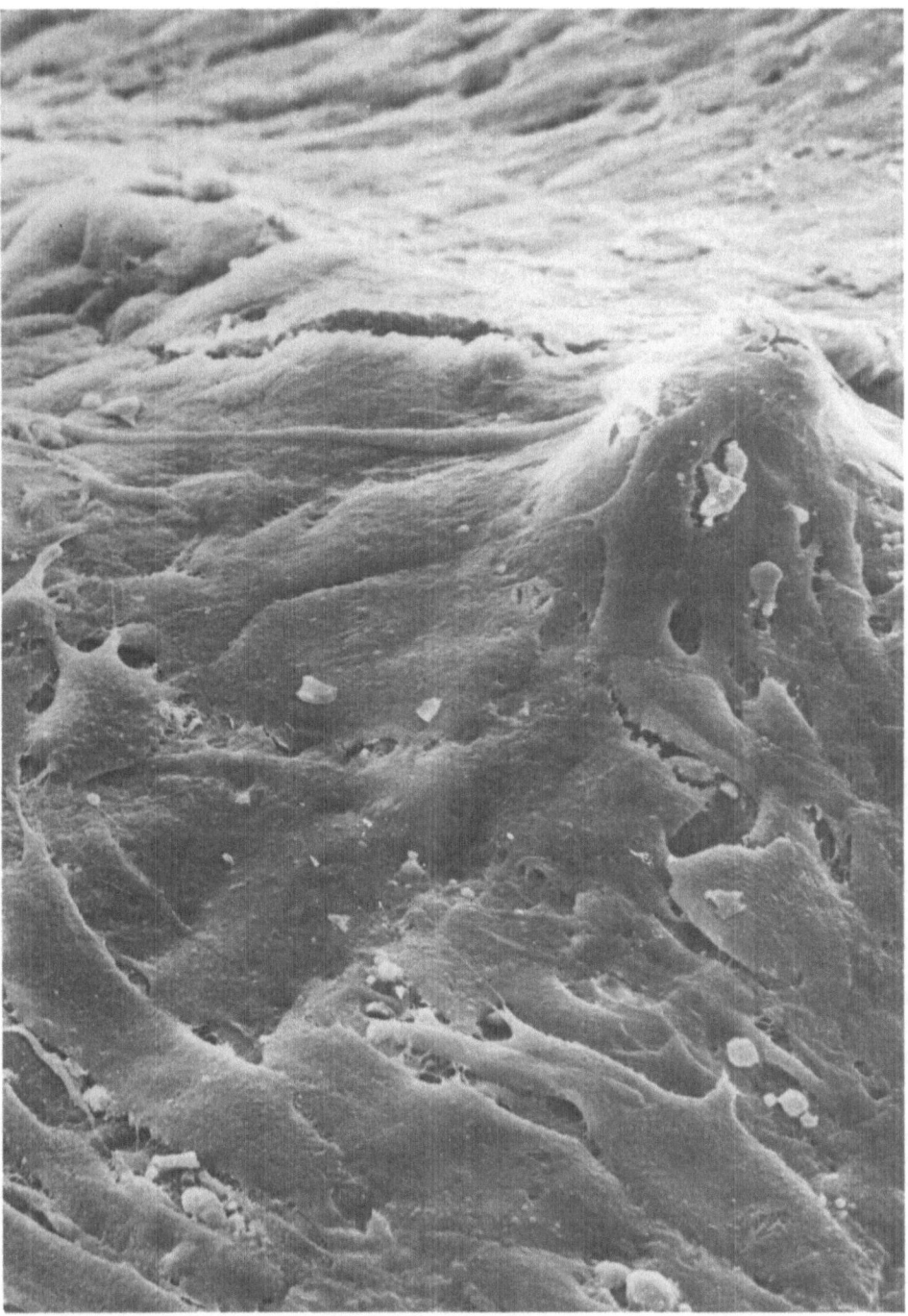

Fig. 3.

Methods for studying the interaction of these cells in culture with homologous I^{125} labeled lipoproteins have been published
elsewhere (5), and provide means for assessment of lipoprotein
binding, uptake and degradation. Binding, measured as surface
bound radioactivity releasable by trypsin, appears to be rapid and
specific. Internalization of lipoproteins presumably by pino-
cytosis is progressive during incubation and can be demonstrated
both by radioautography and by measurement of protein counts in
cell extracts after trypsinization (5). Degradation of iodinated
lipoproteins result in the appearance of water soluble (iodide-
free) protein breakdown products in the medium, which after an
initial delay, increases progressively up to 48 hours (10). It
appears that fibroblasts degrade I^{125} low density lipoproteins
more rapidly than do arterial smooth muscle cells (Fig. 4).

A marked species difference was demonstrated in relation to
specificity of lipoprotein uptake. While homologous high density
lipoprotein (HDL) uptake was approximately the same in human and
rat cells, human cells took up 100 times more lipid-rich very low
density lipoprotein (VLDL) than HDL, in contrast to rat cells
which took up much less VLDL than HDL (Fig. 5). Preliminary results with heterologous lipoproteins indicate that the selectivity
may in part reside in the cells themselves, since rat lipoproteins
were taken up to approximately the same extent as human lipoproteins by human cells (Fig. 5). In studies by Stein and Stein, the
reverse also appears to be true (11). Human LDL were not taken up
to a greater extent than rat LDL by rat cells. In addition, differences in lipoprotein structure may play a role, since human HDL
is taken up more poorly than rat HDL by cells from either species
(11).

Specificity of interaction of homologous lipoproteins with
human skin fibroblasts has been recently demonstrated for LDL by
Goldstein and Brown (12), suggesting that there might be receptors
on arterial smooth muscle cells specific for different lipoproteins.
Studies of inhibition of uptake of I^{125}-LDL into human arterial
smooth muscle cells by an added 50-fold excess of unlabeled lipoproteins indicate that excess LDL, in comparison to excess HDL,
specifically inhibits the uptake of labeled LDL (Fig. 6).

Excess unlabeled VLDL also produces considerable inhibition
of LDL uptake, but excess LDL was three times more effective.
These results suggest that the LDL apoprotein (apolipoprotein B)
is an apoprotein that binds to a specific cell surface receptor;
the difference between inhibition with excess VLDL and LDL appears
to be approximately in proportion to their relative content of
apolipoprotein B. This possibility is supported by studies of
inhibition of uptake of labeled VLDL. Again, excess unlabeled LDL
was more than twice as effective as excess unlabeled VLDL in
inhibiting VLDL uptake (Fig. 7).

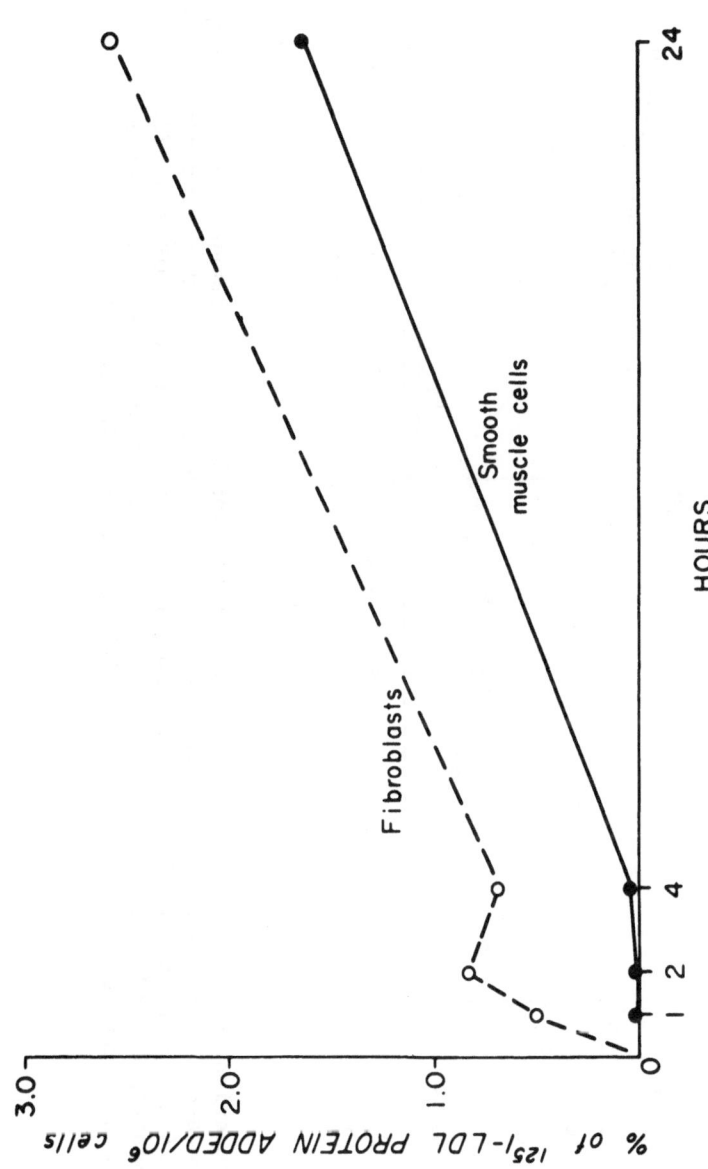

Fig.4. Degradation of ^{125}I-LDL by human arterial SMC and fibroblasts. SMC were obtained from in-timal medial explants, fibroblasts from adventitial explants of renal artery from 29 yr man. Cells after 2nd passage (7.5x10^5, SMC; 3.8x10^5 cells, fibroblasts) were incubated with 12.5μg LDL protein/ml medium containing 10% fetal calf serum. Data expressed as % of ^{125}I-LDL added.

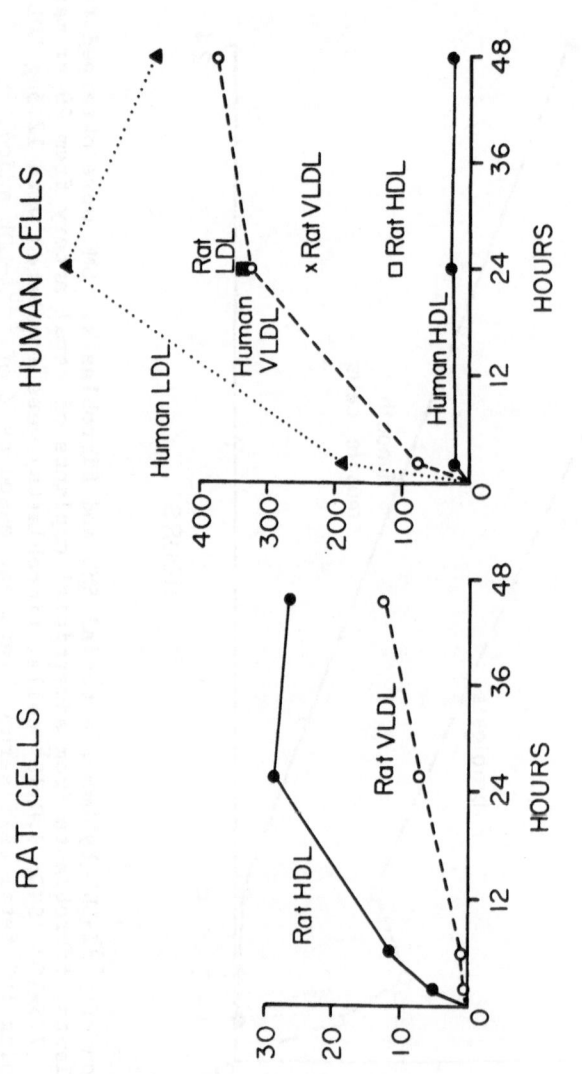

Fig.5. Comparison of uptake of ^{125}I labeled lipoproteins by rat and human cells. Homologous lipo-protein uptake by rat cells (5) and human cells (10) previously published. Superimposed in rt. panel is 24-hr uptake of labeled rat lipoproteins by human cells (1.0×10^6 cells/dish; $7.5 \mu g$ lipo-protein protein added/ml medium supplemented with 10% lipoprotein deficient fetal calf serum). Data is mean of replicate dishes. Note 10-fold difference in ordinate scales.

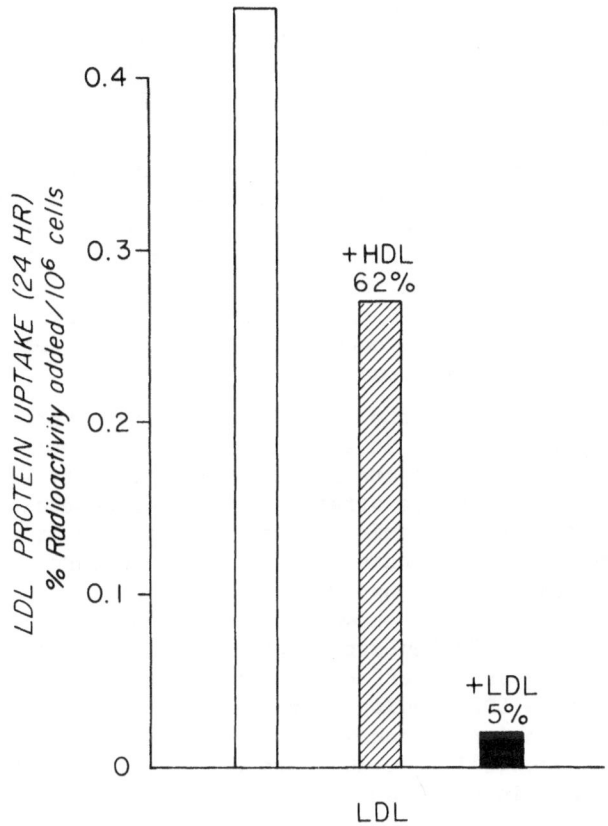

Fig. 6. Inhibition of <u>uptake</u> of ^{125}I LDL into human arterial
smooth muscle cells by addition of 50-fold excess of unlabeled HDL
or LDL. Cells from aorta of 17 yr old donor after the 5th passage
(4×10^5 cells/dish) were incubated with labeled LDL (7.5µg LDL pro-
tein/ml medium containing 10% lipoprotein deficient fetal calf
serum) and unlabeled LDL (solid bar) or HDL (hatched bar) (375µg
lipoprotein protein/ml medium) for 24 hours. LDL protein radioactivity in cells after trypsinization is expressed as % of control
incubation (open bar) without added excess of unlabeled lipoproteins. Data is mean of replicate dishes.

The same conclusion can be derived from studies of surface-binding of labeled lipoproteins by analysis of trypsin-releasable counts. Unlabeled excess LDL was more than twice as effective as unlabeled excess VLDL in inhibiting the binding of both labeled LDL and VLDL to the surface of cultured human arterial smooth muscle cells (Fig. 8). Unlabeled excess HDL failed to inhibit the binding of labeled LDL (92% of control in the presence of HDL). These results are consistent with the hypothesis that specific binding is a prerequisite for uptake.

The age of the cell donor appears to play a role not yet understood. Arterial human smooth muscle cell cultures were obtained from donors ranging in age from 6 months to 72 years. There appears to be a curvilinear inverse relationship between donor age and LDL uptake (Fig. 9). Very young donors appear to accumulate more LDL protein in their cells at 24 hours. Comparison of the ability of cells from young and old donors to degrade lipoproteins is currently under study.

The role of hypoxia on the proliferation and metabolism of arterial smooth muscle cells is of some interest because of the relationship between smoking and lower oxygen delivery to cells. Aortic lesions which resemble atheroma have been produced in experimental animals by systemic hypoxia (13) and arterial lipid accumulation appears to be increased (14,15). Cultured arterial smooth muscle cells grown in hypoxic (5% O_2) conditions instead of the usual room air (20% O_2), showed enhanced proliferation, as previously observed by Hollenberg in chick myocardial cell cultures (16). More striking is the effect of hypoxia on degradation of lipoproteins. While LDL binding is not significantly altered by hypoxia, LDL degradation is consistently impaired and is very apparent by 48 hours (17)(Fig. 10), and may explain the increased content of LDL protein at 48 hours in hypoxic cells.

Thus this system can be used for studying the binding, uptake and degradation of both protein and lipid components of lipoproteins by arterial smooth muscle cells. In addition, the effects of a variety of hormones, metabolites, drugs and experimental conditions on the handling of lipoproteins by these cells can be assessed in tissue culture.

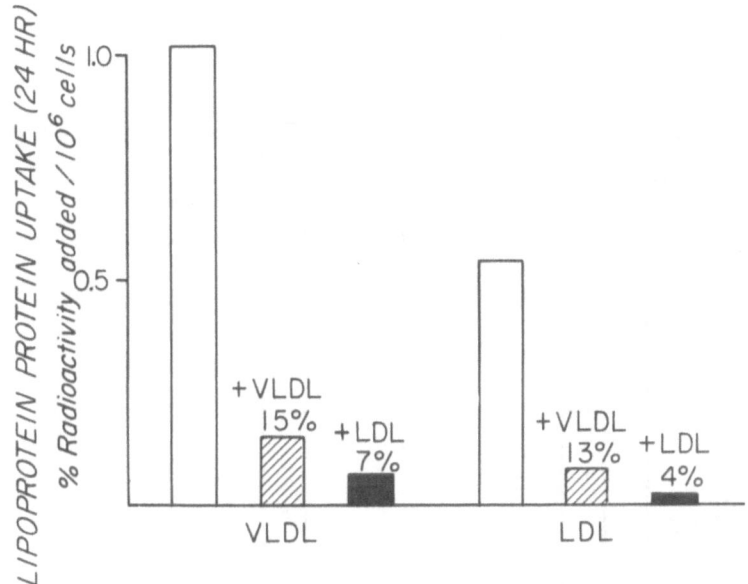

Fig. 7. Inhibition of uptake of ^{125}I VLDL and ^{125}I LDL into human arterial smooth muscle cells by addition of a 50-fold excess of unlabeled VLDL or LDL. Cells from the aorta of a 19 yr old donor after the 3rd passage (2.3×10^6 cells/dish) were incubated with labeled VLDL (left half of figure) or labeled LDL (right half of figure), both 7.5μg lipoprotein protein/ml medium containing 10% lipoprotein deficient fetal calf serum, together with unlabeled LDL (solid bars) or unlabeled VLDL (hatched bars)(375μg lipoprotein protein/ml medium) for 24 hours. Data expressed as in Fig. 6.

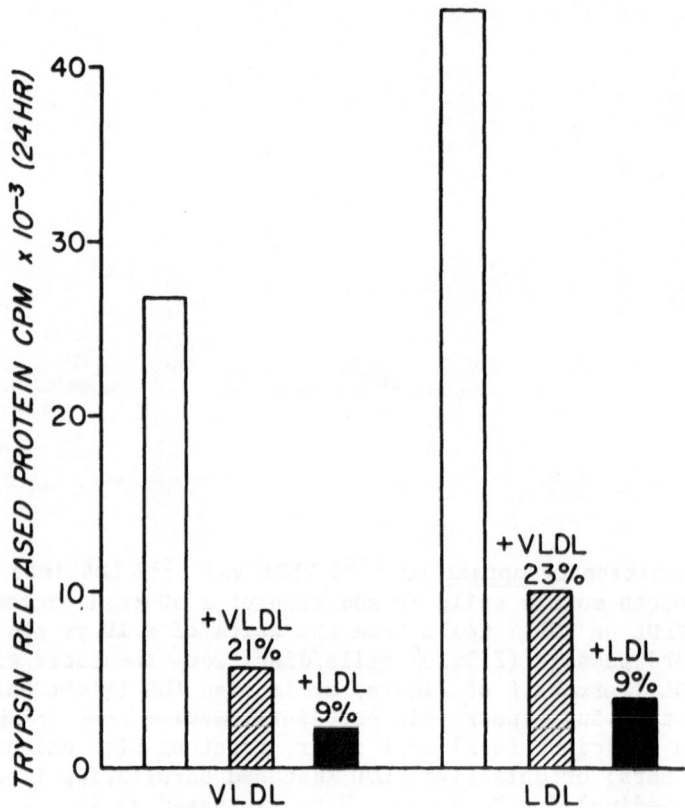

Fig. 8. Inhibition of surface binding of ^{125}I VLDL and ^{125}I LDL to human arterial smooth muscle cells by addition of a 50-fold excess of unlabeled VLDL or LDL. Same experiment as in Fig. 7, except trypsin-released protein radioactivity is measured as an index of surface binding.

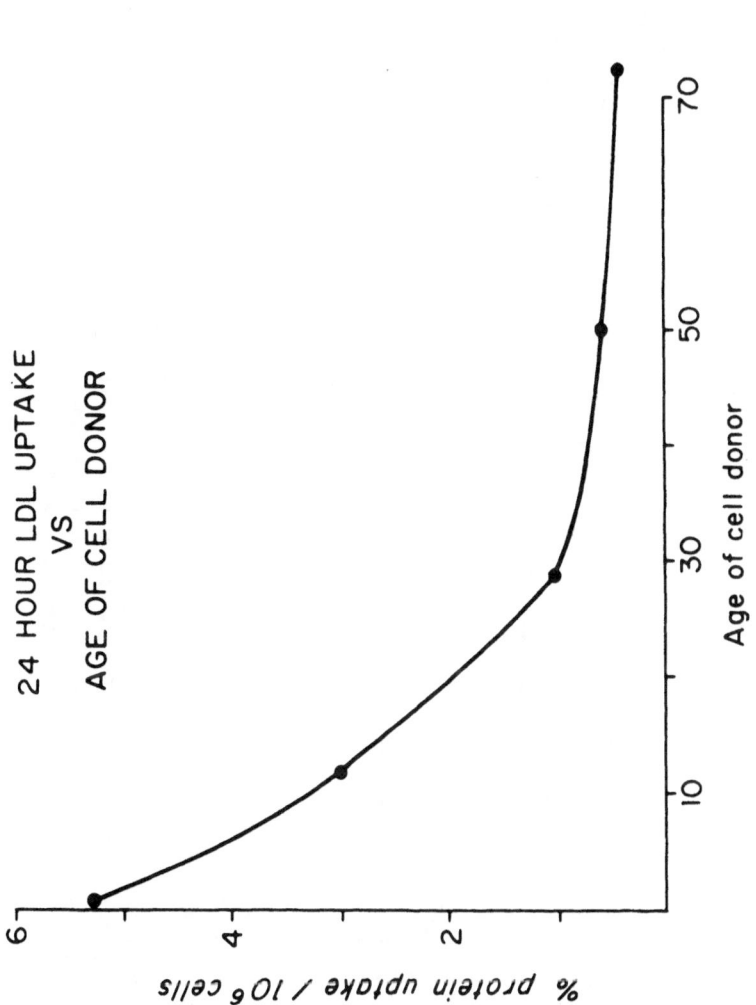

Fig. 9. Net uptake of ^{125}I LDL at 24 hours in human arterial smooth muscle cells cultured from donors of different ages. Cells incubated with 7.5μg LDL protein/ml medium containing 10% lipo-protein deficient fetal calf serum. Date is mean of replicate dishes.

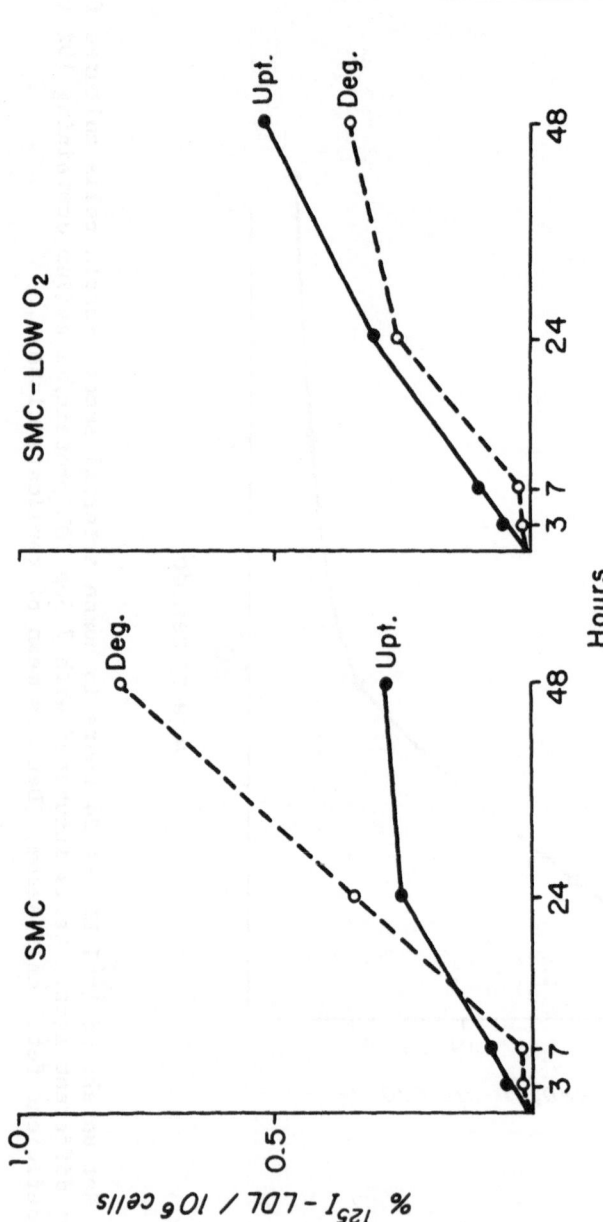

Fig.10. Comparison of ^{125}I LDL protein uptake and degradation by human arterial smooth muscle cells as a function of incubation time with cells exposed to usual room air (20% O_2, 5% CO_2) (left panel) or hypoxic (5% O_2, 5% CO_2)(right panel) conditions. Cells from the aorta of a 6 yr old donor after the 3rd passage (0.9x10⁶ cells/dish) were incubated with labeled LDL (7.5μg LDL protein/ml medium containing 10% lipoprotein deficient fetal calf serum). Uptake (solid line) represents protein radioactivity in cells after trypsinization. Degradation (dashed line) reflects release on non-iodide, TCA soluble radioactivity into the medium. Data is expressed as % of ^{125}I LDL protein added and points represent mean values from replicate dishes.

REFERENCES

1. Geer, J.C., M.D. Haust. 1972. Smooth Muscle Cells in Athero-sclerosis. (V. 2 of: Monographs on Atherosclerosis. Ed. by O.J. Pollak, H.S. Simms and J.E. Kirk). S. Karger, N.Y.

2. Parker, F. 1960. An electron microscopic study of experimental atherosclerosis. Am. J. Path. 36:19-53.

3. Ross, R. and J.A. Glomset. 1973. Atherosclerosis and the ar-terial smooth muscle cell. Science 180:1332-1339.

4. Ross, R. 1971. The smooth muscle cell. II. Growth of smooth muscle in culture and formation of elastic fibers. J. Cell Biol. 50:172-186.

5. Bierman, E.L., O. Stein and Y. Stein. 1974. Lipoprotein uptake and metabolism by rat aortic smooth muscle cells in tissue culture. Circ. Res. 35:136-150.

6. Bierman, E.L., O. Stein and Y. Stein. Unpublished data.

7. Weinstein, D., T.E. Carew and D. Steinberg. 1974. Uptake of low density lipoprotein by porcine aortic smooth muscle cells with inhibition of cholesterol synthesis. Circ. Res. 50:III-70.

8. Ross, R., J.A. Glomset, B. Kariya and L. Harker. 1974. A platelet-dependent serum factor that stimulates the prolifera-tion of arterial smooth muscle cells in vitro. Proc. Nat. Acad. Sci. USA 71:1207-1210.

9. Stout, R.W., E.L. Bierman and R. Ross. 1975. Effect of insulin on the proliferation of cultured primate arterial smooth muscle cells. Circ. Res. 36:319-327.

10. Bierman, E.L. and J.J. Albers. 1975. Lipoprotein uptake by cultured human arterial smooth muscle cells. Biochim. Biophys. Acta 388:198-202.

11. Stein, O. and Y. Stein. 1975. Comparative uptake of rat and human serum low density and high density lipoproteins by rat aortic smooth muscle cells in culture. Circ. Res. 36:436-443.

12. Goldstein, J.L. and M.S. Brown. 1974. Binding and degrada-tion of low density lipoproteins by cultured human fibroblasts. J. Biol. Chem. 249:5153-5162.

13. Helin, P. and I.B. Lorenzen. 1969. Arteriosclerosis in rabbit aorta induced by systemic hypoxia. Angiology 20:1-12.

14. Astrup, P. and K. Kjeldsen. 1973. Carbon monoxide, smoking, and atherosclerosis. Med. Clin. N. Amer. 58:323.

15. Webster, W.S., T.B. Clarkson and H.B. Lofland. 1968. Carbon monoxide-aggravated atherosclerosis in the squirrel monkey. Exp. Mol. Path. 13:36-50.

16. Hollenberg, M. 1971. Effect of oxygen on growth of cultured myocardial cells. Circ. Res. 28:148-157.

17. Albers, J.J. and E.L. Bierman. 1975. Effect of hypoxia on uptake and degradation of low density lipoproteins by cultured human arterial smooth muscle cells. Circulation 52:II-60.

ACKNOWLEDGEMENT

Previously unpublished studies were supported by NIH Grants HD-04872, AM-06670, and Grant AHA-75-747 from the American Heart Association. Scanning electron microscopy was performed by Dr. Phillip H. Smith.

THE REMOVAL OF CELLULAR LIPIDS FROM LANDSCHÜTZ ASCITES CELLS AND

SMOOTH MUSCLE CELLS IN CULTURE

R.L. Jackson, O. Stein, M.C. Glangeaud, M. Fainaru,
A.M. Gotto, and Y. Stein

Baylor College of Medicine, Houston, Texas, and
Hadassah University Hospital, Jerusalem, Israel

INTRODUCTION

Although the function of the plasma high density lipoproteins
(HDL) is unknown, Glomset (1,2) has postulated that plasma HDL and
plasma lecithin:cholesterol acyltransferase (LCAT) play an important role in the transport of unesterified cholesterol from other
lipoproteins and peripheral tissues to the liver. It is postulated that the cholesterol exchanges in an non-enzymic manner between plasma lipoproteins and membranes and HDL. The unesterified
cholesterol in the HDL is then esterified by the plasma enzyme,
LCAT. The cholesteryl esters formed are then transported via HDL
to the liver where they are either converted to bile acids and se-
creted in the bile or incorporated into lipoproteins and released
into the circulation. Evidence that cells can, indeed, lose their
membrane cholesterol to the plasma lipoproteins and, in particular
HDL, has been demonstrated by a number of investigators (3-7).
Stein and Stein (5) found that [^{3}H]cholesterol was removed from
Landschütz ascites cells incubated in the presence of either LDL
or HDL. However, HDL was much more effective in removing cellular
sterol. Although lipid-free HDL (apoHDL) was also effective, the
release of sterol was greatly increased when apoHDL were mixed
with either rat liver phosphatidylcholine or sphingomyelin. In
these earlier studies (5), no attempt was made to use the isolated
apoproteins or phospholipids of known composition. In the present
communication, we have used purified apoproteins from both the
high density and very low density lipoproteins (VLDL) and have
measured the removal of cellular lipids from both Landschütz ascites cells and smooth muscle cells. The findings provide evidence
that the various apoproteins differ in their ability to remove
cellular lipids.

MATERIALS AND METHODS

Isolation of Lipoproteins and Apoproteins

HDL were prepared from normal fasting donors by ultracentri-fugation of plasma between d 1.063-1.210 g/ml. The HDL were de-lipidated and subjected to chromatography on Sephadex G-150 in 5.4 M urea as described previously (8). The homogeneity of the two major apoproteins of HDL, apoA-I and apoA-II, was determined by polyacrylamide gel electrophoresis in urea and by amino acid analysis (8). The major VLDL apoproteins, apoC-I, apoC-II and apoC-III, were isolated from plasma of fasting patients with Type IV or V hyperlipoproteinemia (9). After delipidation of the VLDL (10), the apoproteins were fractionated on Sephadex G-150 and DEAE-cellulose as described by Brown et al. (10).

Tissue Culture Methods

Male albino mice of the Hebrew University strain were used in the study. The animals were inoculated with Landschütz ascites tumor cells, and 6-8 days after the inoculation they were injected intraperitoneally with the [^{3}H]cholesterol. After a further two days, the ascites cells were removed and suspended in 10 volumes of Krebs-Henseleit phosphate buffer, pH 7.4, containing 200 mg% glucose; the cells were pelleted by centrifugation and washed four additional times. The preparation of labeled cholesterol and the conditions for growth of ascites cells have been described in de-tail elsewhere (5). Aortic smooth muscle cells were obtained from male rats of the Hebrew University strain and were cultured ac-cording to the method of Ross (11). The cells were incubated with [^{3}H]cholesterol or [^{3}H]choline as described previously (6). Gen-erally, the cells used in the study were between the fourth and seventh passage.

Preparation of Apoprotein-Phospholipid Mixtures

Rat liver phosphatidylcholine and sphingomyelin were prepared as described previously (5). Phospholipids of known fatty acyl composition were obtained from commercial sources. To prepare apoprotein-phospholipid mixtures, the phospholipids were taken to dryness with a stream of nitrogen and 0.1 M Tris HCl, pH 8.0, containing 0.9% NaCl was added to give 3 µmoles of phospho-lipid per ml. The apoprotein-phospholipid mixtures were then sub-jected to ultrasonic irradiation in a Braun-Sonic 300 instrument using a microtip (4 mm in diameter) at maximal scale for 2 min at 0°, under nitrogen.

Other Procedures

[^{3}H]cholesterol and [^{3}H]phosphatidylcholine were extracted from cells by previously described methods (5). Radioactivity was determined using an Autogamma scintillation spectrometer.

RESULTS

Almost complete isotopic equilibration of the [^{3}H]cholesterol was achieved with the ascites cells in 2-4 days. Using these labeled cells, the effectiveness of albumin and the plasma lipo-proteins to remove cellular cholesterol was studied. As shown in Table I, the removal of cholesterol was a temperature-dependent process. HDL promoted the efflux of cholesterol to a much greater extent than did either albumin or LDL. Furthermore, the HDL lipids appeared to be a necessary prerequisite for the removal of cell cholesterol; HDL was 7 x more effective than apoHDL.

Table I

Release of [^{3}H]cholesterol from ascites cells by human plasma lipoproteins or albumin

Cholesterol acceptor	% Cholesterol released	
	4°	37°
Albumin	0.2	1.4
HDL	0.1	30.0
ApoHDL	0.6	4.4
LDL	0.7	10.9

Ascites cells (7 x 10^7) were incubated with the appropriate cholesterol acceptor (3.2 mg/ml) in a total volume of 0.3 ml. After 2 hrs at the indicated temperatures, the cells were pelleted and the cholesterol released was determined as described in the Materials and Methods. The percent released was calcu-lated taking the total radioactivity in the cells as 100%. Counts released into the medium in the absence of added mixtures were subtracted from each experimental value.

To determine if the removal of cholesterol from cellular membranes might differ from each of the HDL apoproteins and for different kinds of lipid, HDL apoproteins were fractionated on
Sephadex and the ascites cells were exposed to the various purified fractions. As shown in Table II, apoA-II and the unfractionated apoC proteins were more effective in removing cellular cholesterol than was apoA-I. However, the addition of rat liver
phosphatidylcholine or sphingomyelin to any one of the proteins
greatly increased the release of cellular cholesterol; phosphatidylcholine or sphingomyelin alone were ineffective.

Table II

Release of [^{3}H]cholesterol from ascites cells by
purified human HDL apoproteins and apoprotein-lipid mixtures

Cholesterol acceptor	% Cholesterol released		
		+ PC	+ SM
ApoHDL	3.2	N.D.	N.D.
ApoA-I	0.9	6.3	9.0
ApoA-II	2.1	9.4	9.4
ApoC	1.7	8.8	10.8
PC	1.5		
SM	2.2		

Ascites cells (4 x 10^6) were incubated with the various ac-
ceptors (0.5 mg/ml) in a final volume of 0.2 ml for 2 hrs at
37°. The cholesterol released was determined as described
in Methods. N.D., not determined.

In the studies described in Table II, the fatty acyl chains
of the phosphatidylcholine were of an unknown composition. Therefore, to determine whether the removal of cholesterol was effected
by the kind of fatty acyl chain, phospholipids of known composition were mixed with the isolated apoproteins and then these mixtures with the ascites cells. As shown in Table III, there was
comparatively more [^{3}H]cholesterol removed using disaturated phosphatidylcholines than mono- or diunsaturated ones. Furthermore,
apoA-II and apoC-III were the most effective in removing cellular
cholesterol.

The removal of cellular cholesterol was also determined in
rat aortic smooth muscle cells grown in culture. In general, the

Table III

Release of [^{3}H]cholesterol from ascites cells with
mixtures of purified human HDL apoproteins and phosphatidylcholine

Cholesterol acceptor	% Cholesterol released				
	di 14:0	di 16:0	di 18:0	di 18:1	di 18:2
ApoA-I	7.3	7.4	7.8	1.3	5.2
ApoA-II	11.5	7.3	8.2	5.0	13.5
ApoC-I	6.0	11.1	12.0	6.9	8.9
ApoC-II	4.1	7.0	7.8	2.5	6.0
ApoC-III	13.0	14.8	16.8	9.0	7.5

Apoproteins were incubated with the various phosphatidylcholines
in a molar ratio of 50:1 (lipid:protein). For di 14:0, di 18:1,
and di 18:2, the incubation temperature was 23°. For di 16:0 and
di 18:0, the temperature was 42°. After incubation for 12 hrs,
the phospholipid-apoprotein mixtures (3 nmoles) were incubated
with ascites cells (4 x 10^6) for 2 hrs at 37° and the cholesterol
released was determined as described in Methods.

pattern of cholesterol released from the cultured cells was similar to that observed in ascites cells. As shown in Table IV, the
release of [^{3}H]cholesterol from rat aortic smooth muscle cells by
human apoA-I was greatly increased by the addition of rat liver
phosphatidylcholine or sphingomyelin to the apoprotein. The addition of both phosphatidylcholine and sphingomyelin to apoA-I did
not cause an additive effect in the release of the cellular cholesterol.

It also seemed of interest to determine whether the apoproteins differed in their ability to release cellular phospholipids.
In these experiments, the cells were previously labeled with
[^{3}H]choline; more than 85% of the label was in phosphatidylcholine. As shown in Table V, the removal of [^{3}H]phosphatidylcholine
was most effective with apoA-I and apoC-I. When the apoproteins
were added to ascites cells as phospholipid-apoprotein mixtures,
little or no cellular phosphatidylcholine was released.

To determine if the differences of the apoproteins to remove
cholesterol and phosphatidylcholine might be related to the adsorption of the apoproteins to the cells, each apoprotein was labeled with ^{125}I and their adsorption to ascites cells was

Table IV

Release of [^{3}H]cholesterol from rat aortic
smooth muscle cells by human apoA-I and phospholipids

Cholesterol acceptor	% Cholesterol released
ApoA-I	1.9
ApoA-I plus PC	17.0
ApoA-I plus SM	20.5
ApoA-I plus PC and SM	21.6
PC alone	10.3
SM alone	3.3

ApoA-I (0.5 mg/ml) and either rat liver phosphatidylcholine (0.5 mg/ml) or sphingomyelin (0.5 mg/ml) or
combined (0.25 mg/ml each) were sonicated together as
described in the Methods. The phospholipid-apoprotein complexes were then added to the culture media
(2.0 ml) and the cells were exposed to the apoprotein-lipid mixture for 24 hrs. The cholesterol released was determined as described previously (6).

Table V

Release of [^{3}H]phosphatidylcholine from
ascites cells by human HDL apoproteins

Phospholipid acceptor	% Phospholipid released
ApoA-I	1.08
ApoA-II	0.42
ApoC-I	1.12
ApoC-II	0.22
ApoC-III	0.26

Ascites cells were labeled with [^{3}H]choline as described in the Methods. To 4×10^4 cells were added
each apoprotein (3 nmoles) in a final volume of 0.3
ml. After 2 hrs at 37°, the amount of [^{3}H]phospha-
tidylcholine released was determined as described
previously (7).

determined. As shown in Table VI, apoA-II and apoC-III were adsorbed to ascites cells more effectively than apoA-I. Treatment of the cells with trypsin prior to exposure to the apoproteins did not appreciably change the amounts of iodinated apoprotein bound to the cells. Of the counts remaining in the washed cells, approximately 50% was released by trypsin (Table VI).

Table VI

Adsorption of human HDL apoproteins to ascites cells

Apoprotein	n moles added	n moles bound	n moles after trypsin
ApoA-I	10.00	0.31	0.19
ApoA-II	10.00	0.95	0.57
ApoC-III	10.00	0.85	0.48

Ascites cells (4 x 10^6) were incubated with the apoprotein (3 nmoles) for 2 hrs at 37° in a final volume of 0.3 ml. After incubation, the cells were washed extensively and the counts remaining in the washed cells were determined. The washed cells were incubated with 0.5 ml of 0.05% trypsin for 6 min. at 37°. After washing, the trypsin-treated cells were then counted.

DISCUSSION

In the present study, it was shown that plasma HDL and purified HDL apoproteins mixed with phospholipids removed cellular sterol from Landschütz ascites cells and smooth muscle cells in culture. In contrast, the lipid-free apoproteins were much less effective. Of the various apoproteins and phospholipids used, apoC-III and saturated phospholipids were more effective in releasing [^{3}H]cholesterol than apoA-I. Furthermore, apoC-III was adsorbed to cells to a greater extent than apoA-I. In an attempt to explain these differences, we then determined the effects of the isolated apoproteins on the removal of cellular phospholipids. In these experiments, apoA-I was 4 x more effective than apoC-III. None of the apoprotein-phospholipid mixtures removed cellular phospholipid. Although the exact mechanisms for the removal of cholesterol and phospholipids are unknown, the differences between apoA-I and apoC-III may be related to the phenomenon of

phospholipid transfer. It is well known that phospholipids can exchange between the plasma lipoproteins and various tissues (12,13).
It is also known that cholesterol does not bind to an apoprotein
unless the protein is first complexed with phospholipid (14).
Based on this information, we propose that the removal of cholesterol is related to the transfer of phospholipid and that phospholipid is transferred more readily between the membrane and apoC-III-
phospholipid mixtures than between the membrane and apoA-I-phospho-
lipid mixtures. This interpretation would suggest that apoA-I-
phospholipid complexes are more stable in solution than in the membrane. It would also suggest that the phospholipid in apoC-III
complexes can more readily be transferred to the membrane and as a
result of the transfer, cholesterol is removed. The structural
properties of apoA-I and apoC-III that account for these differences in the removal of phospholipid and cholesterol are of considerable interest and are under active investigation.

Acknowledgements - This work was supported in part by Health, Edu-
cation and Welfare Research Grants HL-14194, RR-00350, HL-05435/34
and 17269-01, by a grant from the John A. Hartford Foundation, Inc.,
by the Delegation Generale à la Recherche Scientifique et
Technique of the French Government, and from the Ministry of
Health, the Government of Israel. R. L. Jackson is an Established
Investigator of the American Heart Association. The authors are
also indebted to Ms. Debbie Mason for her assistance in the preparation of the manuscript.

REFERENCES

1. Glomset, J. A. 1968. The plasma lecithin:cholesterol acyl-
    transferase reaction. J. Lipid Res. 9:155-167.

2. Glomset, J. A. 1972. Plasma lecithin:cholesterol acyltrans-
    ferase: In: Blood Lipids and Lipoproteins: Quantitation,
    Composition, and Metabolism. Ed. by G. J. Nelson, Wiley-In-
    terscience, New York, pp. 745-787.

3. Bates, S. R. and G. H. Rothblat. 1974. Regulation of cellu-
    lar sterol flux and synthesis by human serum lipoproteins.
    Biochim. Biophys. Acta 360:38-55.

4. Bjornson, L. E., C. Gniewkowski and H. J. Kayden. 1975. Com-
    parison of exchange of α-tocopherol and free cholesterol be-
    tween rat plasma lipoproteins and erythrocytes. J. Lipid Res.
    16:39-53.

5. Stein, O. and Y. Stein. 1973. The removal of cholesterol from Landschütz ascites cells by high-density apolipoprotein. Biochim. Biophys. Acta 326:232-244.

6. Stein, Y., M. C. Glangeaud, M. Fainaru and O. Stein. 1975. The removal of cholesterol from aortic smooth muscle cells in culture and Landschütz ascites cells by fractions of human high-density apolipoprotein. Biochim. Biophys. Acta 380:106-118.

7. Jackson, R. L., A. M. Gotto, O. Stein and Y. Stein. 1975. A comparative study on the removal of cellular lipids from Landschütz ascites cells by human plasma apolipoproteins. J. Biol. Chem. 250:7204-7209.

8. Jackson, R. L. and A. M. Gotto. 1972. A study of the cystine-containing apolipoprotein of human plasma high density lipoproteins: Characterization of cyanogen bromide and tryptic fragments. Biochim. Biophys. Acta 285:36-47.

9. Fredrickson, D. S. and R. I. Levy. 1972. Familial hyper-lipoproteinemia. In: The Metabolic Basis of Inherited Disease. Ed. by J. B. Stanbury, J. B. Wyngaarden and D. S. Fredrickson, McGraw-Hill, Inc., New York, pp. 545-614.

10. Brown, W. V., R. I. Levy and D. S. Fredrickson. 1970. Further separation of the apoproteins of the human plasma very low density lipoproteins. Biochim. Biophys. Acta 200: 573-575.

11. Ross, R. 1971. Smooth muscle cell: II. Growth of smooth muscle in culture and formation of elastic fibers. J. Cell Biol. 50:172-186.

12. Illingworth, D. R., O. W. Portman, A. L. Robertson and W. A. Magyar. 1973. The exchange of phospholipids between plasma lipo-proteins and rapidly dividing human cells grown in tissue culture. Biochim. Biophys. Acta 306:422-436.

13. Illingworth, D. R. and O. W. Portman. 1972. Exchange of phospho-lipids between low and high density lipoproteins of squirrel monkeys. J. Lipid Res. 13:220-227.

14. Scanu, A., J. Toth, C. Edelstein, S. Koga and E. Stiller. 1969. Fractionation of human serum high density lipoprotein in urea solutions. Evidence for polypeptide heterogeneity. Biochemistry 8:3309-3316.

INDEX

463